Second Edition

Mechanical Ventilation
Clinical Application

Second Edition

Mechanical Ventilation
Clinical Application

Vijay Deshpande MS RRT FAARC
Emeritus Professor
Georgia State University
Atlanta, Georgia, USA

Visiting Faculty
School of Allied Health Sciences
Manipal University
Manipal, Karnataka
India

TR Chandrashekar MD
Intensivist
Liver Transplantation
Department of SGE and LT
Bangalore Medical College and Research Institute
Superspeciality Hospital
Bangalore

CBS Publishers & Distributors Pvt Ltd
New Delhi • Bengaluru • Chennai • Kochi • Kolkata • Mumbai
Bhopal • Bhubaneswar • Hyderabad • Jharkhand • Nagpur
• Patna • Pune • Uttarakhand • Dhaka (Bangladesh)

Disclaimer

Science and technology are constantly changing fields. New research and experience broaden the scope of information and knowledge. The authors have tried their best in giving information available to them while preparing the material for this book. Although, all efforts have been made to ensure optimum accuracy of the material, yet it is quite possible that some errors might have been left. The publisher, the printer and the authors will not be held responsible for any inadvertent errors or inaccuracies.

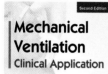

Mechanical Ventilation
Clinical Application
Second Edition

ISBN: 978-81-239-2537-0

Copyright © Authors and Publisher

Second Edition: 2015
Reprint: 2017, 2018, 2020
First Edition: 2012

All rights reserved. No part of this book may be reproduced or transmitted in any form or by any means, electronic or mechanical, including photocopying, recording, or any information storage and retrieval system without permission, in writing, from the authors and the publisher.

Published by Satish Kumar Jain and Produced by Varun Jain for
CBS Publishers & Distributors Pvt Ltd
4819/XI Prahlad Street, 24 Ansari Road, Daryaganj, New Delhi 110002, India.
Ph: 23289259, 23266861, 23266867   Website: www.cbspd.com

Fax: 011-23243014   e-mail: delhi@cbspd.com; cbspubs@airtelmail.in.
Corporate Office: 204 FIE, Industrial Area, Patparganj, Delhi 110092
Ph: 4934 4934   Fax: 4934 4935   e-mail: publishing@cbspd.com; publicity@cbspd.com

Branches

- **Bengaluru:** Seema House 2975, 17th Cross, K.R. Road, Banasankari 2nd Stage, Bengaluru 560 070, Karnataka
  Ph: +91-80-26771678/79   Fax: +91-80-26771680   e-mail: bangalore@cbspd.com
- **Chennai:** No. 7, Subbaraya Street, Shenoy Nagar, Chennai 600 030, Tamil Nadu
  Ph: +91-44-26680620, 26681266   Fax: +91-44-42032115   e-mail: chennai@cbspd.com
- **Kochi:** 42/1325, 1326, Power House Road, Opposite KSEB Power House, Ernakulam 682 018, Kochi, Kerala
  Ph: +91-484-4059061-65   Fax: +91-484-4059065   e-mail: kochi@cbspd.com
- **Kolkata:** No. 6/B, Ground Floor, Rameswar Shaw Road, Kolkata-700014 (West Bengal), India
  Ph: +91-33-2289-1126, 2289-1127, 2289-1128   e-mail: kolkata@cbspd.com
- **Mumbai:** 83-C, Dr E Moses Road, Worli, Mumbai-400018, Maharashtra
  Ph: +91-22-24902340/41   Fax: +91-22-24902342   e-mail: mumbai@cbspd.com

Representatives

• Bhopal	0-8319310552	• Bhubaneswar	0-9911037372	• Hyderabad	0-9885175004
• Jharkhand	0-9811541605	• Nagpur	0-9421945513	• Patna	0-9334159340
• Pune	0-9623451994	• Uttarakhand	0-9716462459	• Dhaka (Bangladesh)	01912-003485

Printed at Rashtriya Printes, Dilshad Garden, Delhi, India

to
my wife Shobha
for her patience and understanding
and
Deven
for the love and joy he brings to his grandfather

Prof Vijay Deshpande

my parents who made me believe in my abilities.
my wife Dr. Kavitha for being in my life.
my lovely daughters Sneha, Vandana and Keertana for
bringing joy to my life.

Dr TR Chandrashekar

Preface to the Second Edition

Mechanical ventilation is an integral part of critically ill patients. Unfortunately, medical education does not find space in the curriculum to discuss mechanical ventilation in details. Most clinicians learn mechanical ventilation at the patient's bedside under the supervision of their experienced seniors. Clinicians involved in managing critically ill patients are expected to be familiar with all aspects of mechanical ventilation. To add to the insult, researchers and manufacturers of mechanical ventilators have introduced various new modes and created an alphabet soup of terminologies. The influx of new modes and their application has an overwhelming effect on clinicians.

The authors have only one intention in writing this book— a user-friendly, succinct description of practical application and academic basis for concepts associated with mechanical ventilation. The first 12 chapters incorporate all practical information including indications, initiation, monitoring, graphics, various basic modes and weaning from ventilation. Although Chapter 5 describes all graphics, some applicable waveforms are repeated. This redundancy in graphs and associated description is deliberately used in certain chapters to maintain continuity and avoid flipping back and forth. Most material is standard information available in books on mechanical ventilation and manufacturer's literature. Every current ventilator is equipped with graphic display and thus a clinician is expected to be proficient is interpreting basic waveforms. A CD, "Essentials of Ventilator Graphics" developed by Dr Ruben Restrepo and Vijay Deshpande, is provided in the pocket on the inside back cover of the book. Readers are permitted to use any slides from this CD for teaching purposes. Chapters 13–22 include academic material from various sources explaining important concepts in mechanical ventilation. Information on PEEP/CPAP, newer modes of ventilation, ARDS management, nutrition, sedation and analgesic use, are discussed in details. Three new chapters have been added in this edition of the book: Chapter 23 "Patient–Ventilator Asynchrony", Chapter 24 "Neurally Adjusted Ventilator Assist" and Chapter 25 "Extracorporeal Membrane Oxygenation".

We hope that all the clinicians taking care of mechanically ventilated patients benefit from this book and it becomes a quick source of information in the ICU.

Vijay Deshpande
TR Chandrashekar

Acknowledgments

Our sincere appreciation to Susan Pilbeam and Theresa Gramlich for being lifelong friends and giving valuable suggestions. Dr Ruben Restrepo, for his contribution as the codeveloper of the CD, "Essentials for Ventilator Graphics". Material from this CD is used liberally in this book and the CD is also provided. Dr Kedar Toraskar, Dr Mayur Patel, Pandurang Tekawade and Sanjay Savarkar for sharing their clinical experiences with ventilated patients. Maquet clinical specialists Jagannathan and Mehul Damania for providing technical and clinical information. Ashim Purohit for his encouragement and trust.

Appreciation to Dr MSN Prasad and Mr Ravi Shankar for assisting with collecting data and partially writing one chapter. We appreciate Prof Mangal Gogte for assistance in proofreading the typescript.

Dr Rajesh Chawla, Dr Kapil Zirpe, Dr Sushama Patil and Jaganathan for timely completing their chapters. Their contribution has added more credibility to this book.

Vijay Deshpande
TR Chandrashekar

Contents

Preface to the Second Edition   vii

1. Indications for Mechanical Ventilation

Acute vs Chronic Respiratory Failure	3
Characteristics of Acute Respiratory Failure	3
Hypercapnic Respiratory Failure	3
Hypoxemic Respiratory Failure	4
Common Causes of ARF	4
Acute on Chronic Respiratory Failure	6
Indications for Mechanical Ventilation	7
Goals of Mechanical Ventilation	8

2. Hypoxemic Respiratory Failure: Prevention and Management

Oxygen Delivery	9
Effect of increased Airway Resistance	11
Effect of Decreased Lung Compliance	12
Hypoxia and Hypoxemia	15
Hypoxemia—Common Causes, and Clinical Signs	17
Management of Hypoxemia—Responsive and Refractory	18
Cardiovascular Effects of Hypoxemia	20

3. Acid Base Disorders and ABG Interpretation

Henderson–Hasselbach Equation	21
Lactic Acidosis	28
Keto Acidosis	31
Anion Gap	31
Metabolic Alkalosis	33
ABGs Associated with COPD	36

4. Terms and Definitions Related to Mechanical Ventilation

Negative Pressure Ventilation	41
Positive Pressure Ventilation	43
Positive Pressure Ventilation—Volume and Pressure Ventilation	43
Essential Parameters in Mechanical Ventilation	44
Interrelationship between Flow, Time, Volume and Respiratory Frequency	46

5. Essentials of Ventilator Waveforms

Scalars and Loops	49
Flow–Time, Pressure–Time and Volume–Time	49
Pressure–Volume and Flow–Volume Loop	49
Analysis of Scalar Graphics	51
Basics of Flow-Volume Loop	62
Modes of Mechanical Ventilation	64

6. Initiation of Mechanical Ventilation

Initiation of Gas Flow	69
Phases and Parameters of Ventilation	70
Triggering, Limiting and Cycling	72

Volume Ventilation	74
Setting Inspiratory Flow	75
Monitoring Pressures	77
Pressure Targeted Ventilation	80
Drawbacks in Volume and Pressure Ventilation	82
Dual Modes of Ventilation	83

7. Basic Modes of Ventilation

Control Ventilation	88
Assisted Ventilation	89
Modes and Alarms in Volume Ventilation	91
Modes and Alarms in Pressure Ventilation	93
SIMV	93
PSV	96
CPAP	98
SIMV + PSV + CPAP	100
PSV + CPAP (BiPAP)	100

8. Volume vs Pressure Targeted Ventilation

Drawbacks of Volume Ventilation	101
Volume Ventilation in ALI and ARDS	103
Limitations of Pressure Ventilation	105
Type of Pressure Ventilation and Modes	107
Flow-Time Scalar in PCV	108

9. Dual-Controlled Modes of Ventilation

Dual-Controlled Modes—Within-a-Breath	113
Dual Controlled Modes—Breath-to-Breath	114
Volume Support, PRVC and Auto Mode	116
Adaptive Support Ventilation	118

10. Initial Settings

Tidal Volume in Volume Ventilation	120
Tidal Volume in Pressure Ventilation	121
Frequency	122
Inspiratory Flow Settings	123
PEEP and FiO_2	124

11. Patient Monitoring and Abnormal Ventilator Waveforms

Initial Assessment—Volume Ventilation	125
PIP and Alarm Settings	127
Plateau Pressure (P_{Plat})	128
Transairway Pressure (P_{TA})	128
Static and Dynamic Compliance	129
Interrelationships between Ventilator Pressures	131
Cuff Pressure	132
Mean Airway Pressure	133
Common Abnormal Waveforms	135
Auto-PEEP	136
Air Leak	138
Inadequate Flow	139

12. Weaning from Mechanical Ventilator

Patient's Readiness to Wean	143
Rapid Shallow Breathing Index (RSBI)	146
Muscle Strength	147
Ventilatory Drive	148

13. Positive End-Expiratory Pressure and Continuous Positive Airway Pressure

Types of PEEP	155
PEEP in Preventing VILI	158
Effects of PEEP	160
PEEP and FiO_2	167
Stress Index	168

14. Mechanical Ventilation

COPD	
Goals of Mechanical Ventilation in COPD	172
Goals for Ventilator Settings in COPD	172
Applied PEEP in COPD	179
Asthma	184
Ventilator Settings	185
Use of NPPV	185
Severe Brain Injury	186
Goals of Mechanical Ventilation in Brain Injury	186
Role of PEEP	187
PEEP and ICP	188
Chest Trauma	189
Flail Chest	189
Pulmonary Contusion	190
Practical Approach to Mechanical Ventilation in Chest Trauma	190
Bronchopleural Fistula	191
Neuromuscular Disease	192
Guillain-Barre' Syndrome	194
Myasthenia Gravis	194
Chronic Neuromuscular disease	194

15. Non Invasive Ventilation

Definition and Clinical Advantages	197
Different Interfases	198
Leak Compensation	201
Goals of NPPV	203
Ventilators and Modes used in NPPV	204
Aerosol Delivery, FiO_2 and Humidification during NPPV	205
Applications of NPPV	206
Immunosuppression	209
Asthma	209
Monitoring and weaning from NPPV	212

16. ARDS and Ventilatory Challenges

Definition	215
Causes of ARDS	217
Pathophysiology	218
Rationale for PEEP Use Prone Positioning	220
Lung Protective Strategies	221
Ventilatory Strategies used in ARDS	222
Modes of Ventilation	222
Inverse Ratio Ventilation and BiLevel	222
FiO_2 and Oxygen Toxicity	223
Permissive Hypercapnia	224
Prone Positioning	227
Recruitment maneuvers	228
Lung Protective Ventilation	231

17. Hazards of Mechanical Ventilation

Ventilator Induced Lung Injury (VILI)	233
Pathogenesis	234

Types of VILI	236
Volutrauma	236
Atelectrauma	236
Biotrauma	237
Pulmonary Barotrauma	240
Lung Protective Ventilation	241
Oxygen Toxicity	241
Prevention	242
Ventilator Associated Pneumonia	244
Definition	244
Etiology and Pathophysiology	244
Diagnosis	245
Clinical Features	246
Preventive Measures	248
Treatment	250

18. Newer Modes of Mechanical Ventilation

Dual Control Modes	253
Rationale for Newer Modes	
Adaptive Support Ventilation (ASV)—Hamilton Ventilator	260
Proportional Assist Ventilation (PAV +)—Covedien Puritan Bennett	265
Airway Pressure Release Ventilation (APRV)—Drager Ventilator	265
Smartcare—Drager Ventilation	268

19. Sedation, Analgesics and Neuromuscular Blockers in Mechanical Ventilated Patients

Spectrum of Comfort, Distress and Sedation	271
Analgesics	273
Assessment of Pain in Mechanically Ventilation Patient	273
Sedation management	278
Delirium management	281
Neuromuscular Blocking Agents	283

20. Nutritional Assessment and Management in Mechanically Ventilated Patients

Assessment of Nutritional Requirements in Mechanically Ventilated Patient	286
Anthropometric	286
Laboratory	286
Indirect Calorimetry	286
Predictive Equations	286
Enteral Feeding	287
Bowel Disturbances	290
GI bleeding	290
Pulmonary Failure	290
Contraindications	290
Parental Nutrition	291
Pharmaconutrition	292

21. Aerosol Therapy and Humidification

Types of Aerosol Delivery Devices	296
Nebulisers	296
Small Volume Nebulisers (SVN)	296
Ultrasonic Nebulisers (USN)	298
Meter Dose Inhalers (MDI)	298
MDI position in the ventilator circuit	298
Spacer	299
Factors Affecting Aerosol Therapy during Mechanical Ventilation Humidification	300
Density of Inhaled Gas	301
Endotracheal tube size	301
Ventilator Mode and setting	301
Technique for delivering Aerosols during Mechanical Ventilation	302

Care of spacers and nebulizers	303
Assessing Bronchodilator response	303
Aerosol Delivery during NPPV	303
Aerosolized Drugs	303
Bronchodilators	303
Surfactants	304
Other drugs	304
Humidfication	305
Definitions	306
Physiologic and Thermodynamic Basics	307
Mucocilliary Elevator	308
Types of Humidifiers	
Passive-Heat Moisture Exchangers (HME)	310
Heated Humidifiers	311

22. Heart–Lung Interaction during Mechanical Ventilation

Pertinent Basics Cardiovascular and Respiratory Physiology	318
Relationship between Airway pressure and Pleural Pressure	318
Realtionship between Flow and Pressure	318
Pressures acting on the circulatory system	319
Detreminants of Cardiac Performance	320
Frank-Starling law	321
Heart Lung Interactions	321
Cadiovascular effects due to changes in Thoracic Pressure	322
On the left Ventricle	323
Left Ventricular Afterload	323
Intratjoracic Aortic Transmural Pressure	324
Cardiovascular Effects due to changes in Lung Volume	325
On the Right Ventricular Aftreload	325
Hypoxic Pulmonary vasoconstriction	326
On Pulmonary Vascular Resistance	326
Mechanical Compression of the Heart due to Increased Lung Volume s	327
Autonomic Tone	328
Humoral Effects	328
Ventricular interdependence and LV diastolic function	328
Spontaneous Breathing	329
Positive Pressure Ventilation	329

23. Patient–ventilator Asynchrony

Patient-Ventilator Asynchrony (PVA)	332
Patient factors	332
Ventilator related factors	334
Types of Asynchrony	335
Trigger Asynchrony	335
i. Ineffective or Missed Trigger	336
ii. Double Triggering	338
iii. Auto- triggering	339
Flow Asynchrony	340
Termination Asynchrony	341
Expiratory Asynchrony	342
Markers of PVA	343

24. Neurally Adjusted Ventilator Assist (NAVAA)

Neurally Adjusted Ventilatory Assist (NAVA)	345
NAVA concept	345
Neuro-ventilator Coupling	346
Measurement of Electrical Signal from the Diaphragm	347
Edi Catheter	347
Verification of Proper Positioning of the Edi Catheter	349
NAVA Level	350
Trigger Level	352

Triggered Breath Delivery	352
Breath Cycling – Beginning of Expiration	353
Indications for NAVA	354
Contra-indications for NAVA	354
Weaning from NAVA	354

25. Extracorporeal Membrane Oxygenation (ECMO)

Indications for ECMO	357
Contra-indications	358
Contiguration of ECMO	358
Components of ECMO	360
ECMO therapy	363
Suggested Reading	*369*
Index	*373*

INDICATIONS FOR MECHANICAL VENTILATION

Respiratory failure and impending respiratory failure are grounds for instituting mechanical ventilation. Respiratory failure results from inadequacy in alveolar ventilation, blood oxygenation and/or tissue oxygenation (Fig 1.1). Impending respiratory failure is also sometimes termed respiratory insufficiency. It differs from frank respiratory failure in that the diagnostic tests such as arterial blood gases (ABG) do not verify acute respiratory failure and yet, clinically the patient is very close to it. The patient exhibits signs of increased work of breathing, dyspnea, use of accessory muscles and sometimes, paradoxical breathing, whereas in respiratory failure the diagnostic tests support the conclusion as Respiratory Failure (Fig 1.2). Criteria for instituting mechanical ventilation include apnea, acute respiratory failure, impending respiratory failure and severe oxygenation defect associated with increased work of breathing (Fig 1.3).

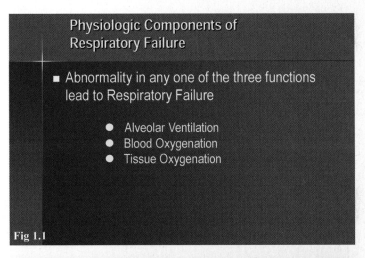

Fig 1.1

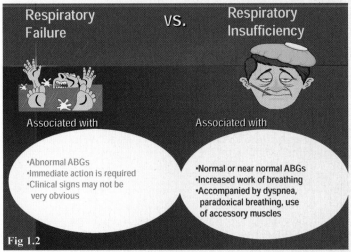

Fig 1.2

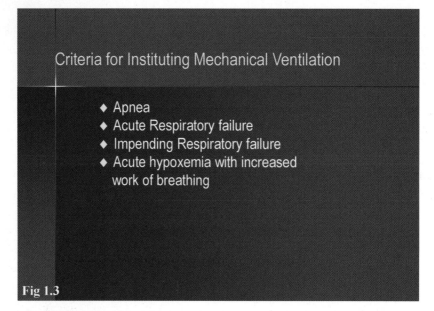

Fig 1.3

Recognition of Respiratory Distress

Assessment of patients in respiratory distress may reveal altered level of consciousness, changes in skin texture and color. Patient may demonstrate physical signs of distress such as nasal flaring, use of accessory muscles and abnormal abdominal as well as chest wall movement (Fig 1.4).

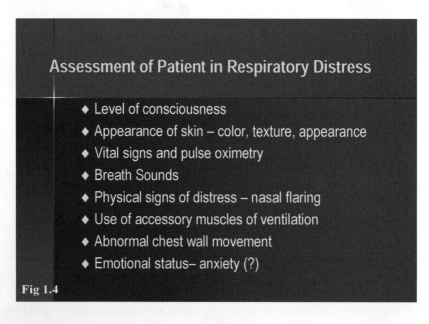

Fig 1.4

Concurrent evaluation of vital signs, pulse oximetry, breath sounds can provide valuable information. Patient's emotional condition such as anxiety may aggravate the underlying cause. Specific clinical manifestations depend on the type of underlying problem.

Indications for Mechanical Ventilation

Respiratory Failure—Acute vs Chronic

Respiratory failure by definition is the inability of the respiratory system to maintain normal delivery of oxygen to the cells and removal of CO_2 from the cells. Respiratory failure is associated with hypoxemia (partial pressure of oxygen in arterial blood (PaO_2) less than 60 mm Hg) and/or hypercapnea (pressure of carbon dioxide in arterial blood ($PaCO_2$) greater than 50 mm Hg) breathing room air. Respiratory failure can be acute or chronic where acute failure requires immediate attention and chronic failure does not require aggressive treatment. Essentially, acute respiratory failure (ARF) can be described as a life-threatening inability of the cardiopulmonary system to maintain adequate gas exchange at the pulmonary level. Pathogenesis of ARF is associated with Lung failure (inadequate gas exchange) and/or Ventilatory failure (inadequate ventilation). Additionally, underlying physiology describes acute respiratory failure in three primary categories (Fig 1.5).

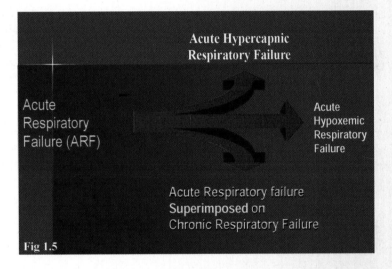

Fig 1.5

Types of Acute Respiratory Failure (ARF)
a. Hypercapnic respiratory failure
b. Hypoxemic respiratory failure
c. Acute respiratory failure superimposed on chronic respiratory failure

The two common types of ARF—hypoxemic respiratory failure and hypercapnic failure result from lung failure or ventilatory failure. Acute respiratory failure superimposed on chronic respiratory failure is associated with exacerbation of Chronic Obstructive Pulmonary Disease.

Characteristics of the Three Types of ARF:

Hypercapnic Respiratory Failure

Acute hypercapnic respiratory failure also referred to as acute ventilatory failure results from failure of the respiratory system to maintain CO_2 homeostasis. Characteristically elevated $PaCO_2$ (above 50 mm Hg) and acidotic pH (< 7.25) are landmarks of acute hypercapnic respiratory failure. Patients in this situation demonstrate dyspnea and tachypnea or hypopnea based on the underlying pathology. Tachycardia and hypertension are also associated with hypercapnic respiratory failure. Neurologically, patients with hypercapnic ARF exhibit somnolence and complain of headache (Fig 1.6) due to elevated $PaCO_2$ which induces increased cerebral blood flow.

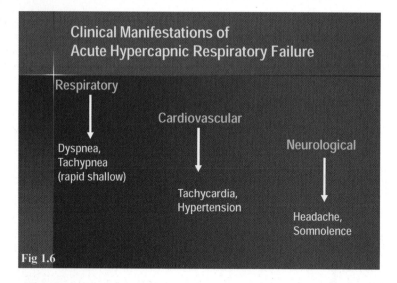

Fig 1.6

Hypoxemic Respiratory Failure

On the other hand, hypoxemic respiratory failure results from inadequate oxygen delivery to the blood. Sustained hypoxemia promotes hyperventilation which leads to respiratory muscle fatigue and subsequent hypoventilation results in hypercapnia and acidosis. Many patients in acute respiratory failure develop both hypoxemia and hypercapnia. Patients in hypoxemic respiratory failure are generally hyperventilating in an attempt to improve oxygen delivery from lungs to blood. Clinically, these patients have dyspnea and tachycardia. They are restless and disoriented (Fig 1.7).

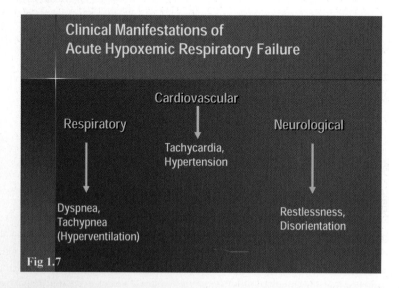

Fig 1.7

Common Causes of Acute Respiratory Failure

Common disorders associated with acute hypercapnic respiratory failure are listed in Fig 1.8. Representative ABGs indicate acute alveolar hypoventilation or hypercapnea ($PaCO_2 > 50$ mm Hg)

Indications for Mechanical Ventilation

with concomitant decrease in pH (uncompensated respiratory acidosis). This obvious ventilation failure requires ventilatory support. Acute hypoxemic failure results from failure of gas exchange due to lung consolidation, acute respiratory distress syndrome (ARDS), sepsis or trauma. Notice representative ABGs in Fig 1.9 exhibiting acute hyperventilation secondary to hypoxemia despite delivery of 100% oxygen (refractory hypoxemia).

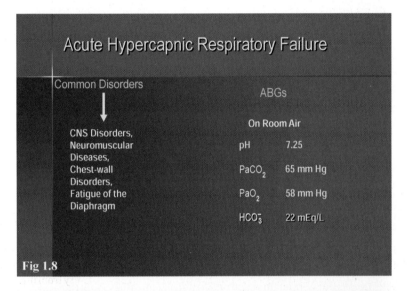

Fig 1.8

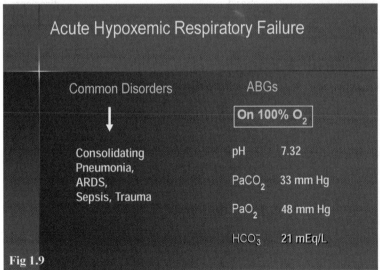

Fig 1.9

Sequence of Hypoxemic Respiratory Failure

The chain of events that precipitate hypoxemic failure begins with refractory hypoxemia which promotes tachycardia and hyperventilation. Tachycardia results in increased myocardial work. Sustained hyperventilation leads to diaphragmatic fatigue reducing diaphragmatic excursion. In order to maintain adequate alveolar ventilation, the patient's respiratory rate increases.

This rapid shallow breathing promotes respiratory acidosis (increased $PaCO_2$ and decreased pH). Hypercapnic Respiratory Failure ensues and the patient becomes a candidate for mechanical ventilation (Fig 1.10).

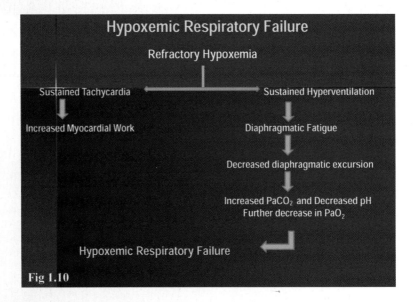

Fig 1.10

Acute Respiratory Failure Superimposed on Chronic Respiratory Failure

Patients with long term chronic ventilatory failure are periodically subjected to acute exacerbation of the chronic lung disease. Added insult to the chronic failure by congestive heart failure, pulmonary emboli and bacterial or viral infections, also promote acute exacerbation. In the emergency department they exhibit acute respiratory failure component superimposed on the underlying chronic failure (Fig 1.11). Increased $PaCO_2$ is responsible for the acidosis, thus hypercapnic failure. However, the degree of hypercapnea does not reflect the level of pH. At a level of $PaCO_2$ of 80 mm Hg, a much lower pH is expected. The higher than normal serum bicarbonate level indicates an underlying long standing disorder. Clinically, this situation is called Acute Respiratory Failure Superimposed on Chronic Respiratory Failure. Care should be taken during weaning these patients. Trying to bring their ABG to normal $PaCO_2$ of a normal adult can be detrimental to these patients since their baseline $PaCO_2$ is higher than textbook normal for adults. Treatment regimen for patients in such situations involves noninvasive ventilation. Avoidance of traditional invasive mechanical ventilation is strongly recommended by many sources. When these patients are extubated, $PaCO_2$ rises to their chronic hypercapnic level. The adjustment of bicarbonate during weaning to normal bicarbonate levels may not be able to compensate for the rise in $PaCO_2$, this leads to acidosis (renal compensation takes a few days to optimize) and extubation fails. Traditional invasive mechanical ventilation is used in patients who fail noninvasive ventilation or have contraindications for noninvasive ventilation.

Concurrent evaluation of vital signs, pulse oximetry, breath sounds can provide valuable information.

Indications for Mechanical Ventilation

Patient's emotional condition such as anxiety may aggravate the underlying cause. Specific clinical manifestations depend on the type of underlying problem.

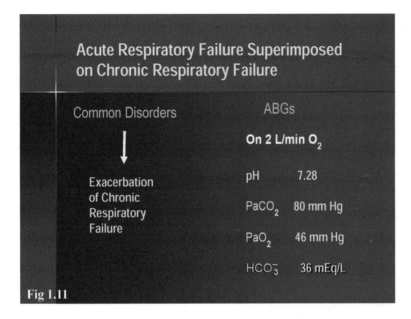

Fig 1.11

Indications for mechanical ventilation and their generic causes include:

1. Apnea
2. Acute hypercapnic respiratory failure
   a. Exacerbation of Neuromuscular Disorders
   b. Drug overdose (Paralytic, Narcotic)
   c. Brain or Brainstem Injury
   d. Central Sleep Apnea
   e. Ingestion of poisonous material such as Organophosphates
3. Acute hypoxemic respiratory failure
   a. Refractory Hypoxemia
   b. Consolidating Pneumonia
   c. Large Atelectasis
   d. ARDS
   e. Persistent hyperventilation leading to respiratory muscle fatigue
4. Acute respiratory failure superimposed on chronic respiratory failure
   a. Exacerbation of COPD (Noninvasive Ventilation is preferred)
   b. Exacerbation in Chronic Restrictive Disorders (Pulmonary Fibrosis - rare)

Goals of Mechanical Ventilation

Initiation of mechanical ventilation facilitates clinicians to increase lung volumes and manipulate pulmonary gas exchange. Patient's work of breathing is reduced as the ventilator assumes all or part of the work of breathing. Figure 1.12 lists the goals of mechanical ventilation.

Goals of Mechanical Ventilation

Increase Lung Volume
- To prevent or treat atelectasis with lung inflation
- To restore Functional Residual Capacity (FRC)

Support or Manipulate Pulmonary Gas Exchange
- Achieve normal alveolar ventilation
- Maintain oxygen delivery

Reduce Work Of Breathing

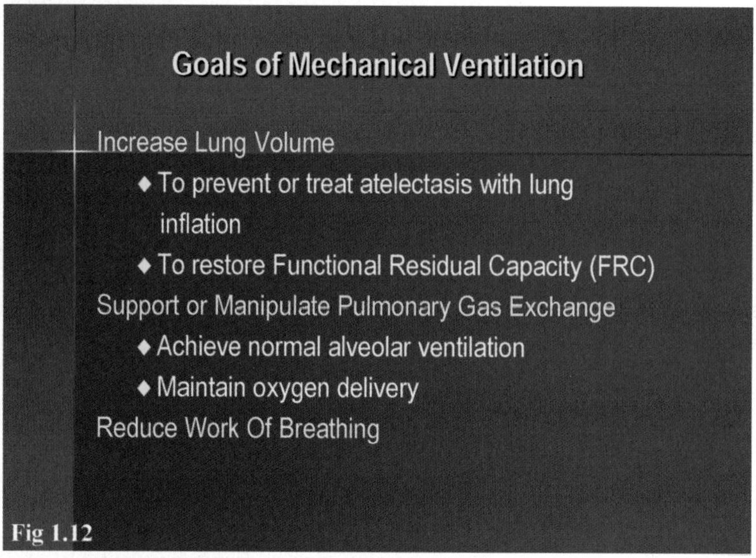

Fig 1.12

★★★

HYPOXEMIC RESPIRATORY FAILURE: PREVENTION AND MANAGEMENT

Oxygen Delivery

Delivery of oxygen to cells depends on two parameters: QT (cardiac output), and CaO_2 (content of oxygen in the arterial blood). Mathematically, the cellular delivery of oxygen is expressed as $QT \times CaO_2$. Figure 2.1 shows parameters that determine the delivery of oxygen to cells. Heart rate and Stroke Volume regulate cardiac output to supply adequate blood flow to tissues in most physiological situations. Whereas, CaO_2 provides the measure of oxygen content in arterial blood. This oxygen is primarily combined to hemoglobin (98%) and is released to cells at capillary tissue membrane. The adequacy of oxygen delivery depends on both the cardiac output and CaO_2. Cardiac output depends on heart rate and stroke volume. Physiologically, cardiac output is adjusted to support the demand of oxygen and the supply to tissues. Demand of oxygen is denoted by $\dot{V}O_2$ whereas supply is the difference between the content of oxygen in the arterial and venous blood ($CaO_2 - CvO_2$) (Fig. 2.2).

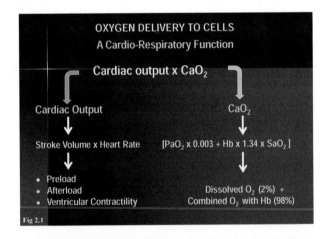

Fig 2.1

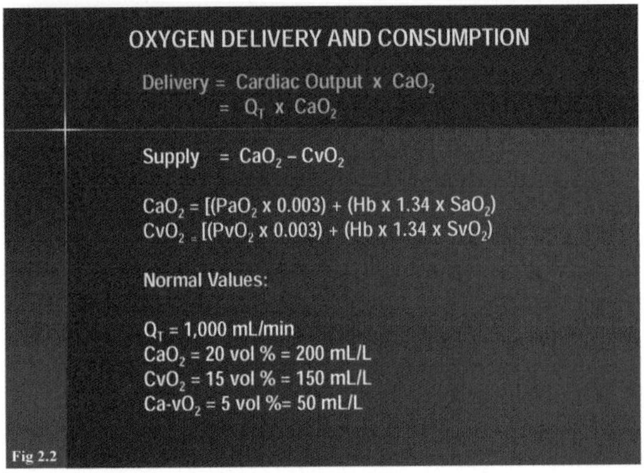

Fig 2.2

Pulmonary disorders and need for oxygenation

Almost all pulmonary disorders affect tissue oxygenation levels via hypoxemia and/or hypoxia. Thus, oxygen therapy is essential in respiratory abnormalities. Oxygen therapy is indicated in treating hypoxemia, to reduce work of breathing and to support myocardial work.

Whether it is secondary to infection or trauma or any other cause, pulmonary diseases/disorders exhibit one or more clinical manifestations such as increased airways resistance, decreased respiratory system compliance and/or pulmonary deadspace (Fig 2.3). In all these situations oxygen therapy is essential. Emphysema is the only disease where lung compliance is increased (decreased recoiling force) causing slow or prolonged expiration.

Pulmonary Disorders
Result in one or more of the following physiological manifestations

- Increased Airway Resistance
- Decreased Lung Compliance
- Increased Lung Compliance (Emphysema)
- Shunt or Shunt like effect
- Deadspace

Fig 2.3

During ventilation, lung characteristics such as airways resistance and lung compliance can change. By definition, gas physics describes resistance through tubing as pressure gradient (ΔP) per unit flow i.e. ΔP/flow and is expressed in cm H_2O/L/min or cm H_2O/L/sec. Normal airways resistance in a spontaneously breathing person is approximately 0.6 – 2.4 cm H_2O/L/sec. Whereas, compliance reflects ease of distensibility measured by volume change per unit pressure change or $C = \Delta V/ \Delta P$ and measured in L/cm H_2O or mL/ cm H_2O (Fig 2.4).

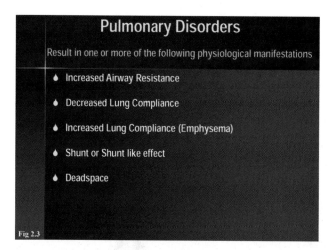

Airway Resistance
- Measure of work required to move air through the airways
- Resistance = $\dfrac{\text{Pressure}}{\text{Flow}}$ = $\dfrac{cmH_2O}{L/sec}$
- primarily influenced by airway diameter
- Normal R_{aw} = 0.6 – 2.4 cmH_2O/L/sec

Compliance
- Measure of work required to deliver the tidal volume to the lungs.
- Compliance = $\dfrac{\Delta \text{Volume}}{\Delta \text{Pressure}}$ = L / cm H_2O
- Normal Lung Compliance = 0.1 L/cmH_2O (100 ml/cmH_2O)
- High compliance easier - to inflate
- Low compliance - harder to inflate

Fig 2.4

Increased Airways Resistance

Obstructive diseases are characterized by increased airways resistance resulting in decreased expiratory flow rates measured by spirometry. Figure 2.5 lists etiologies in common obstructive diseases. Obstruction of the airways in asthma is secondary to bronchospasm that narrows the airways and decreases expiratory flow rates. In bronchitis, bronchiectasis and cystic fibrosis increased secretions are responsible for the increased airways resistance. Inflammation, as in bronchitis and inhalation of noxious gases can also cause narrowing of the airways. Increase in airways resistance to gas flow is inversely proportional to the 4th power of airway radius,

$$R_{aw} \propto 1/r^4$$

Thus reduction in airway diameter has a profound effect on airway resistance.

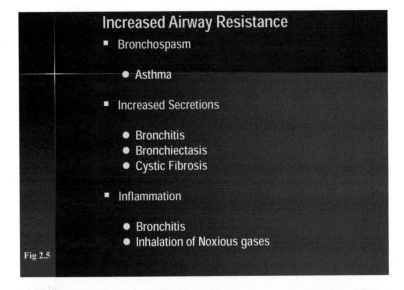

Fig 2.5

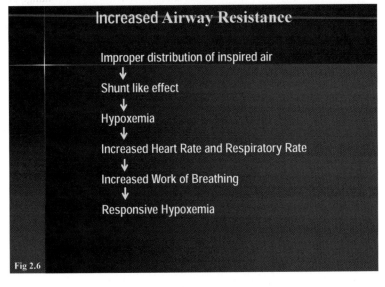

Fig 2.6

Increased airways resistance is associated with improper distribution of inspired air and a shunt like effect (Fig 2.6). Inspired air follows the path of least resistance and thus, the partially obstructed areas receive lesser amount of air. This results in inadequate oxygenation of the venous blood in these areas. Ensuing venous admixture in pulmonary vein and left atrium promotes hypoxemic hypoxia (Fig 2.7). Clinically this can be verified by tachycardia, hyperventilation and decreased PaO_2 or SpO_2. This type of hypoxemia responds to oxygen therapy. Administration of supplemental oxygen increases alveolar partial pressure of oxygen (PaO_2) in these areas, improving PaO_2, thus relieving hypoxemia.

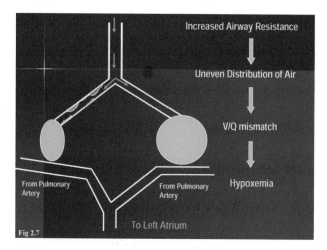

Fig 2.7

Decreased Lung Compliance

By definition in pulmonary physiology, lung compliance is a measure of ease of distensibility of the lung. Compliance is reciprocal of elastance which reflects the recoiling force of the lung. The higher the elastance, lower is the compliance, and stiffer the lung.

Restrictive disorders listed in Fig 2.8 are commonly observed in patients admitted to hospitals. In these diseases/disorders, as compliance decreases, functional residual capacity (FRC) of the lung decreases reducing lung volume. In severe cases lung collapses (Atelectasis) resulting in intrapulmonary shunting and refractory hypoxemia.

Decreased Lung Compliance
- Atelectasis
- Pneumonia
- Pneumothorax
- Pulmonary Edema
- Pleural Effusion
- Neuromuscular Diseases
- ARDS
- Chest Trauma
- Picwickian Syndrome
- Flail Chest

Fig 2.8

Decreased Lung Compliance
- Stiffer lung units
  ↓
- Intrapulmonary Shunt
  ↓
- Hypoxemia
  ↓
- Increased Heart Rate and Respiratory Rate
  ↓
- Increased Work of Breathing
  ↓
- Refractory Hypoxemia (need for CPAP/PEEP)

Fig 2.9

Figure 2.9 describes the sequence of physiological manifestations of decreased lung compliance. As the compliance decreases, the lung units reduce in volume. When it decreases below the minimal opening volume, lung units collapse. Atelectasis promotes intrapulmonary shunting and refractory hypoxemia. To open stiffer lungs require higher pressure gradient. During spontaneous breathing, decreased lung compliance necessitates increased work on the respiratory muscles to inflate the lung in order to receive adequate tidal volume. Venous blood circulating around the collapsed part of the lung units does not take part in gas exchange. Thus the blood returning to left atrium from these shunted areas has the same content of oxygen as venous blood. If the atelectatic area is large, the venous admixture is also large enough to cause significant decrease in PaO_2 and SpO_2 (hypoxemia). Upon initiating oxygen therapy, the shunted area with no communication with ventilated alveoli, does not receive any oxygen. This results in refractory hypoxemia (Figs 2.10 and 2.11).

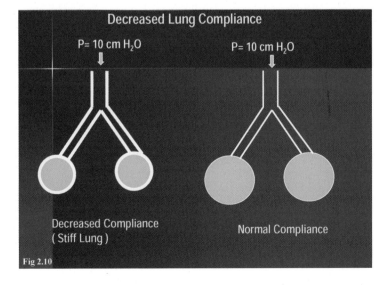

Fig 2.10

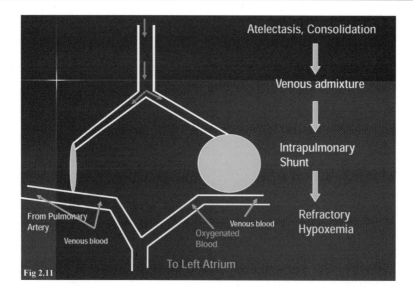
Fig 2.11

Improvement in oxygenation can be accomplished, in many cases, by treating the underlying disorder and re-opening the collapsed lung areas. Application of positive pressure is commonly used to expand the collapsed lung. Appropriate level of continuous positive airway pressure (CPAP) is used if hyperinflation therapy is inadequate. If CPAP is ineffective the patient's respiratory rate continues to increase secondary to hypoxemia. Increased work of breathing results in diaphragmatic fatigue and acute respiratory failure. This sequence leading to hypoxemic respiratory failure indicates need for mechanical ventilation.

Initial steps are always taken to prevent hypoxemic respiratory failure. In situations of V/Q mismatch supplemental oxygen therapy generally improves oxygenation. Treatment with bronchodilators, bronchial hygiene techniques or inhaled steroids indicated by the underlying cause is also employed. Figure 2.12 identifies the therapy to be used in specific situations listed.

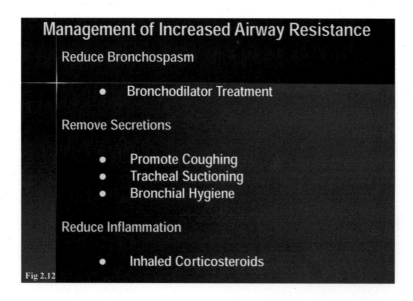
Fig 2.12

Hypoxemic Respiratory Failure: Prevention and Management

Similarly actions are taken to prevent hypoxemic respiratory failure in restrictive disorders. It is common to initiate noninvasive treatment regimen involving deep breathing exercises, incentive spirometry and CPAP. Use of intermittent positive pressure breathing(IPPB) has lost its popularity due to lack of evidence. Patients not responding to these interventions require mechanical ventilation (Fig 2.13).

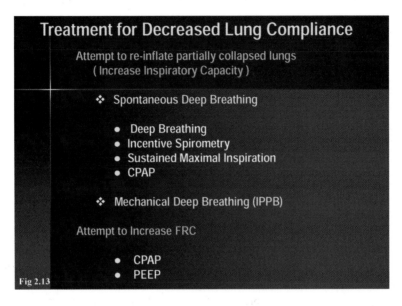

Fig 2.13

Hypoxia and Hypoxemia

Dissolved oxygen constitutes a very small amount (2%) of oxygen whereas oxygen combined with hemoglobin amounts to 98% of the total content. Any reduction in cardiac output, PaO_2 or hemoglobin leads to inadequate tissue oxygenation known as Hypoxia. Although used interchangeably, hypoxia and hypoxemia are not the same. Hypoxia is referred to clinical deprivation of cellular oxygen revealed from tachycardia, hyperventilation and hypertension. Hypoxemia, on the other hand, simply indicates that the partial pressure of oxygen in the arterial blood is less than normal. $PaO_2 < 80$ mm Hg or $SpO_2 < 92\%$ (Fig 2.14).

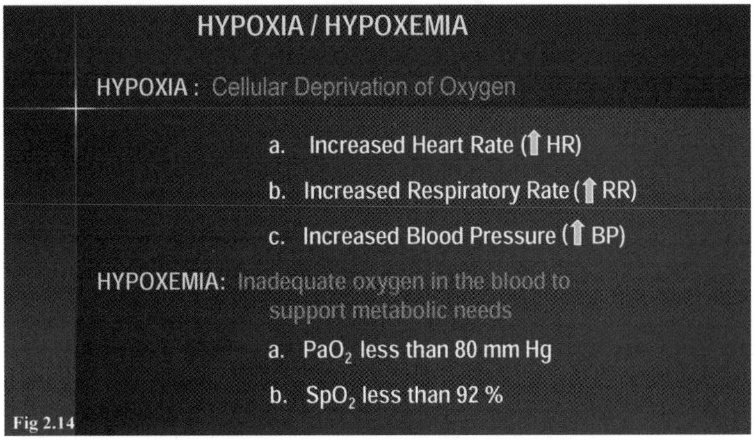

HYPOXIA / HYPOXEMIA

HYPOXIA: Cellular Deprivation of Oxygen
a. Increased Heart Rate (↑ HR)
b. Increased Respiratory Rate (↑ RR)
c. Increased Blood Pressure (↑ BP)

HYPOXEMIA: Inadequate oxygen in the blood to support metabolic needs
a. PaO_2 less than 80 mm Hg
b. SpO_2 less than 92 %

Fig 2.14

These clinical manifestations—tachycardia, hyperventilation (tachypnea) and hypertension are considered as homeostatic responses to cellular inadequacy of oxygen.

Conventionally, hypoxia are classified from their etiology such as low PaO_2 (hypoxemic hypoxia), low hemoglobin (anemic hypoxia), inadequate cellular perfusion secondary to decreased cardiac output (circulatory hypoxia) and inability for the cells to remove oxygen from the arterial blood (histotoxic hypoxia). Clinically, recognition of the underlying cause of hypoxia facilitates selecting proper treatment (Fig 2.15).

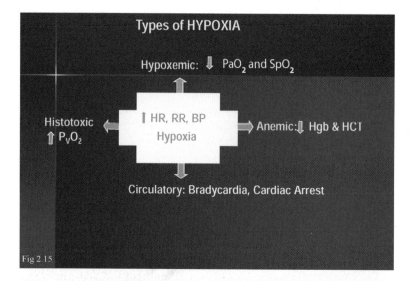

Fig 2.15

Table 2.1 demonstrates that in Hypoxemic Hypoxia, the PaO_2 and SpO_2 (saturation of hemoglobin obtained from pulse oximetry) are decreased. In fact, a decreased PaO_2 and SpO_2 confirms hypoxemic hypoxia and indicates the need for supplemental oxygen. In anemic hypoxia, the PaO_2 and

SpO_2 can be normal, however due to decreased hemoglobin the total content of oxygen (CaO_2) is decreased and thus the inadequate oxygen delivery to the cells leads to tachycardia and hyperventilation. In circulatory hypoxia the underlying problem is decreased cardiac output promoting inadequate supply of oxygen to tissues. Finally, in histotoxic hypoxia, the arterial content of oxygen and cardiac output are normal and yet, the cells are deprived of oxygen due to cellular abnormality to remove oxygen across the capillary-cellular interface. Interestingly, PaO_2 is decreased only in hypoxemic hypoxia and can be normal in other types of hypoxia. Thus, cellular adequacy of oxygenation involves evaluation of PaO_2 or SpO_2, hemoglobin level and adequacy in cardiac output.

Table 2.2 exhibits the effect of decreased hemoglobin on oxygen transport. Compared to hypoxemic hypoxia where the SaO_2 is only 80% the total content of oxygen is higher than in anemic hypoxia where the PaO_2 and SaO_2 are normal. The total oxygen content is significantly reduced (10 vol% compared to 16.3 vol%).

	Normal Oxygenation	Hypoxemic Hypoxia	Anemic Hypoxia
PaO_2	90 mm Hg	45 mm Hg	90 mm Hg
SaO_2	98%	80%	98%
Hb	15 g/dL	15 g/dL	7.5 g/dL
CaO_2	200 ml/L (20 vol%)	163 ml/L (16.3 vol%)	100 ml/L (10 vol%)
% change		−18.6%	−49.5%

Table 2.2

Common causes of hypoxemia are listed in Fig 2.16

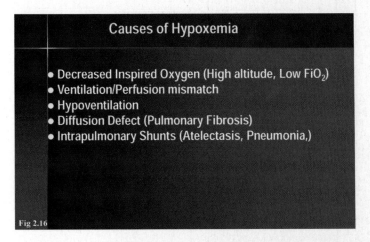

Causes of Hypoxemia

- Decreased Inspired Oxygen (High altitude, Low FiO_2)
- Ventilation/Perfusion mismatch
- Hypoventilation
- Diffusion Defect (Pulmonary Fibrosis)
- Intrapulmonary Shunts (Atelectasis, Pneumonia,)

Fig 2.16

Acute hypoxemia is suspected when tachycardia, hyperventilation and/or tachypnea are present. If hypoxemia is not treated, oxyhemoglobin continues to desaturate ($HbO_2 + H^+ \rightleftarrows HHb^+ + O_2$). Resulting deoxyhemoglobin (HHb^+) imparts bluish coloration to gums, fingertips, lips etc. This condition is known as cyanosis and requires immediate delivery of supplemental oxygen. Neurologically, acute hypoxemia promotes restlessness and confusion (Fig 2.17).

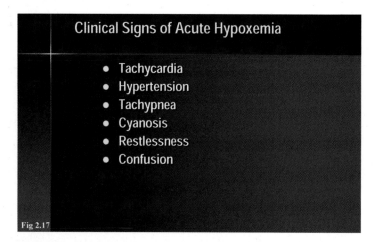
Fig 2.17

Hypoxia can be managed by identifying the type of underlying cause

Clinically, low PaO_2 and/or low SpO_2 confirm hypoxemia. Associated tachycardia and hyperventilation verify hypoxemic hypoxia. Upon initiation of supplemental oxygen, patients correctable V/Q mismatch respond to the oxygen therapy and the PaO_2, SpO_2, as well as heart rate and respiratory rate return to normal levels. However, if PaO_2 and SpO_2 return to normal levels and yet, tachycardia and hyperventilation persists, anemic hypoxemia may be suspected. An evaluation of hemoglobin and hematocrit is recommended (Fig 2.18).

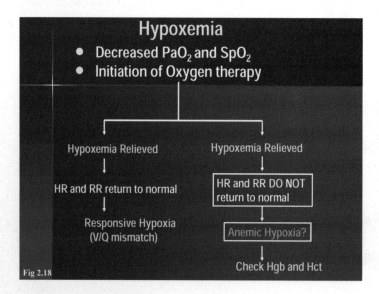
Fig 2.18

Hypoxemic Respiratory Failure: Prevention and Management

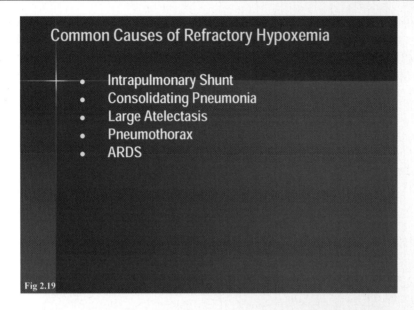

Fig 2.19

In presence of intrapulmonary shunting as observed in disorders such as atelectasis, consolidating pneumonia and acute respiratory distress syndrome (ARDS), PaO_2 and SpO_2 do not return to normal levels despite supplemental oxygen therapy. This situation where hypoxemia is not relieved by oxygen therapy is referred to as refractory hypoxemia. Figure 2.19 lists the common causes of refractory hypoxemia. Chest radiogram provides further information on the underlying cause. Based on the underlying cause a treatment regimen can be employed. Consolidation due to pneumonia or atelectasis is treated by therapy such as continuous positive airway pressure (CPAP) to open collapsed lung (Fig 2.20).

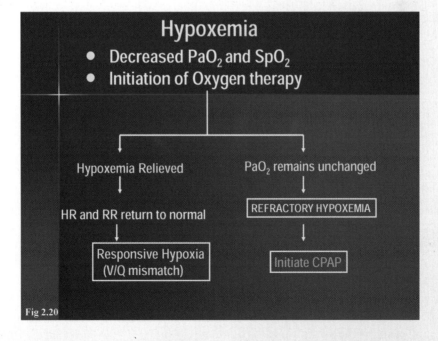

Fig 2.20

One more clinical manifestation of hypoxemia must be recognized. Hypoxemia promotes pulmonary vasoconstriction leading to pulmonary hypertension. Figure 2.21 lists cardiovascular effects of hypoxemia. Thus, hypoxemia should be treated appropriately, as soon as possible.

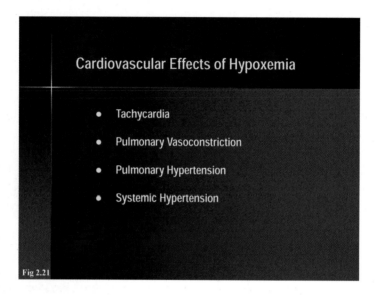

Fig 2.21

Sustained hyperventilation secondary to refractory hypoxemia can promote diaphragmatic fatigue leading to hypoventilation. Hypoventilation further decreases PaO_2. This condition, associated with hypoxemia (low PaO_2), hypercapnia (high $PaCO_2$) and low pH, is characterized as Respiratory Failure. Thus, sustained refractory hypoxemia leads to hypoxemic respiratory failure and may require mechanical ventilation (Fig 2.22).

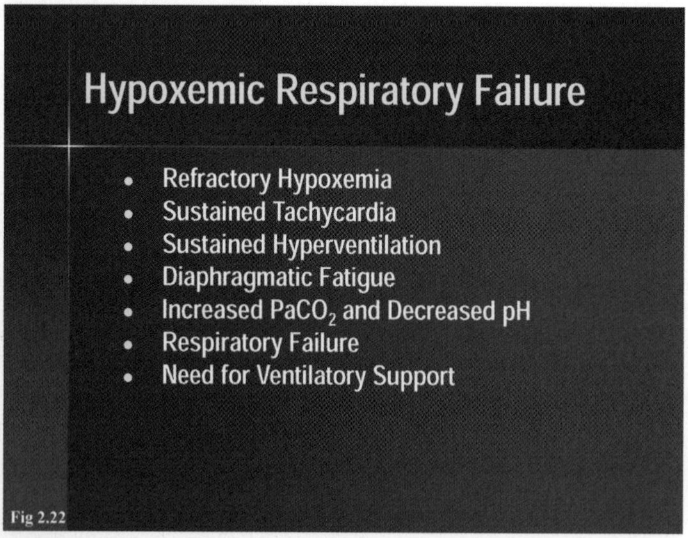

Hypoxemic Respiratory Failure

- Refractory Hypoxemia
- Sustained Tachycardia
- Sustained Hyperventilation
- Diaphragmatic Fatigue
- Increased $PaCO_2$ and Decreased pH
- Respiratory Failure
- Need for Ventilatory Support

Fig 2.22

★★★

ACID BASE DISORDERS AND ABG INTERPRETATIONS

Survival of cells depends primarily on temperature, pH of the surrounding fluid, nutrients available and adequacy of capillary blood flow. Precision in hydrogen ion concentration (pH) plays an important role in making the cells function normally. The amount of hydrogen ions in the arterial blood reflects the concentration around the cells. Homeostatic mechanisms maintain the required environment around the cells for proper function. Acid base balance is controlled by the lungs, the kidneys and the buffer system.

A. When hydrogen ions (H^+) are added in the body fluids, the buffers combine with free floating H^+, thereby decreasing their concentration.

B. An increase in the concentration of H^+ promotes the following:

1. The lungs increase their excretion of CO_2 (hyperventilation).
2. The kidneys accelerate excretion of hydrogen ions.

C. The combined action of buffers, lungs, and kidneys maintains optimal hydrogen ion concentration, or pH, necessary for proper metabolism.

Although detailed description of acid base physiology is beyond the scope of this book, specific important concepts are identified.

Henderson–Hasselbach Equation

A commonly described physiologic equation, Henderson–Hasselbach equation, expresses the combined relationship of H^+, HCO_3^- and pH.

$$pH = pK + \log \frac{[HCO_3^-]}{[H_2CO_3]}$$

$$= pK + \log \frac{[HCO_3^-]}{PaCO_2 \times 0.03}$$

Substituting normal values, for pK, $PaCO_2$, HCO_3^-

$$pH = 6.1 + \log \frac{24}{40 \times 0.03}$$

$$= 7.4$$

where, pK is the pH of the reaction at equilibrium and is constant for a given reversible chemical reaction, $[HCO_3^-]$ is the bicarbonate concentration and 0.03 is the solubility coefficient for CO_2 in plasma.

Significance of the Henderson–Hasselbach equation:

A. pH varies directly with the ratio of HCO_3^-/H_2CO_3.
B. HCO_3^-/H_2CO_3 ratio is normally 20:1.
C. For a given bicarbonate concentration, as the PCO_2 increases, the pH decreases.
D. For a given PCO_2 value, as the HCO_3^- increases, the pH increases.

Recognize that the homeostasis maintains precise concentration of 40 nanomoles in the arterial blood. 40 nanomoles is extremely small, 40×10^{-9} or 0.000,000,040 moles of hydrogen ions $[H^+]$. Any small deviation in $[H^+]$ can have a profound effect on the cellular environment and results in physiologic response.

Figure 3.1 shows the relationship between hydrogen ion concentration and pH.

[H⁺] at different levels of pH

pH	$[H^+]$ (moles/L)	$[H^+]$ (nanomoles/L)
6.0	10^{-6}	1000
7.0	10^{-7}	100
7.4	$10^{-7.4}$	40
8.0	10^{-8}	10

pH and nano mole concentration of Hydrogen ions in clinical range

8.0	7.7	7.4	7.1	7.0	pH
10	20	40	80	100	nano moles (10^{-9} moles)

Fig 3.1

In disease states, lungs and kidneys, attempt to bring the disturbed acid base balance to normal level. In critically ill patients requiring mechanical ventilation, the clinician has to manipulate ventilator settings to provide assistance to the physiological efforts. This requires a thorough understanding of the interpretation of arterial blood gases.

Figure 3.2 shows the normal values of the common parameters measured by the blood gas machine and their normal values.

NORMAL ARTERIAL BLOOD GAS VALUES

Parameter	Absolute Normal	Normal Range
pH	7.40	7.35 – 7.45
$PaCO_2$	40 mm Hg	35 – 45 mm Hg
HCO_3^-	24 mEq/L	22 – 26 mEq/L
Base Excess	0	±2
PaO_2	100 mmHg	80 – 100 mm Hg
SaO_2	97%	> 95%
Hemoglobin	14 gram%	12 – 15 gram%

Fig 3.2

Interpretation of ABGs

NORMAL VALUES

PaO_2	80 – 100 mm Hg
$PaCO_2$	35 – 45 mm Hg
pH	7.35 – 7.45
HCO_3^-	22 – 26 mEq/L

Fig 3.3

The four parameters used to interpret a blood gas results are PaO_2, $PaCO_2$, pH and HCO_3^- (Fig 3.3). Since, lungs and kidneys maintain acid base balance by managing elimination of CO_2 and H^+, any abnormality in the pH value can be attributed to the abilities of these two organs. A disorder precipitated by abnormal lung function is referred to as respiratory disorder and that secondary to kidney function is called metabolic disorder. Secondly, since there are only two types of acid base imbalances, acidosis and alkalosis, by evaluating pH, $PaCO_2$ and HCO_3^- the clinician can determine the type of acid base imbalance. Figure 3.4 indicates how to determine the underlying respiratory or metabolic abnormality.

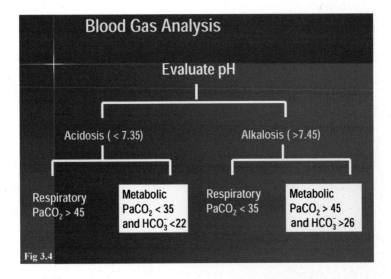

Fig 3.4

Lungs adjust alveolar ventilation as required by the current acid base status. In acidosis, lungs accelerate elimination of CO_2 via hyperventilation. In neuromuscular diseases, lung function is impaired and causes hypoventilation. It is imperative that a clinician must determine the degree of ventilation during patient assessment.

Ventilation is assessed from minute ventilation, deadspace ventilation and alveolar ventilation. The relationship of these three terms is expressed by a common equation:

Alveolar ventilation = Minute ventilation – Deadspace ventilation

$$V_A \times f = (V_T \times f) - (V_D \times f)$$
$$= (V_T - V_D) f$$

Lung performance is described from the degree of alveolar ventilation as normal ventilation, hypoventilation and hyperventilation. Figure 3.5 illustrates the relationship between $PaCO_2$ and alveolar ventilation and Fig 3.6 shows determination of type of ventilation from $PaCO_2$ levels.

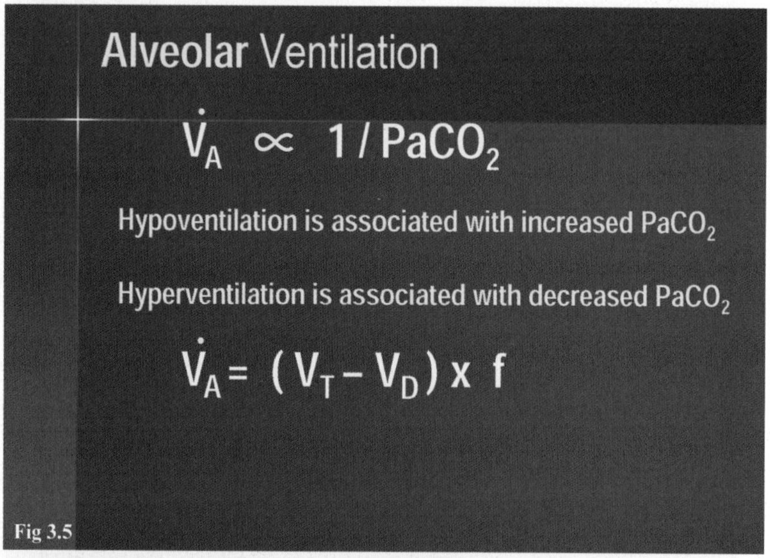

Alveolar Ventilation

$$\dot{V}_A \propto 1/PaCO_2$$

Hypoventilation is associated with increased $PaCO_2$

Hyperventilation is associated with decreased $PaCO_2$

$$\dot{V}_A = (V_T - V_D) \times f$$

Fig 3.5

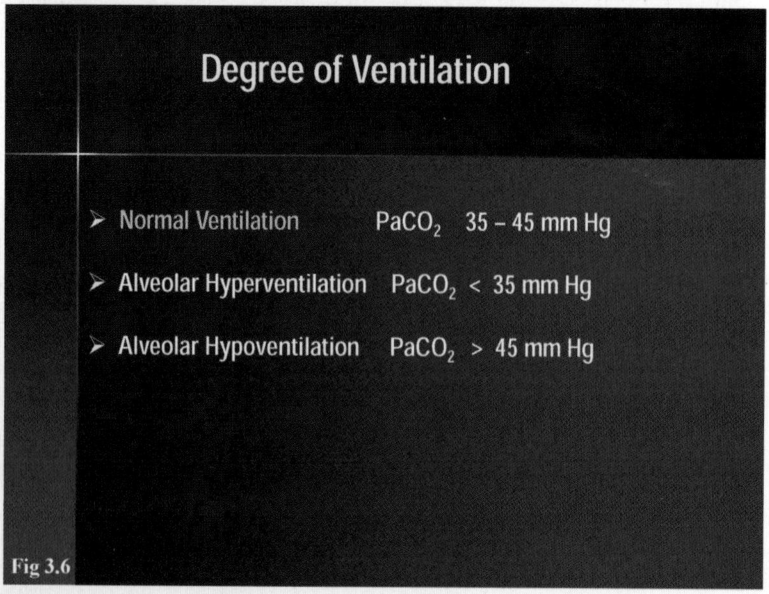

Degree of Ventilation

- Normal Ventilation — $PaCO_2$ 35 – 45 mm Hg
- Alveolar Hyperventilation — $PaCO_2$ < 35 mm Hg
- Alveolar Hypoventilation — $PaCO_2$ > 45 mm Hg

Fig 3.6

Acid Base Disorders and ABG Interpretations

In their management of acid base balance, lung and kidneys attempt to compensate the underlying imbalance. In respiratory acidosis, the kidneys accelerate the excretion of H^+ and retention of HCO_3^- to compensate for acidosis whereas in respiratory alkalosis the H+ excretion is minimized. Similarly, the respiratory compensation during metabolic acidosis is exhibited by hyperventilation and in severe metabolic alkalosis lungs tend to hypoventilate.

Figure 3.7 describes the definitions of acute and chronic disorders and the compensatory activity of lungs and kidneys.

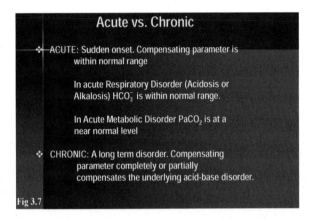

Fig 3.7

Now it is time to evaluate arterial blood gas values, interpret and recommend a corrective action for the underlying disorder. In reality, the patient's other clinical parameters, underlying disease state and compensatory levels should be assessed before making a treatment decision.

IN THIS CHAPTER, THE CASES THAT FOLLOW ARE SIMPLE ABG VALUES AND ARE EXPLAINED IN THE CONTEXT OF ACADEMIC INTERPRETATION

Blood gas analysis can be interpreted in two ways, academic interpretation and clinical interpretation. For example, ABG in Fig 3.8A, the values show alkalotic pH, a less than normal $PaCO_2$ and normal HCO_3^-. The PaO_2 indicates hypoxemia (< 80 mm Hg). Thus, academically this ABG is interpreted as **uncompensated respiratory alkalosis with hypoxemia.** Clinical interpretation is simply a quick communication within the clinicians to express the values in clinically related terms. The ABG in Fig 3.8A is also interpreted as **Acute Alveolar Hyperventilation with hypoxemia.**

BLOOD GAS INTERPRETATION

	A	B
pH	7.52	7.52
$PaCO_2$	28 mm Hg	28 mm Hg
PaO_2	55 mm Hg	85 mm Hg
HCO_3^-	23 mEq/l	23 m Eq/l
FiO_2	0.21	0.21

Fig 3.8

Upon interpreting ABG, the clinician is expected to identify the underlying cause and treat it accordingly. For ABGs in Fig 3.8A, causes of acute hyperventilation must be identified. It is known that hypoxemia, hyperthermia, anxiety or inappropriate ventilator settings can promote hyperventilation (Fig 3.9). In ICU, hypoxia and anxiety are the most common causes of hyperventilation. Hyperventilation secondary to hypoxemic hypoxia can simply be treated by initiating supplemental oxygen or increasing FiO_2 on the ventilator. The patient will also hyperventilate in anemic hypoxia. However, in anemic hypoxia the PaO_2 is within normal limits with hemoglobin level < 12 gm%. Similarly, hyperthermia, anxiety and pain related hyperventilation exhibit normal PaO_2. Fig 3.8B represents values associated with hyperventilation secondary to anemia, anxiety and pain. Thus, uncompensated respiratory alkalosis can be much effectively interpreted as Acute Alveolar Hyperventilation. The clinicians address acute alveolar hyperventilation by identifying the underlying cause and treat it. Later in Chapter 7, importance of recognizing the degree of ventilation will be discussed in view of making changes in ventilator parameters.

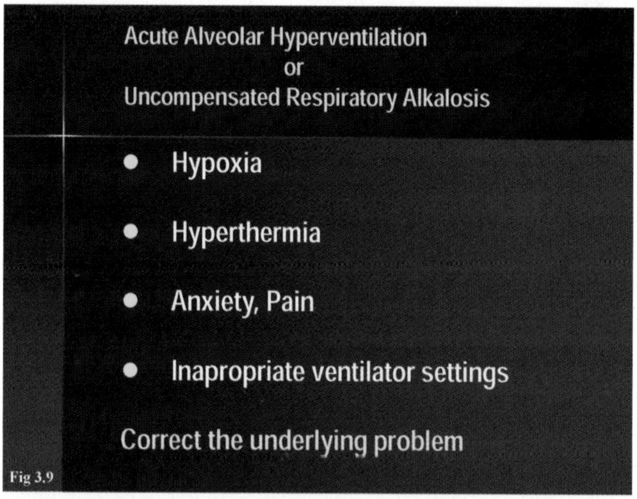

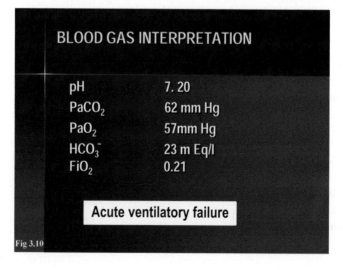

Fig 3.9

Fig 3.10

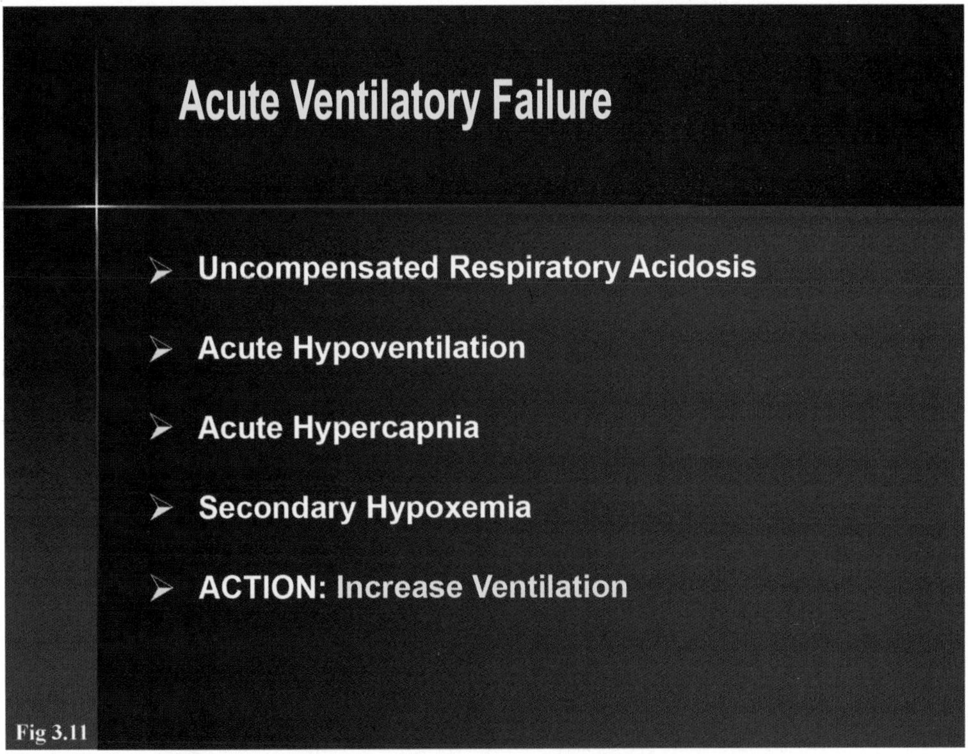

Acute Ventilatory Failure

- Uncompensated Respiratory Acidosis
- Acute Hypoventilation
- Acute Hypercapnia
- Secondary Hypoxemia
- ACTION: Increase Ventilation

Fig 3.11

The ABG in Fig 3.10 is an example of **Acute Ventilatory Failure.** Academically, this ABG is interpreted as **uncompensated respiratory acidosis or acute alveolar hypoventilation or even, acute hypercapnia (Fig 3.11).** These interpretations are consistent with acidotic pH resulting from increased $PaCO_2$ with normal level of HCO_3^-. Higher than normal $PaCO_2$ is associated with hypoventilation and is also referred to as hypercapnia. The clinical interpretation **Acute Ventilatory Failure** implies that the ventilatory system has failed to provide adequate ventilation as indicated by increased $PaCO_2$ and decreased pH. There is no renal compensation which confirms acute situation. Interpretation as acute ventilatory failure also assists the clinician to respond by increasing alveolar ventilation. The patient exhibiting ABGs in Fig 3.10 is generally ventilated via non-invasive ventilation e.g. (BiPAP) or intubated and placed on an invasive ventilator.

Metabolic acidosis is also one of the challenging patient situations in ICU. Figure 3.12 shows a severely decreased pH (acidosis). However, $PaCO_2$ is decreased and thus, is not responsible for the acidosis. In fact, this degree of hyperventilation (decreased $PaCO_2$) should result in severe respiratory alkalosis. Thus, the acidosis is non-respiratory or metabolic acidosis.

This is also confirmed from decreased HCO_3^- which is the primary cause of acidosis in this case. Hyperventilation is an effort from the lungs to reverse metabolic acidosis by exhaling as much CO_2 (gas form of acid) as possible. However, the compensatory mechanism has not brought the pH back to normal and thus this ABG is interpreted as Partially Compensated Metabolic Acidosis. What can cause metabolic acidosis? Fig 3.13 lists the four common causes of metabolic acidosis–**Lactic acidosis, Keto acidosis, Renal failure and Diarrhea.**

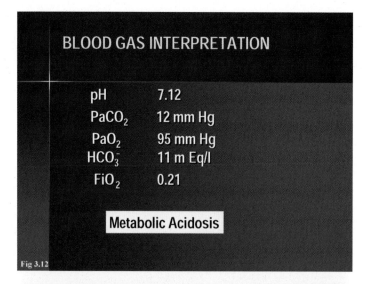
Fig 3.12

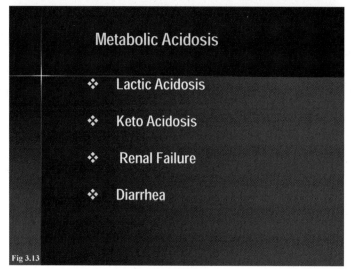
Fig 3.13

Lactic Acidosis

Lactic acidosis results from inadequate availability of oxygen at mitochondria level. The primary engine to generate energy required for survival and maintaining bodily functions is Citric Acid Cycle also known as Kreb's cycle. In 1937 Krebs proposed a specific metabolic pathway within the cells to account for the oxidation of the basic components of food – carbohydrates, protein and fats – for energy. The Krebs' cycle takes place inside the mitochondria or 'power plant' of cells and provides energy required for the organism to function. During metabolism, Glucose molecules go through Glycolysis, an anaerobic degradation of Glucose to Pyruvic acid which is further converted to Acetyl Co-enzyme A (Fig 3.14). In presence of oxygen, Acetyl Co-A goes through Kreb's cycle (Citric Acid cycle). In simple terms, the Krebs' cycle metabolizes acetyl coenzyme A into citric acid and then runs through a complex series of biological oxidations, producing free hydrogen ions. Each molecule of citric acid that rotates through the Krebs' cycle, generates 38 molecules of ATP for tissue fuel.

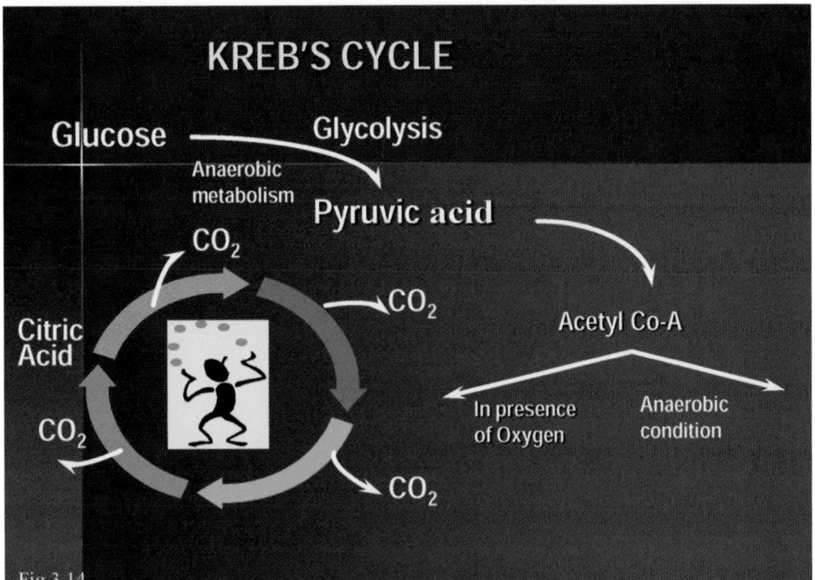

Acid Base Disorders and ABG Interpretations

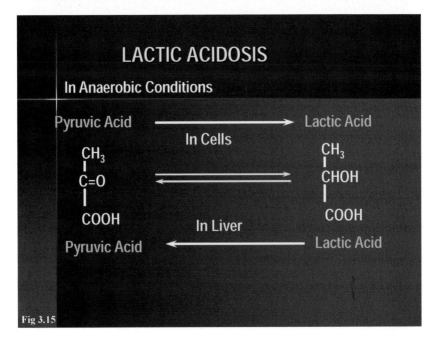

Fig 3.14

Fig 3.15

During this aerobic metabolic process every conversion produces CO_2 as a by-product which, being gaseous, is exhaled by the lungs. In absence of oxygen the conversion of Acetyl Co-A is stopped and an alternative pathway is selected by the metabolic system to generate energy. This anaerobic pathway uses cellular energy and converts Pyruvic acid into Lactic Acid. Concentration gradient moves Lactic Acid from cells to blood and to the Liver, where enzymatic reaction reconverts it back to Pyruvic Acid (Fig 3.15).

Lactate Measurement
Assessment of adequacy of Oxygen Delivery

- $CaO_2 \times CO$ = Oxygen Delivery
- $ScVO_2$ reflects Oxygen consumption
- Increased Lactate levels indicate Anaerobic metabolism
- Decreased ATP production
- May lead to cell death
- Lacti-Time, a prognostic indicator

Fig 3.16

Since Lactic acidosis results from inadequate oxygen delivery to cells, Lactate measurement can verify or rule out anaerobic metabolism (Fig 3.16). $ScVO_2$, venous saturation of oxygen, reflects oxygen consumption by the cells. Figure 3.17 shows the levels of $ScVO_2$ and their significance in oxygen delivery and consumption. When oxygen delivery is decreased and is unable to provide normal oxygen consumption, lactic acidosis ensues. In many institutions lactate measurement is frequently done when anaerobic metabolism is suspected. As discussed earlier, lactates are converted back to pyruvic acid. The time required for the lactates to return to normal is associated with mortality. Prolonged lactate clearance results in increased mortality. Inability to bring elevated lactate level to normal level has 100% mortality. Lacti-time is a prognostic test. Longer lacti-time is a serious condition and is addressed immediately.

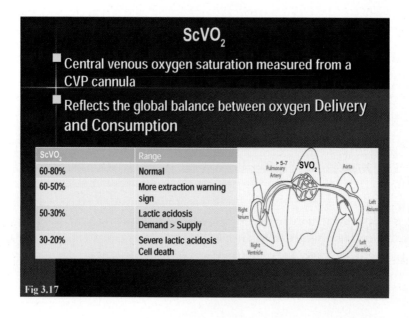

$ScVO_2$

- Central venous oxygen saturation measured from a CVP cannula
- Reflects the global balance between oxygen Delivery and Consumption

$ScVO_2$	Range
60-80%	Normal
60-50%	More extraction warning sign
50-30%	Lactic acidosis Demand > Supply
30-20%	Severe lactic acidosis Cell death

Fig 3.17

KETO ACIDOSIS

Normally, glucose metabolism involves conversion of Pyruvic acid through Kreb's cycle producing energy and by-product CO_2 which is exhaled. In inadequate or absence of Insulin, Pyruvic acid conversion is inhibited. Therefore, cells experience accumulation of Pyruvic acid. Concentration gradient allows pyruvic acid to enter the blood and migrates to the Liver where it is converted into Acetoacetyl Co–A. Subsequent degradation produces three products, Acetoacetic acid, Beta hydroxyl butyric acid and Acetone (Fig 3.18). All these three products contain organic keto group (C=O). Acetoacetic acid and beta hydroxyl butyric acid are organic acids and cannot be exhaled and thus precipitate ketoacidosis. The third product, Acetone, is a low boiling organic compound and barely exists in liquid form at room temperature. At body temperature Acetone is in gaseous condition and finds its way out through respiratory system and imparts a peculiar smell. In clinical settings clinicians recognize this "Acetone Breath" and recognize that the patient has developed KETO ACIDOSIS. The patent is treated according to the protocol for treatment of diabetic patients.

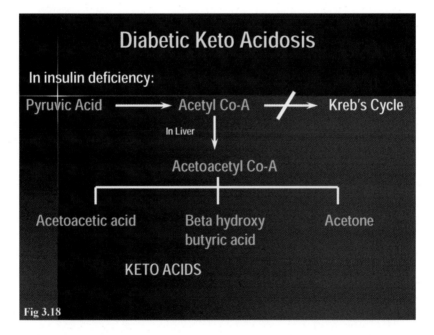

Fig 3.18

The other two causes of metabolic acidosis, renal failure and diarrhea are relatively common in ICU. In renal failure, blood urea nitrogen (BUN), is elevated and creatinine clearance is decreased. Patients experiencing diarrhea lose HCO_3^- which results in acidosis. These two causes are treated symptomatically with appropriate diagnostic tests and medications.

ANION GAP

The normal electrolyte concentration in plasma is shown in Fig 3.19. The total number of anions (negatively charged ions) and cations (positively charged ions) are always in equal concentration, approximately 154 mEq/L, to maintain electro-neutrality.

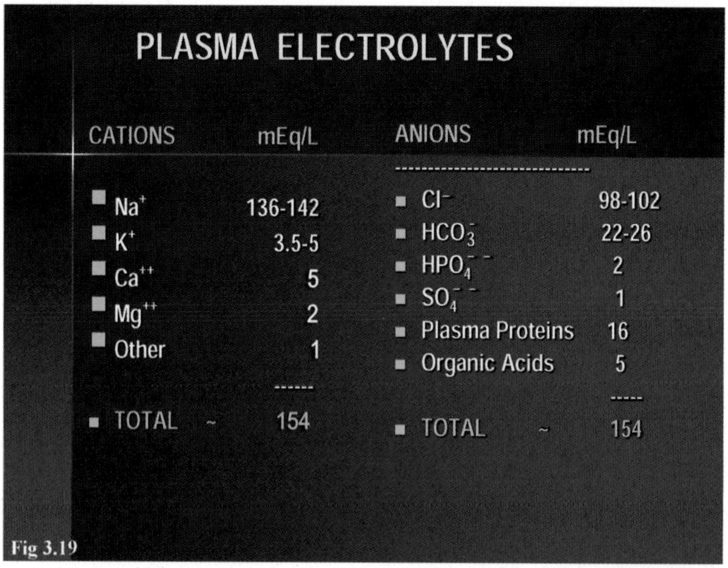

PLASMA ELECTROLYTES

CATIONS	mEq/L	ANIONS	mEq/L
Na^+	136-142	Cl^-	98-102
K^+	3.5-5	HCO_3^-	22-26
Ca^{++}	5	HPO_4^{--}	2
Mg^{++}	2	SO_4^{--}	1
Other	1	Plasma Proteins	16
		Organic Acids	5
TOTAL ~	154	TOTAL ~	154

Fig 3.19

The most abundant positive ion is sodium (Na^+) whereas, chloride (Cl^-) and HCO_3^- are abundant negative ions in plasma. The difference between these three ions, provide a quick diagnosis of metabolic acidosis. As shown in Fig 3.20, the difference in measured concentration of Na^+ and (Cl^- + HCO_3^-) is used as an index of type of metabolic acidosis.

Anion Gap = (Na^+) − (Cl^- + HCO_3^-)

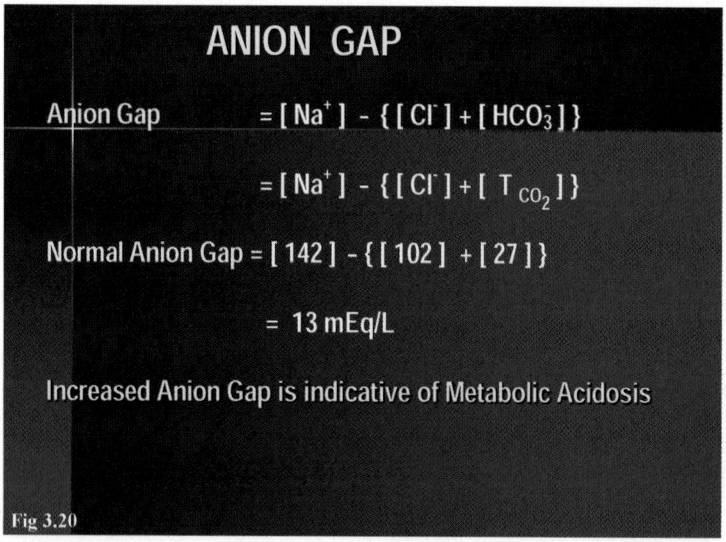

ANION GAP

Anion Gap $= [Na^+] - \{[Cl^-] + [HCO_3^-]\}$

$= [Na^+] - \{[Cl^-] + [T_{CO_2}]\}$

Normal Anion Gap $= [142] - \{[102] + [27]\}$

$= 13 \text{ mEq/L}$

Increased Anion Gap is indicative of Metabolic Acidosis

Fig 3.20

Figure 3.21 shows the distribution of the three ions in two common metabolic acidosis and the anion gap levels. Metabolic acidosis with normal anion gap is associated with loss of HCO_3^- as in diarrhea. Whereas, metabolic acidosis with high anion gap is observed in diabetic ketoacidosis, lactic acidosis and renal failure. Lactate measurement verifies or rules out lactic acidosis.

Acid Base Disorders and ABG Interpretations

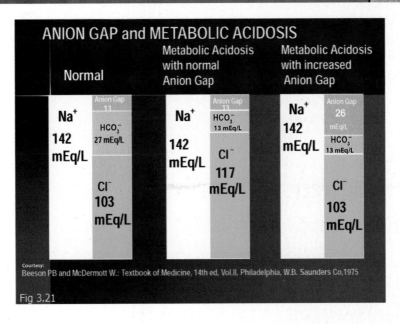

Fig 3.21

METABOLIC ALKALOSIS

A typical ABG in metabolic alkalosis is represented in Fig 3.22. Observe alkalotic pH and elevated HCO_3^- with $PaCO_2$ slightly higher than normal. This level of $PaCO_2$ should push the pH in acidosis, however the actual pH is alkalotic. This is consistent with metabolic alkalosis with partial respiratory compensation. It is claimed that metabolic alkalosis is a rule rather than exception in ICUs. Figure 3.23 lists the common causes of metabolic alkalosis- N-G tube suctioning, IV fluids, diuretics, administration of corticosteroids. Protracted vomiting NG tube drainage remove stomach acids and precipitate metabolic alkalosis. Administration of IV fluids without K^+ supplement, loop diuretics, corticosteroid regimen eliminate potassium (K^+) and causes hypokalemia.

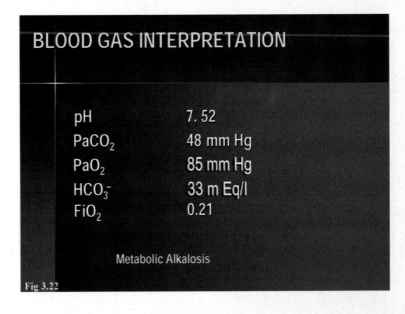

Fig 3.22

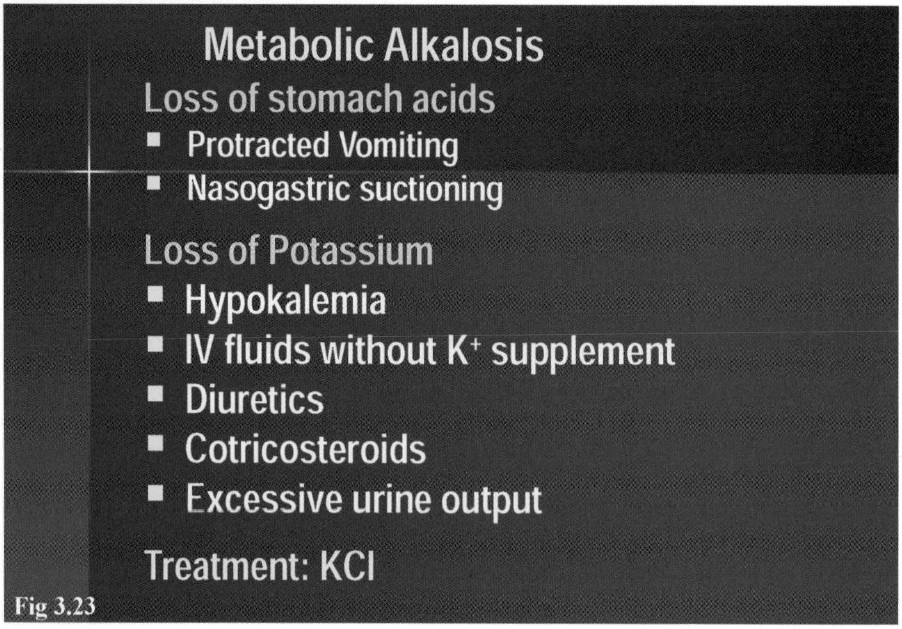

Metabolic Alkalosis
Loss of stomach acids
Protracted Vomiting
Nasogastric suctioning
Loss of Potassium
Hypokalemia
IV fluids without K+ supplement
Diuretics
Cotricosteroids
Excessive urine output
Treatment: KCl

Fig 3.23

Causes of Metabolic Alkalosis

H+ and K+ exchange at the kidneys
Kidneys do not allow Na+ excretion. Only 1% of body sodium is excreted producing 1,500 ml urine output in a day.
At the proximal tubules, 80% of Na+ is reabsorbed with Cl⁻ Remaining Na+ is reabsorbed at the distal tubules in exchange for K+ or H+.
Proximal Tubules
Peritubular Capillary Blood
Tubular Cell
Luminal Fluid
80%
Na+
Cl⁻
Na+
Cl⁻
Na+
Cl⁻
Distal Tubules
Peritubular Capillary Blood
Tubular Cell
Luminal Fluid
Na+
Na+
Na+
20%
H+
H+
K+
K+
When H+ is low, K+ must go

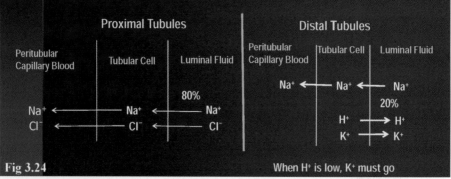

Fig 3.24

Sodium (Na^+) reabsopation at Proximal and Distal Tubules

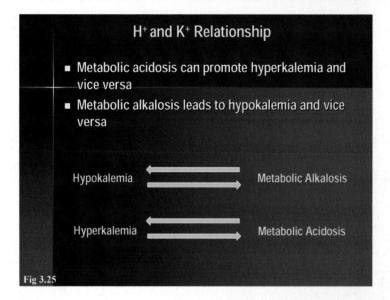

Fig 3.25

Hypokalemia is the most common cause of Metabolic Alkalosis. Figure 3.24 explains the mechanism of renal tubular events. Reabsorption of sodium is accomplished at two levels, 80% is reabsorbed at the proximal tubules along with abundant Cl^- in the luminal fluid. The remaining 20% is reabsorbed at the distal convoluted tubules in exchange for H^+ or K^+. In presence of hypokalemia, distal tubules prefer to exchange H^+ for Na^+ and preserve K^+. This leads to metabolic alkalosis. Conversely, in presence of alkalosis kidneys promote K^+ excretion and hold on to H^+. Opposite occurs in hyperkalemia and metabolic acidosis (Fig 3.25). Since most K^+ is inside the cells, only small amount is measured in plasma. Normal potassium level is 3.5–5 mEq/L. Potassium is a crucial electrolyte for cardiac and neural function. Changes in K^+ level can profoundly affect cardiac electrical function as shown in Fig 3.26. Hyperkalemia can be life threatening and must be addressed immediately.

Effects of varying K+ levels on ECG

Serum K+ Level mEq/L	Electrocardiogram
10	Ventricular Fibrillation
9	Atrial Standstill, (Intraventricular Block)
8	Prolonged P-R Interval, High T Wave, Depressed S-T segment
7	High T Wave
3.5-5	NORMAL ECG
3.0 <	Low T wave, High U wave

Fig 3.26

ABG's associated with COPD

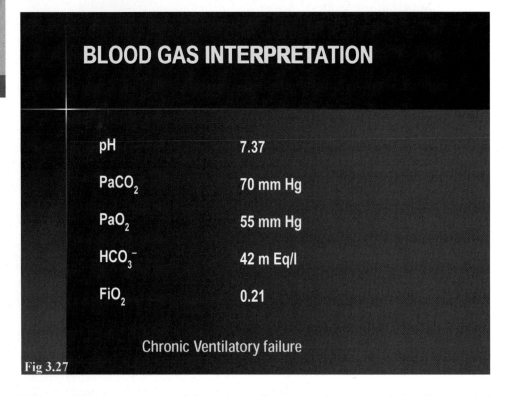

Fig 3.27

Managing COPD patients is one of the major challenges in pulmonary medicine. Titrating their medicines, oxygen, bronchodilators and managing frequent exacerbation is routinely addressed in COPD patients. Many COPD patients are CO_2 retainers. Figure 3.27 reveals a typical ABG of a stable end stage COPD patient. Observe normal pH, elevated $PaCO_2$ (Hypercapnia) and elevated HCO_3^-. High level of $PaCO_2$ affects the level of oxygenation indicated by decreased PaO_2 (Hypoxemia). The degree of elevated HCO_3^- provides a clue in this academic example, that this patient's kidneys are retaining HCO_3^- for a very long time, perhaps many years - a chronic condition. The acid base status is consistent with Hypercapnia, and yet not acidotic due to complete compensation by elevated HCO_3. High bicarbonate and $PaCO_2$ reveal Chronic Failure with moderate Hypoxemia. Thus, the ABG is expressed as "Chronic Ventilatory Failure" implying pH within normal limits, high level of $PaCO_2$ compensated by elevated HCO_3^-. This patient does not require any specific treatment to bring the $PaCO_2$ down to normal level (35–45 mm Hg) of non-COPD patients. The patient is settled in his new state of equilibrium and may need assistance in maintaining his oxygen level. Generally, these patients are given low amount of supplemental oxygen (0.5–2.0 L/min) to retain their hypoxic drive (a controversial issue). Excessive amount of oxygen is claimed to obviate hypoxic drive and promote further hypoventilation (Oxygen induced hypoventilation). A short summary of Chronic Ventilatory Failure is listed in Fig 3.28. Although, this patient may be stable, minor disorder such as infection, increased secretions, bronchospasm can lead to exacerbation.

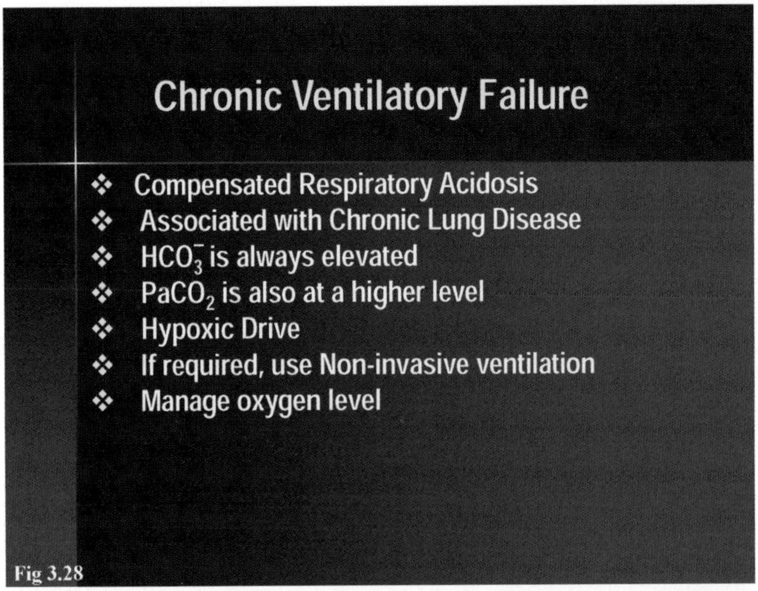

Chronic Ventilatory Failure

- Compensated Respiratory Acidosis
- Associated with Chronic Lung Disease
- HCO_3^- is always elevated
- $PaCO_2$ is also at a higher level
- Hypoxic Drive
- If required, use Non-invasive ventilation
- Manage oxygen level

Fig 3.28

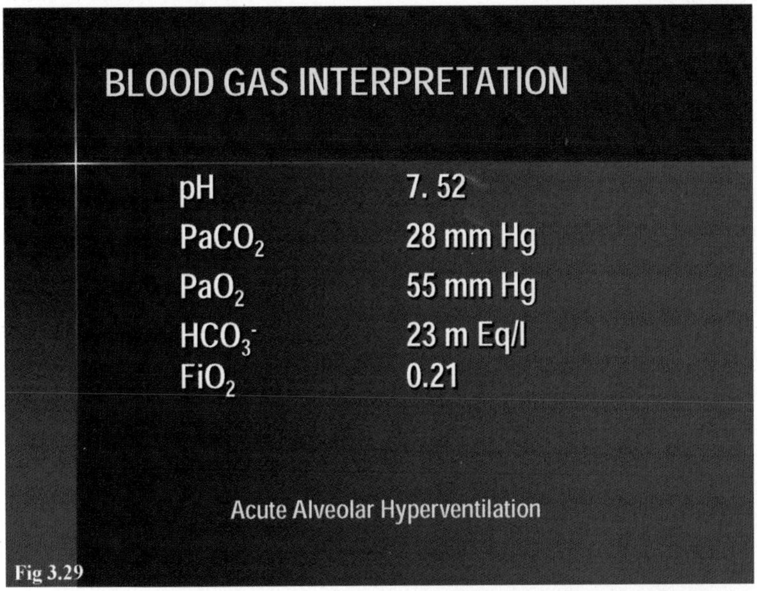

BLOOD GAS INTERPRETATION

pH	7.52
$PaCO_2$	28 mm Hg
PaO_2	55 mm Hg
HCO_3^-	23 m Eq/l
FiO_2	0.21

Acute Alveolar Hyperventilation

Fig 3.29

Interpretation of ABGs' for an exacerbated COPD patient can be tricky, especially the terms used for proper communication within the clinicians taking care of the patient. As discussed before in this chapter, ABGs drawn on a non-COPD patient (Fig 3.29) demonstrate acute alveolar hyperventilation as indicated by increased pH, decreased $PaCO_2$ and normal HCO_3^-. The patient is also hypoxemic which may have caused acute hyperventilation. If similar situation occurs in an end-stage COPD patient, the ABGs' may be confusing. Figure 3.30 shows the ABG for a COPD patient in exacerbation. **On the face value, academically, this ABG is consistent with uncompensated Metabolic Alkalosis (wrong interpretation).**

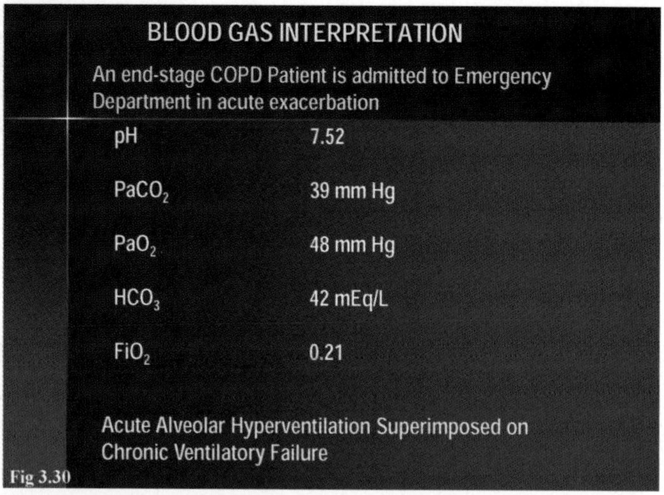

BLOOD GAS INTERPRETATION

An end-stage COPD Patient is admitted to Emergency Department in acute exacerbation

pH	7.52
$PaCO_2$	39 mm Hg
PaO_2	48 mm Hg
HCO_3	42 mEq/L
FiO_2	0.21

Acute Alveolar Hyperventilation Superimposed on Chronic Ventilatory Failure

Fig 3.30

On examination it can be seen that the high level of HCO_3^- is not acutely elevated, but over a long span (Chronic) since, the patient is known to be an end-stage COPD patient. Thus, high bicarbonate level is existing for a long time. It is conceivable that before exacerbation, in stable condition, the patient must have had very high $PaCO_2$ (approximately 70 mmHg and pH in normal range). Due to exacerbation promoting hypoxemia, the patient must have increased his respiratory rate and alveolar hyperventilation decreased the $PaCO_2$ from high level to a low level (39 mmHg). This level of $PaCO_2$ is not normal for this patient. This is equivalent to alveolar hyperventilation for a CO_2 retainer. Interpretation for this ABG is, unfortunately, long – **ACUTE ALVEOLAR HYPERVENTILATION SUPERIMPOSED ON CHRONIC VENTILATORY FAILURE.** Recognise that this interpretation clarifies that an advanced COPD patient with underlying hypercapnia is hyperventilating due to hypoxemia. $PaCO_2$ level can be deceiving. An incorrect interpretation of Metabolic Alkalosis may induce a clinician to give KCL to correct Hypokalemic alkalosis which can be detrimental to this patient. The treatment for this patient is to correct the underlying problem- Hypoxemia. Along with oxygen therapy (with an air-entrainment mask), bronchodilator therapy and any other treatments for co-morbid diseases is recommended.

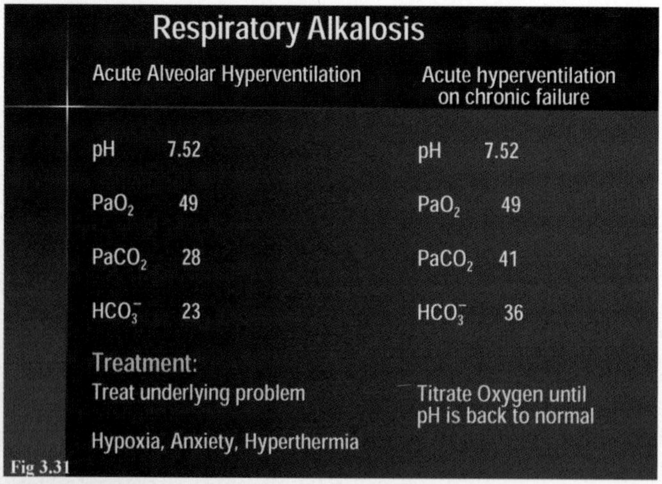

Respiratory Alkalosis

Acute Alveolar Hyperventilation		Acute hyperventilation on chronic failure	
pH	7.52	pH	7.52
PaO_2	49	PaO_2	49
$PaCO_2$	28	$PaCO_2$	41
HCO_3^-	23	HCO_3^-	36
Treatment:			
Treat underlying problem		Titrate Oxygen until pH is back to normal	
Hypoxia, Anxiety, Hyperthermia			

Fig 3.31

Acid Base Disorders and ABG Interpretations

Figure 3.31 explains the difference in interpreting ABGs in a non-COPD patient and an advanced COPD patient both being hypoxemic and hyperventilating. The treatment is the same, to correct hypoxemia which will reduce or eliminate hyperventilation and the acid base status will return to normal level. Notice, that the oxygen therapy for the COPD patient is aimed at precise concentration of oxygen to prevent excessive delivery of oxygen (obviate hypoxic drive). As small precise doses of oxygen are delivered via air-entrainment mask, the PaO_2 increases which is expected to reduce the degree of hyperventilation ($PaCO_2$ rises and pH decreases).

Currently COPD patients in exacerbation are placed on non-invasive ventilation with a mask.

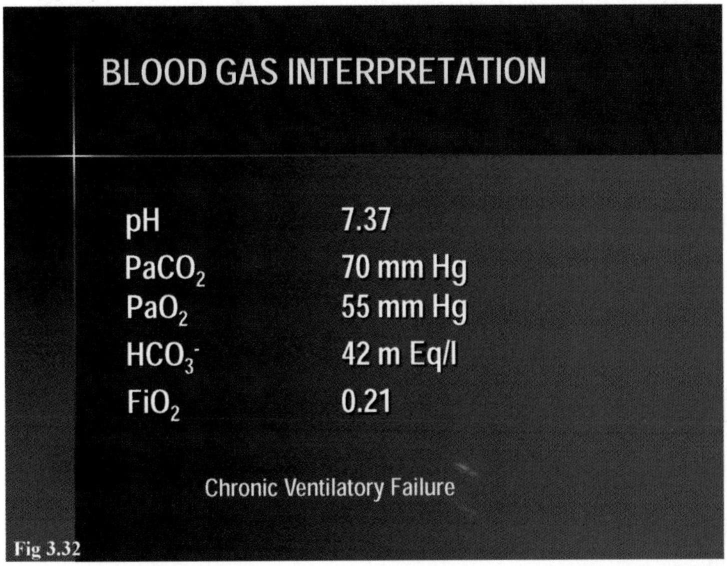

BLOOD GAS INTERPRETATION

pH	7.37
$PaCO_2$	70 mm Hg
PaO_2	55 mm Hg
HCO_3^-	42 m Eq/l
FiO_2	0.21

Chronic Ventilatory Failure

Fig 3.32

Similarly, acute hypercapnia superimposed on chronic ventilator failure must be evaluated appropriately. Again, Fig 3.32 shows ABGs representing Chronic Ventilatory Failure with normal pH in spite of high $PaCO_2$ which is compensated by chronically elevated HCO_3^-. Upon exacerbation, the patient may decrease ventilation and the level of hypercapnia can increase. In this example, Fig 3.33, pH is acidotic with very high $PaCO_2$ (90 mmHg). Thus there is an acute component of hypercapnia superimposed on chronic failure. This ABG is interpreted as Acute Ventilatory Failure superimposed on Chronic Ventilatory Failure. It must be appreciated that this verbose definition is essential for the clinicians to select appropriate management regimen. A $PaCO_2$ level of 90 mm Hg generally warrants mechanical ventilation. Use Non-invasive ventilation. If invasive ventilation is used, ascertain that the $PaCO_2$ level in NOT titrated to a normal range of 35-35 mm Hg. The patient has a different value of normal $PaCO_2$ level–much higher than 35-45 mm Hg. Figure 3.34 again compares Acute Ventilatory Failure and Acute Failure superimposed on Chronic Failure in terms of hypothetical ABG values and treatments. patient may decrease ventilation and the level of hypercapnia can increase. In this example, Fig 3.33, pH is acidotic with very high $PaCO_2$ (90 mmHg). Thus, there is an acute component of hypercapnia superimposed on chronic failure. This ABG is interpreted as Acute Ventilatory Failure superimposed on Chronic Ventilatory Failure. It must be appreciated that this verbose definition is essential for the clinicians to select appropriate management regimen.

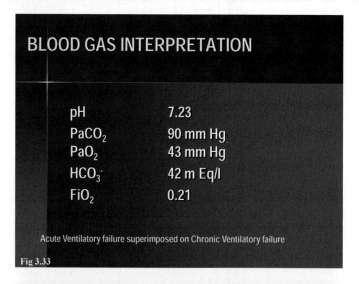

Fig 3.33

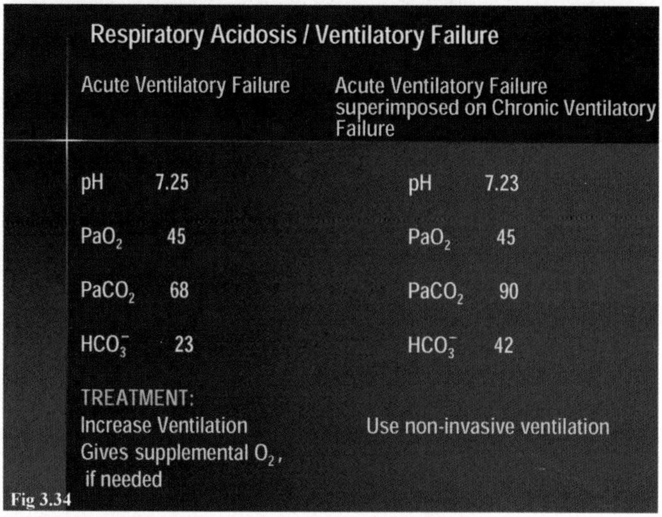

Fig 3.34

Arterial blood gas interpretation is essential for all clinicians working in ICU. Proper understanding of acid base balance is expected of all ICU clinicians. This chapter has scratched the surface of acid base physiology. The emphasis was to provide explanation of interpretations of commonly encountered abnormal ABGs. More detailed interpretation of mixed acid–base problems can be found in most Physiology books.

★★★

TERMS AND DEFINITIONS RELATED TO MECHANICAL VENTILATION

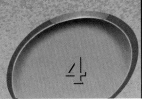

In mechanical ventilation the delivery of air to the lungs is accomplished in two ways–by providing positive pressure at the airways or creating sub-atmospheric pressure at the chest wall. Secondly, these delivery methods can be given invasively or non-invasively (Fig 4.1).

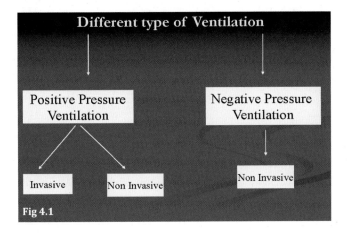

Fig 4.1

Negative Pressure Ventilation

This type of ventilation, not requiring tracheal intubation, is also known as non-invasive ventilation (NIV). A negative extra-thoracic pressure is applied to the chest wall.

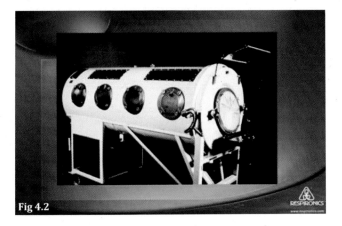

Fig 4.2: Iron lung, an early developed negative pressure ventilator. The patient is placed in the cabinet with his head outside. A pump creates extrathoracic negative pressure increasing thoracic volume and thus, decreases intrathoracic pressure. Inspiration occurs. This type of ventilation is also non-invasive ventilation, since the patient does not require tracheal intubation.

This causes a rise in the chest wall resulting in decreased intra-thoracic pressure and creates a pressure gradient from the mouth to alveoli. Inspiration occurs (Figs 4.2 and 4.3).

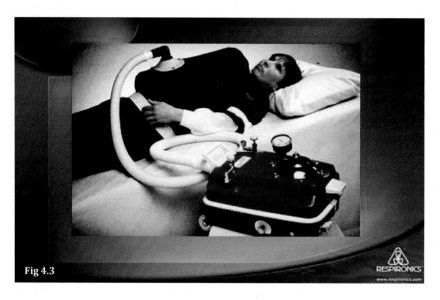

Fig 4.3

Fig 4.3: Chest Curraise represents another negative pressure ventilator where a negative pressure is generated by a suction pump at the chest. Chest wall is lifted to create negative extrathoracic volume providing negative intrathoracic pressure to promote inspiration.

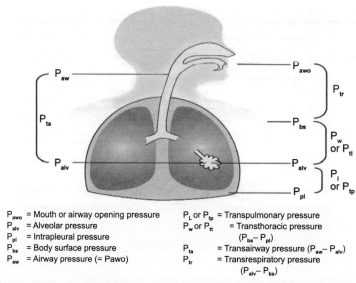

P_{awo} = Mouth or airway opening pressure
P_{alv} = Alveolar pressure
P_{pl} = Intrapleural pressure
P_{bs} = Body surface pressure
P_{aw} = Airway pressure (= Pawo)

P_L or P_{tp} = Transpulmonary pressure
P_w or P_{tt} = Transthoracic pressure
              ($P_{bs} - P_{pl}$)
P_{ta} = Transairway pressure ($P_{aw} - P_{alv}$)
P_{tr} = Transrespiratory pressure
              ($P_{alv} - P_{bs}$)

Courtesy: Wilkins RL, Stoller JK, Kacmarek RM: Egan's Fundamentals of Respiratory Care, 9th Edition, St. Louis, 2009, Mosby.

Fig 4.4

Terms and Definitions Related to Mechanical Ventilation

Airway Opening Pressure (P_{awo})

Other terms: Mouth Pressure (P_m), Airway Pressure, Mask Pressure, Proximal Airway Pressure, Upper-airway Pressure. Since the baseline pressure is atmospheric, in pulmonary medicine P_{awo} is normally considered as Zero or Atmospheric. In situations such as positive pressure ventilation the P_{awo} is positive and during tracheal suction it is negative.

Body Surface Pressure (P_{bs}) is also zero or atmospheric in normal conditions. P_{bs} increases when a patient is placed in a Hyperbaric Chamber for treatment. During Negative Pressure Ventilation P_{bs} is negative.

Intrapleural Pressure (P_{pl}) is always less than atmospheric. It is the pressure in the potential space between the parietal and visceral pleura. It is difficult to reach this space to measure P_{pl}. A special balloon catheter is inserted in the esophagus to obtain Esophageal Pressure which is a close estimation of the pleural pressure. P_{pl} is approximately -5 cm H_2O at the end expiration during normal spontaneous breathing and becomes more negative (~ -10 cm H_2O) at the end of inspiration.

Alveolar Pressure (P_{alv}) or Intrapulmonary Pressure is directly dependent on the pleural pressure (P_{pl}). During normal spontaneous breathing, at the end expiration when P_{pl} is -5 cm H_2O, the alveolar pressure (P_{alv}) is the same as P_{awo} or mouth pressure with no gas flow. At the beginning of exhalation P_{alv} is greater than atmospheric ($\sim +3-4$ cm H_2O) promoting exhalation. During mechanical ventilation P_{alv} is obtained from plateau pressure (Pp). This will be discussed in details in later chapters.

Transairway Pressure (P_{TA}) is the pressure gradient between P_{awo} and P_{alv}. P_{TA} is the pressure gradient required to generate airflow against the frictional resistance. In situations of increased airway resistance (PRAW) the transairway pressure needs to be increased to overcome airway resistance to ventilate the lung.

Transpulmonary pressure (P_L), the gradient between alveolar pressure and pleural pressure ($P_L = P_{alv} - P_{pl}$). During exhalation, the alveolar pressure decreases. However, P_L at end exhalation does not allow alveoli to close, thus, it is also referred to as Alveolar Distending Pressure. PL is essential to open alveoli during inspiration. In spontaneous breathing, contraction of the diaphragm increases the negative intrapleural pressure (more negative) resulting in increased P_L and expansion of the lung. In mechanical ventilation application of positive pressure at the airway opening increases P_{alv} and thus, increases P_L which results in lung expansion.

Positive Pressure Ventilation

A positive pressure (greater than atmospheric) is applied to the mouth (P_{awo}) providing a positive pressure gradient from mouth to alveoli (P_{TA}) resulting in inspiration. This can be applied with a mask (non-invasive) or with a tracheal tube (invasive). Current ICU ventilators are primarily positive pressure ventilators.

Volume Ventilation

Generally referred to as Volume Targeted Ventilation. Tidal volume, set by the clinician, is delivered by the ventilator during each mechanical breath. Ventilating pressure is variable, and depends on the lung characteristics such as airways resistance or lung compliance.

Pressure Ventilation

Also called Pressure Targeted Ventilation. Ventilator uses clinician set ventilating pressure as the target. It delivers this pressure to the patient's airways. Lung characteristics determine the volume delivered to the lung. In situations of increased airways resistance some of the delivered pressure is used up in overcoming the airways resistance. Thus, lesser pressure is available for lung expansion and lesser volume delivery. During pressure ventilation when lung compliance is decreased (stiffer lung), strong elastic forces allow lesser volume to be delivered at the set pressure. Thus, changes in lung characteristics affect volume delivery at the same applied pressure (Table 4.1).

	Tidal Volume (V_T)	Pressure
Volume Ventilation	Clinician Set	Varies as Resistance and Compliance change
Pressure Ventilation	Varies as Resistance and Compliance change	Clinician Set

Table 4.1

Essential Parameters in Mechanical Ventilation

Triggering (Initiation of a breath)

Triggering refers to initiation of a mechanical breath

1. **Patient Triggered or Assisted Ventilation** where a mechanical breath results from an inspiratory effort made by the patient.
2. **Time Triggered or Controlled Ventilation** is a term used when a mechanical breath is generated by a timer allowing delivery of breaths at fixed time intervals.
3. Triggering can be secondary to a negative pressure generated by the patient **(Pressure triggering)** or it results when patient removes a specific amount of flow from the circuit during inspiratory effort **(Flow triggering)**.
4. **Figure 4.5** demonstrates two mechanical breaths, an assist breath indicating a small negative deflection on the P/T scalar before the breath is traced, whereas, the time triggered control breath begins at the baseline.

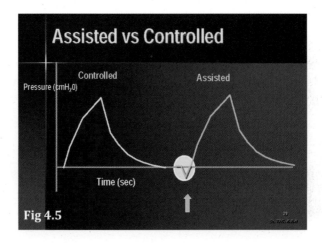

Fig 4.5

Cycling (Termination of a breath)

Termination of a mechanical breath is called "cycling". Cycling parameters are characteristics of different ventilator modes (Figs 4.6A–C).

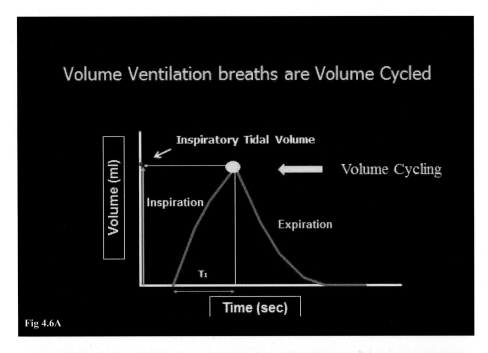

Fig 4.6A

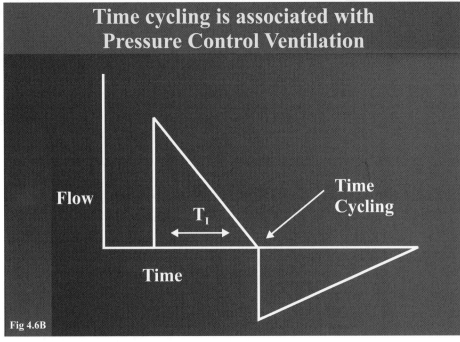

Fig 4.6B

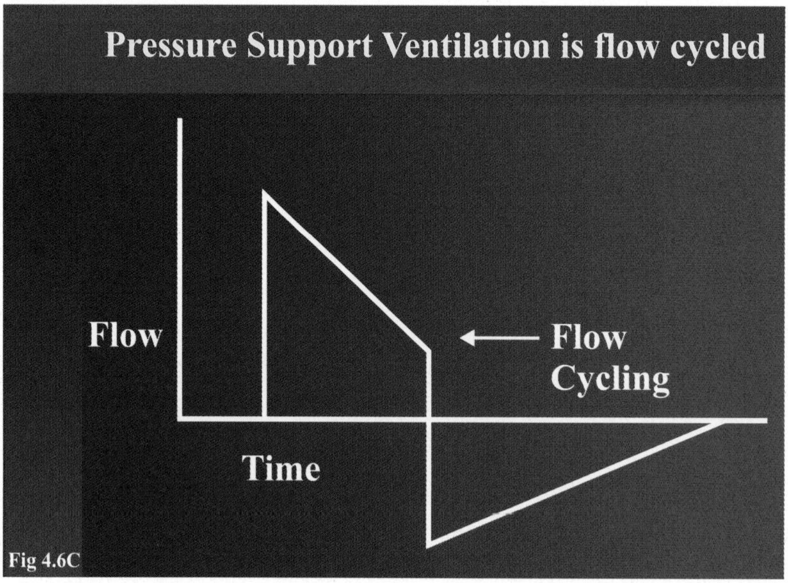

Pressure Support Ventilation is flow cycled

Fig 4.6C

1. *Pressure-Cycled:* Inspiration is terminated when the preset pressure reaches.
2. *Volume-Cycled:* Inspiration is terminated when the preset volume is delivered by the ventilator.
3. *Time-Cycled:* When the preset inspiratory time elapses, inspiration is terminated.
4. *Flow-Cycled:* Inspiration is terminated when flow decreases to a system specific flow rate.

Interrelationship between Ventilator Parameters

Tidal Volume (V_T)

Volume delivered by the ventilator per breath. It is also the average volume inspired by a spontaneously breathing patient per minute (minute volume). Tidal volume can be calculated by dividing minute volume by the respiratory frequency. Measured in milliliters (ml) or Liters (l).

Inspiratory flow rate ($\dot{V}$)

$\dot{V}$ = Inspiratory flow = $V_T \times f$

$V_T = \dot{V} \times T_I$

Respiratory Frequency (*f*)

Number of breaths taken spontaneously or delivered by the ventilator or in combination of spontaneous and mechanical breaths in one minute. Frequency is expressed in number of breaths per minute. *f* = breaths/min.

Minute Volume (V_E)

Volume delivered spontaneously or by the ventilator or in combination of spontaneous and mechanical breaths per minute. It is the volume delivered per breath (tidal volume) times the frequency $V_E = V_T \times f$.

Terms and Definitions Related to Mechanical Ventilation

Inspiratory Flow Rate ($\dot{V}$)

Inspiratory flow rate determines the rate of delivery of tidal volume. How fast or slow the volume is delivered.

$\dot{V}$ = Inspiratory flow = V_T / T_I

Inspiratory time and tidal volumes can be calculated,

$V_T = \dot{V} \times T_I$ and $T_I = V_T$/flow rate

Inspiratory Time (T_I)

This is the time required to deliver the set tidal volume at a given inspiratory flow rate

$T_I = V_T$/flow rate

As the inspiratory flow rate is increased, the volume is delivered in shorter time. Conversely, for a fixed tidal volume slower flow rates will require longer inspiratory time to deliver the volume.

Cycle Time (T_C)

Respiratory Rate or frequency (f) is expressed in cycles or breaths per minute. Thus, time needed to complete one cycle or breath is called cycle time (T_C).

T_C = 60 seconds/ respiratory frequency

   = 60 sec/f

Typical time parameters in mechanical ventilation are Inspiratory Time, Expiratory Time and Cycle Time. They are interrelated.

$T_C = T_I + T_E$

Thus, $T_I = T_C - T_E$

and $T_E = T_C - T_I$

Expiratory Time (T_E)

This is the time used for expiration and is the remainder of the cycle time after the inspiration is completed.

$T_E = T_C - T_I$. For a given cycle time (60 sec/respiratory frequency) as inspiratory time is decreased (by increasing inspiratory flow rate), the expiratory time increases. Conversely, for a given Inspiratory Time and Expiratory Time, as the respiratory frequency is decreased the expiratory time increases.

Inspiratory Time %

This expresses the % of cycle time used for inspiration. If the cycle time is 4 seconds and the T_I% is set at 25%, the actual Inspiratory Time is 25 % of 4 seconds or 1 second.

I–E ratio

An I–E ratio indicates the ratio of inspiratory time to expiratory time i.e. TI:TE. It is conventionally expressed as a ratio with left side of the equation reduced to 1. If the inspiratory time is 2 seconds and expiratory time is 3 seconds, the actual I–E ratio is 2: 3. However, conventionally it is written as, 1: 1.5. Similarly if T_I is 3 seconds and T_E is 6 seconds the I–E ratio is 1: 2 (3 seconds: 6 seconds).

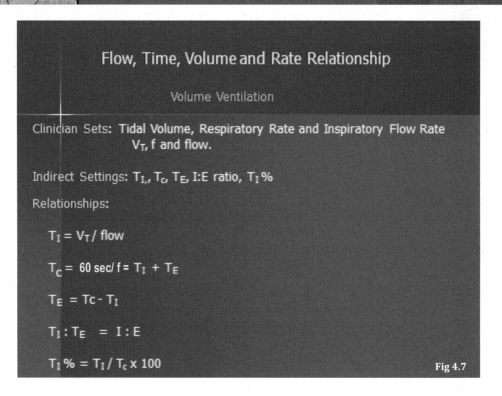

Fig 4.7

Figure 4.7 summarizes the interrelation ship between the above basic parameters. Based on clinical situation clinician is generally involved in making changes in one or more parameters. These changes may have an effect on other parameters. For example, when a clinician changes inspiratory time, it changes inspiratory flow rate and also change expiratory time.

Some of the above material will be repeated in later chapters to re-emphasize the basic concepts.

★★★

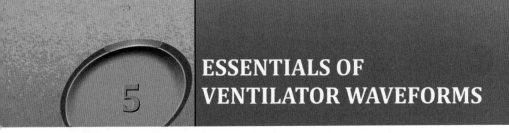

ESSENTIALS OF VENTILATOR WAVEFORMS

The figures in this chapter may look different since they are reproduced directly from the CD which is provided in the back cover pocket.
"Essentials of Ventilator Graphics" developed by Vijay Deshpande, MS, RRT, FAARC and Ruben Restrepo, MD, RRT, FAARC for Respimedu, Inc. in 2000.

INTRODUCTION
The purpose of this chapter is to provide clinicians with the specific knowledge and interpretive skills necessary to recognize various aspects of patient and ventilator interaction, in both text and graphical formats.

DESCRIPTION
This chapter identifies typical tracings and analysis of commonly encountered waveforms during mechanical ventilation. The following waveforms are described in this module:

SCALARS	LOOPS
1. Flow vs Time	1. Pressure-Volume Loop
2. Pressure vs Time	2. Flow-Volume Loop
3. Volume vs Time	

OBJECTIVES
A. **General Objectives**
   1. Identify the variables that make up the scalars and loops.
   2. Differentiate between loops and scalars.
   3. Recognize the most common modes of ventilation on scalar graphics.
B. **Identify on a Flow–Time Curve:**
   1. Inadequate flow.
   2. Different Flow Patterns.
   3. Airway Obstruction vs. Active Exhalation.
   4. Air trapping.
C. **Identify on a Volume–Time Curve:**
   1. Air leak.
   2. Active exhalation.
D. **Identify on a Pressure–Time Curve:**
   1. Mechanical vs Spontaneous Breath.
   2. Patient Cycled or Assisted Breath.
   3. Components of the Pressure Curve.
   4. PIP, P_{plat} and correlation with Airway Resistance (R_{aw}).
E. **Identify on a Pressure–Volume Loop:**
   1. Controlled, Assisted, and Spontaneous Breath.
   2. Opening Pressure.
   3. Hysteresis.
   4. Increased Airway Resistance.
   5. Decreased and Increased Lung Compliance.
   6. Components of Mechanical WOB.
   7. Overdistension.
   8. Inspiratory and Expiratory Inflection Points.
   9. Air leak.

F. Identify on a Flow–Volume Loop:
   1. PIFR/PEFR.
   2. Air Leak.
   3. Air Trapping.
   4. Airway Resistance.
   5. β_2 response.
   6. Inadequate flow.

Abbreviations and Definitions

Throughout this chapter the following words and abbreviations are used:

- PIFR — Peak Inspiratory Flow Rate
- PEFR — Peak Expiratory Flow Rate
- PIP — Peak Inspiratory Pressure
- PEEP — Positive End Expiratory Pressure
- P_{plat} — Plateau Pressure
- R_{aw} — Airway Resistance
- P_{aw} — Airway Pressure
- V_T — Tidal Volume
- T_I — Inspiratory Time, in seconds
- T_E — Expiratory Time, in seconds
- TCT — Total Cycle Time, in seconds
- I–E Ratio — Inspiratory to Expiratory Time Ratio
- Scalar Graphic — A single variable plotted against time
- Loop — Two variables plotted simultaneously
- Hysteresis — Widening of a Pressure–Volume Loop
- Inflection Point — The point of change in the slope of a line
- Tracing — Used interchangeably with loop or curve
- Opening Pressure — The point where pressure delivered begins to induce a corresponding volume change
- WOB — Work of Breathing
- C_L — Lung Compliance
- FRC — Functional Residual Capacity

Ventilator Graphics: *General Concepts*

Ventilator graphics have become an essential tool in managing patients on mechanical ventilators. All newer mechanical ventilators are equipped with a graphic package that displays selected ventilator waveforms facilitating assessment of the patient's condition.

Guidelines for proper interpretation and application of the most common ventilator graphics are described below:

The following waveforms will be described in this module:

SCALARS	LOOPS
1. Flow vs Time 2. Pressure vs Time 3. Volume vs Time	1. Pressure-Volume Loop 2. Flow-Volume Loop

Any single variable displayed against time is known as a **SCALAR** graphic. The three parameters that make up the ventilator graphics, Flow, Volume and Pressure are plotted against Time.

Essentials of Ventilator Waveforms

These three scalars are generally referred to as:
Flow Curve | Volume Curve | Pressure Curve

When viewing scalar graphics, time is conventionally shown on the horizontal (x) axis, whereas, flow, volume, and pressure are plotted on the vertical (y) axis.

The tracings indicate typical Flow vs. Time, Pressure vs. Time and Volume vs. Time scalars during mechanical volume cycled ventilation with a constant (preset) flow. The next few frames discuss scalars and their clinical significance.

LOOPS are the two-dimensional graphic displays of two scalar values. There are two loops available for interpretation. They are:

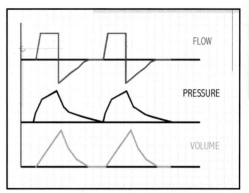

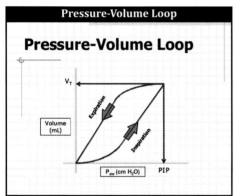

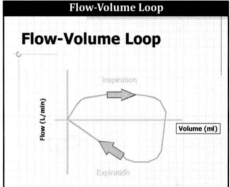

When viewing the Pressure-Volume Loop, pressure is usually displayed on the horizontal (x) axis while volume is displayed on the vertical (y) axis.

When viewing the Flow-Volume Loop, the horizontal (x) axis is used to indicate volume whereas flow is displayed on the vertical (y) axis. As indicated in the flow-volume loop below, the inspiratory curve is plotted above the baseline and expiratory curve is traced below the baseline. However, it is not unusual to see a completely reverse pattern where the inspiratory component is presented below the baseline.

ANALYSIS OF SCALAR GRAPHICS

Each scalar will be discussed individually identifying components of the tracing and commonly observed normal and abnormal patterns.

Flow vs. Time Curve	
Basics of Flow vs. Time Curve	**Recognition of Common Abnormalities**
Spontaneous Breath	Obstruction vs. Active Expiration
Mechanical Breath	Response to Bronchodilators
Typical Flow Patterns	Air Trapping/Auto-PEEP
Inspiratory Flow	
Expiratory Flow	

Spontaneous Breath

Observe that the inspiratory flow is traced above the baseline whereas expiratory flow is indicated below the baseline. The flow/Time curve for a spontaneous breath resembles a SINEWAVE flow pattern.

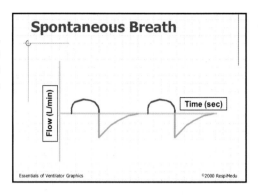

Mechanical Breath

This tracing shows components of a Flow vs. Time curve for a mechanical volume-targeted breath. Observe the following:

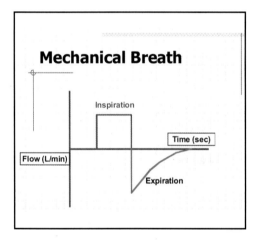

- The inspiratory flow pattern is square, indicating a constant flow delivery. This pattern is selected by the operator on the ventilator

- There is a significant tracing below the baseline representing expiratory flow, which is dependent on the patient's lung characteristics and effort

- Only the Flow vs. Time curve demonstrates a significant tracing below the baseline. The other scalars stay above the baseline except on a Pressure vs. Time curve where a very small deflection occurs below the baseline when the patient initiates inspiration

Typical Flow Patterns

Most ventilators allow a clinician to select a flow pattern that is most suitable to the patient. Typically a SQUARE FLOW, DESCENDING RAMP or DECELERATING FLOW, ASCENDING or ACCELERATING FLOW AND A SINE WAVE FLOW patterns are available. Observe that in each flow pattern illustrated on this frame the maximum flow rate is the same and T_I varies. However, if using a time-cycled ventilator (e.g. Servo 300) the T_I remains constant and flow varies to deliver the preset V_T.

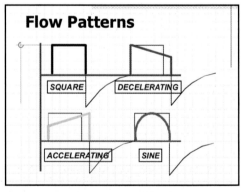

Components of Inspiratory Flow

A SQUARE FLOW PATTERN is used throughout this part to identify each component during the inspiratory phase of a mechanical volume-targeted breath. Observe each phase of the development of the inspiratory flow. Notice the following points and events on the flow vs. time scalar:

Essentials of Ventilator Waveforms

1. Initiation of flow at the beginning of inspiration: At this time the exhalation valve closes to permit a mechanical breath to deliver volume to the patient's lungs.
2. The peak inspiratory flow (PIFR) level is reached instantaneously during a constant flow pattern. The flow remains at this level until the inspiration is terminated.
3. End of inspiratory flow delivery and beginning of expiration: This event occurs when the preset tidal volume is delivered. At this time the exhalation valve opens to allow for passive exhalation.

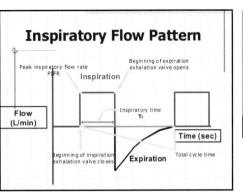

4. Notice Inspiratory Time (T_I), Expiratory Time (T_E) and the Total Cycle Time (TCT) for one mechanical breath.

Components of Expiratory Flow

Expiration, whether from a mechanical breath or a spontaneous breath, is generally a passive maneuver. Both the inspiratory and the expiratory flows reach their peak value instantaneously and both return to the baseline.

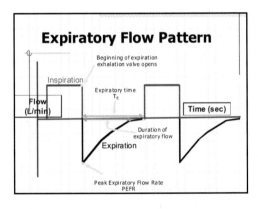

Observe the following points on the expiratory section of the flow/time tracing:

1. Initiation of Expiration
2. Peak Expiratory Flow Rate (PEFR)
3. Duration of Expiratory flow
4. Expiratory Time (T_E)

Notice that the expiratory flow decays to zero before the next mechanical breath is initiated. Thus, the duration of expiratory flow may be shorter than the allocated expiratory time (TCT–T_I).

Recognition of Common Abnormalities

Flow vs. Time scalars help in recognizing certain disorders. Different lung disorders show different flow patterns. These abnormal flow patterns, their causes, and appropriate actions are discussed below:

Airway Obstruction vs. Active Exhalation

Exhalation is normally passive. The expiratory flow pattern and PEFR depend upon the changes in the patient's lung compliance and airway resistance, as well as patient's active efforts to exhale.

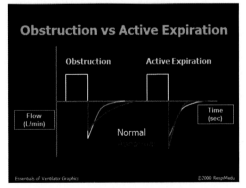

For example, increased airway resistance due to bronchospasm or accumulation of secretions in the airway may result in decreased PEFR and a prolonged expiratory flow. If the patient begins to actively exhale using expiratory muscles, this may result in an increase in PEFR and a shorter duration of expiratory flow.

Response to Bronchodilator

Flow vs. Time tracing can verify clinically suspected bronchoconstriction. In these cases, the PEFR is reduced and expiratory flow returns to the baseline very slowly. Administration of a bronchodilator improves PEFR and allows for an expiratory flow to return to baseline within a normal time.

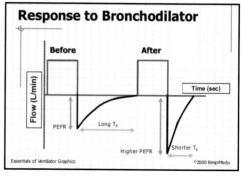

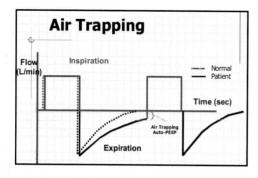

Air-trapping or Auto-PEEP

Normally, expiratory flow returns to the baseline prior to the next breath. In the event that the expiratory flow does not return to the zero line and the subsequent inspiration begins below the baseline, auto-PEEP or air trapping is present.

The presence of auto-PEEP or air trapping may result from:
a. Inadequate expiratory time
b. Too high respiratory rate
c. Long inspiratory time
d. Prolonged exhalation due to bronchoconstriction or loss of recoiling force as observed in advanced Emphysema patients.

Even though auto-PEEP is best detected from the flow-time waveform, its magnitude is not directly measured from the flow-time scalar. A higher inspiratory flow rate (in volume-cycled ventilators) or short T_I (in time-cycled ventilators) allows for a longer T_E and may eliminate auto-PEEP.

Volume vs. Time Curve	
Basics of Volume vs. Time Curve:	**Recognition of Common Abnormalities:**
Components of the Volume vs Time	Air Leak
	Active Exhalation

Basics of Volume vs. Time Curve

Information obtained from a Volume vs Time scalar graph includes a visual representation of:

- Inspiratory tidal volume
- Inspiratory phase
- Expiratory phase
- Inspiratory time

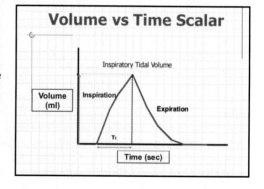

Recognition of Common Abnormalities

The Volume vs. Time scalar can be used to identify the following common abnormalities:

Presence of Air Leak

A leak in the circuit or around the tracheal tube can be detected from the volume/time curve. If the expiratory tracing smoothly descends, and then plateaus, and abruptly drops to the baseline followed by the next tracing, it indicates the presence of a leak in the system. This pattern mandates that the leak should be located and fixed. The volume of the leak can be easily estimated by measuring the distance from the plateau to the end of the expiratory tracing.

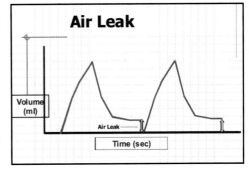

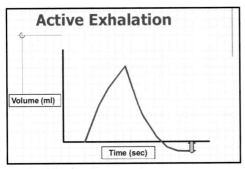

Active Exhalation

Forced exhalation is seen on the volume/time tracing as a tracing that extends below the zero line. It can also occur if the flow transducer is out of calibration.

Pressure vs. Time Curve	
Basics of Pressure vs. Time Curve	**Recognition of Common Abnormalities**
Spontaneous Breath	Increased Airway Resistance
Mechanical Breath	Effect of High Inspiratory Flow
Controlled vs Assisted Breath	Decreased Lung Compliance
Components of Inflation Pressure	Inadequate Inspiratory Flow

Basics of Pressure vs. Time Curve

Spontaneous Breath

Observe that unlike the Flow vs. Time curve, the Pressure vs. Time scalar indicates inspiration below the baseline and expiration is traced above the baseline which is consistent with the normal spontaneous respiratory pattern. Observe that during the inspiratory phase the pressure curve shows a negative deflection and during exhalation goes above the baseline. Compare this with the adjacent mechanical breath demonstrating inspiration above the baseline and no tracing below the baseline since during exhalation the pressure returns to zero.

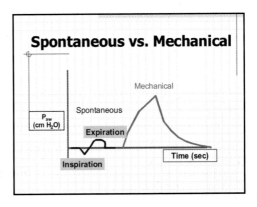

Mechanical Breath

The Pressure vs Time scalar is one of the most useful waveforms in clinical setting. It provides visual representations of the following:

Peak Inspiratory Pressure (PIP) is the maximum pressure achieved during a breath. PIP indicates the pressure required to deliver a set tidal volume during volume ventilation. Increased Airway Resistance (R_{aw}) and/or decreased lung compliance result in an increased PIP.

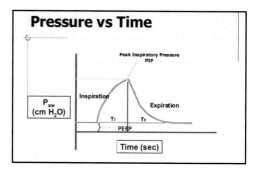

Positive End Expiratory Pressure (PEEP), Since PEEP is a pressure parameter it can be seen only on a Pressure vs Time scalar and a pressure-volume loop. PEEP is present when the baseline pressure is above zero. The tracing also shows the *Inspiratory time and Expiratory time*

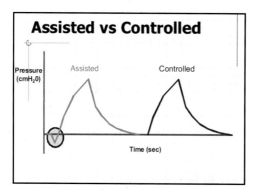

A Pressure vs. Time scalar verifies the triggering mechanism of the mechanical breath. If the breaths are initiated at the baseline at fixed intervals the mode is time triggered or a control mode. In an assist mode the patient initiates the breath by generating a negative pressure. The ventilator sensor recognizes the patient's effort and delivers a mechanical breath. This event can be observed on the Pressure vs. Time scalar where a small negative deflection below the baseline precedes a mechanical breath.

Components of Inflation Pressure

Although dynamic lung mechanics can be observed from a Pressure vs. Time curve, the addition of an inspiratory pause or inflation hold provides information to calculate static mechanics.

Plateau Pressure (P_{plat}) or Alveolar Pressure is obtained upon activation of an Inflation Hold or Inspiratory Pause control. The exhalation valve is kept in a closed position after the tidal volume is delivered and the volume is held in the lungs.

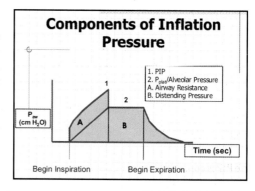

For clinical purposes, the plateau pressure is the same as the alveolar pressure. This measurement provides a means of measuring static lung compliance.

Transairway Pressure (P_{TA} = PIP – P_{plat}) reflects the pressure required to overcome airway resistance. Bronchospasm, airway secretions, and other types of airway obstructions are verified from an increase in the transairway pressure (PIP-P_{plat}).

With inflation hold, the pressure required to overcome the recoiling force (lung compliance) can be determined. The static lung compliance can be obtained by dividing the tidal volume in the lungs by the plateau pressure minus PEEP, if present.

$$C_{static} = \frac{V_T}{PIP-P_{plat}}$$

Essentials of Ventilator Waveforms

Observe the sequence of tracing pressure vs. time curve when the inflation hold (inspiratory pause) is activated. At the beginning, the exhalation valve closes and the ventilator delivers volume to the patient's lungs. During this volume delivery the flow of gas molecules experience frictional resistance. The pressure time curve indicates this pressure generated by flow resistance as initial rise in the pressure. As the gas reaches beyond terminal bronchioles elastic characteristics of the lung oppose the incoming gas. Delivered tidal volume generates pressure required to overcome elastic recoil of the lung. The total pressure is represented by Peak Inspiratory Pressure (PIP). At the end of volume delivery, inspiratory flow stops. Technically, the exhalation valve is supposed to open. However, inspiratory hold activation maintains the exhalation valve in closed position. Thus, the volume in the lungs is balanced by the elastic recoil and the resultant pressure represents Plateau Pressure (P_{plat}). Clinically this is the alveolar pressure. As shown, PIP is higher than P_{plat}, since P_{plat} represents only the pressure required to oppose elastic recoil to deliver volume to the lungs. Flow resistance is absent since the gas flow is stopped. This pressure is known as Transairway Pressure (P_{TA}). As the time set for inspiratory hold elapses, exhalation valve opens and the pressure returns to the baseline. This graph has significant clinical significance as seen in the next two waveforms.

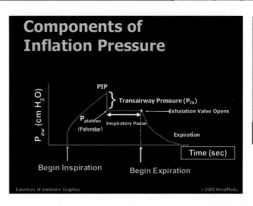

Recognition of Common Abnormalities

PIP vs. P_{plat}

Changes in the pressure vs. time curve have profound clinical significance. Four common clinical situations are demonstrated in the following tracings:

Normal curve: Indicates PIP, P_{plat}, P_{TA}, and T_I.

High Raw: A significant increase in the P_{TA} is associated with increased airway resistance.

High Flow: Notice that the inspiratory time is shorter than normal, indicating a higher inspiratory gas flow rate.

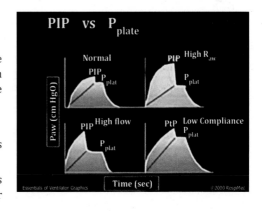

Decreased Lung Compliance: An increase in the plateau pressure and a corresponding increase in the PIP is consistent with decreased lung compliance.

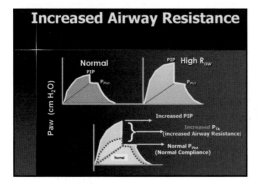

Increased Airway Resistance

As the airway resistance increases due to bronchospasm, secretions or any obstruction, the transairway pressure (PTA) increases as shown by the rise in PIP without any increase in P_{plat}. The gradient PIP–P_{plat} represents PTA.

Clinically, this situation requires airway suctioning, administration of bronchodilators or removal of obstruction such as kink in the inspiratory line of the circuit.

Decreased Lung Compliance

PIP can also increase when the lung compliance decreases. In conditions such as small pneumothoraces or blocked chest tube drainage system, lung compliance decreases. Consequently, P_{plat} or Alveolar Pressure increases causing equivalent increase in PIP. Recognize that the difference between PIP and P_{plat} or P_{TA} is unchanged from the original condition. Suctioning the airways serves no purpose since the airways resistance is normal.

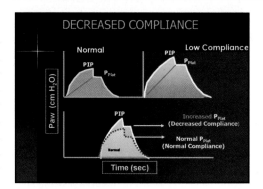

Identification of the underlying cause and eliminating it is essential in this situation.

Inadequate Inspiratory Flow

A Pressure vs. Time curve can also detect inadequate flow that is indicated when the pressure rises very slowly or sometimes is indicated when there is a depression in the inspiratory limb of the pressure contour.

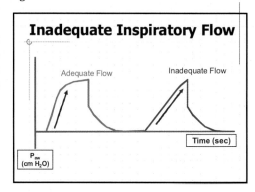

LOOPS

Loops are the two-dimensional graphic displays of two scalar parameters.

Pressure-Volume Loop	
Basics of a Pressure-Volume Loop	**Recognition of Common Abnormalities**
Type of Breath	Decreased Lung Compliance
Spontaneous-Assisted-Controlled	Increased Airway Resistance
FRC and Pressure-Volume Loop	Alveolar Overdistension
Components of a Pressure-Volume Loop	Increased Work of Breathing
PEEP and the P-V Loop	Inappropriate Sensitivity
Inflection Points (Upper and Lower)	Inadequate Inspiratory Flow
Type of Breath	Air Leak
Work of Breathing	

Observe the direction of the tracing of the loop. When the tracing is counterclockwise, the breath delivered is a mechanical breath. On the other hand, a clockwise tracing indicates a spontaneous breath. The angle, shape and size of the loop impart pertinent information to the clinician. In an assisted mechanical breath the tracing begins clockwise indicating patient's spontaneous effort and resumes in counterclockwise fashion for the mechanical delivery.

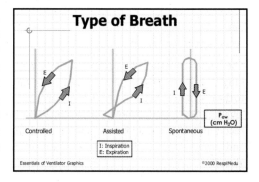

Essentials of Ventilator Waveforms

FRC and P-V Loop

It is important to recognize that the beginning point on a Pressure-Volume loop is the FRC level since, the breath is delivered at end-expiratory level (FRC). When PEEP is added, the FRC level increases or moves up the compliance curve.

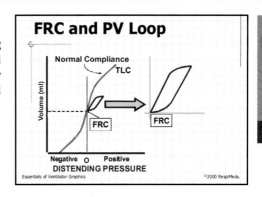

Component of a P-V Loop

A Pressure-Volume loop traces changes in pressures and corresponding changes in volume. Inspiration begins from the FRC level and terminates when the preset parameter (volume or pressure) is achieved. The tracing continues during expiration and returns to FRC at end of exhalation. PIP and delivered tidal volume can readily be obtained from the Pressure-Volume loop.

PEEP

When PEEP is applied, the Pressure-Volume curve shifts to the PEEP level on the horizontal scale (Pressure scale).

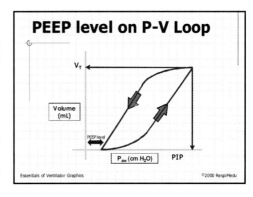

Inflection Point

Inflection point, in geometry, represents sudden change of direction in a graphical tracing.

Physiologically, the inflection points on P-V loop are associated with sudden changes in alveolar opening and closing. The lower inflection point represents the opening pressure, whereas the upper inflection point, in this graph, represents recoiling characteristics.

The higher the opening pressure, the stiffer the lung, as indicated by the curve moving laterally to the right along the pressure axis. Setting PEEP levels at the level of the lower inflection point is recommended to optimize alveolar recruitment and prevent repeated opening and closing of alveoli.

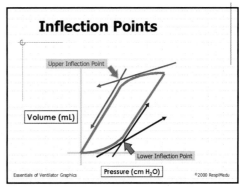

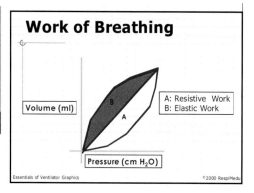

Work of Breathing

The major advantage of a Pressure-Volume loop is that it provides a quick assessment of the elastic as well as resistive work of breathing.

Since, work of breathing is calculated from the product of pressure and volume

(WOB = Pressure × Volume). The shaded area represents elastic work of breathing.

Decreased Lung Compliance

A shift of the curve to the right of a Pressure-Volume loop indicates decreased lung compliance and a shift to the left is associated with an increased compliance. Observe the pressure required to deliver the same tidal volume in the three graphs.

Notice that in Volume-Targeted Ventilation the PIP is the changing variable.

Volume Targeted Ventilation

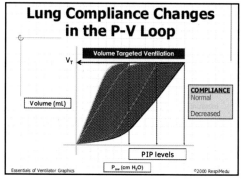

Pressure-Targeted Ventilation

In Pressure-Targeted Ventilation where the PIP is kept constant and V_T is the changing variable.

Observe as dynamic compliance varies, so does the delivered volume. Essentially, as lung becomes stiffer, the delivered volume decreases for the given present pressure.

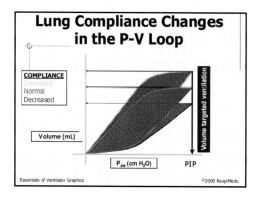

Increased Airways Resistance

An increased Airway resistance is associated with the abnormal widening of the inspiratory tracing. Patients with obstructive disorders exhibit a wide Pressure-Volume loop. This abnormal widening of the shape of the P-V loop is referred to as an increased "Hysteresis".

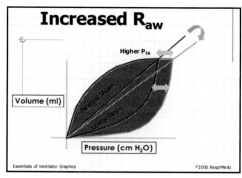

Alveolar Overdistension

Alveolar distension is a common observation made during ventilation of patients with ARDS on a volume-targeted mode. Alveolar overdistension is detrimental to patients. The classic sign, known as "Beak Effect" or "Duckbill" shows an increase in airway pressure without any appreciable increase in volume. A switch to pressure targeted ventilation, at appropriate safe pressure level, or a reduction in V_T are indicated.

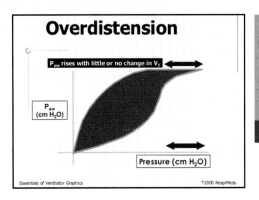

Increased WOB

Inadequate Sensitivity

Normally the Pressure-Volume loop traces in a counterclockwise direction. A clockwise tracing prior to the initiation of a mechanical breath indicates patient's effort. Adjusting the sensitivity can minimize this effort. Inadequate sensitivity setting promotes increased triggering WOB. On the P-V loop it exhibits a significant clockwise deflection of the tracing with the pressure decreasing significantly (>5 cm H_2O) below the baseline pressure.

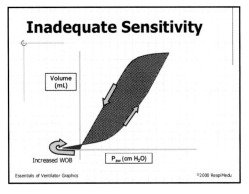

Inadequate Inspiratory Flow Rate

Inappropriate inspiratory flow rates are recognized from a scooped out pattern. In some situations, the patient makes inspiratory effort in the middle of the mechanical breath exhibiting a "notch" on the inspiratory curve.

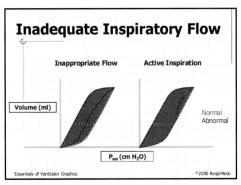

Air Leak

On Volume/Time scalar when the expiratory curve does not return to the baseline, a leak in the system is present.

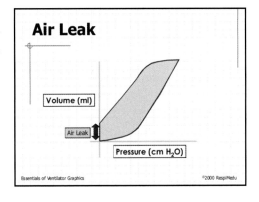

Mechanical Ventilation

Flow-Volume Loop

Basics of Pressure-Volume Loop	Recognition of Common Abnormalities
Components of a Flow-Volume Loop	Air Leak
	Auto-PEEP/Air Trapping
	Increased Airway Resistance
	Airway Secretions/Accumulation of Condensate

Basics of Flow-Volume Loop

Components of a Flow-Volume Loop

There is no set convention in assigning the inspiratory and expiratory quadrants on a Flow-Volume loop. Some ventilators produce flow-volume loop with inspiration on the upper half and expiration on the lower half. Other ventilators plot inspiration on the lower side of the volume axis and expiration on the upper side. A flow-volume loop provides the following information

1. PIFR
2. PEFR
3. TIDAL VOLUME
4. END EXPIRATION AND BEGINNING OF INSPIRATION

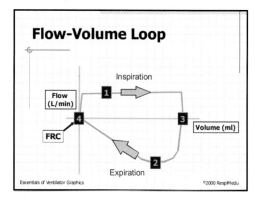

Recognition of Common Abnormalities

Air Leak

Ideally, expired volume should be equal to the inspired volume. With an air leak, however, expired volume is less than inspired volume. This is commonly observed in situations such as leak around the endotracheal tube, and in the ventilator circuit. A leak can be identified from a flow-volume loop when the volume does not return to the FRC (zero volume level). The deficit of volume indicates the magnitude of air leak.

Auto-PEEP

In an air trapping or auto-PEEP situation the *flow does not return to the zero level*. Since the next inspiration must begin from the zero flow level, the tracing jumps abruptly, from the trapped level to the zero level and proceeds with next breath.

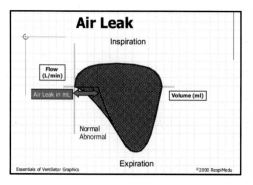

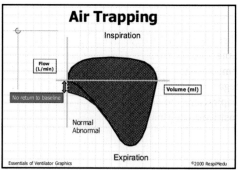

Essentials of Ventilator Waveforms

Increased Airway Resistance

An increased airway resistance due to bronchospasm, such as in asthma, is shown on a flow-volume loop as a scooped out pattern on the expiratory tracing and a decreased PEFR. Effective administration of bronchodilator will show an improvement on both the configuration of the expiratory tracing and the PEFR. A continued scooped out appearance and a low PEFR indicates ineffectiveness of the bronchodilator therapy.

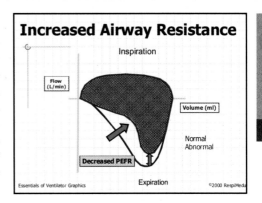

Airway Secretions and Accumulation of Condensate in the tubing

The presence of secretions in the large airways, as well as excessive fluid condensation in the ventilator circuit, appear as a distinctive pattern in the flow-volume loop known as a "saw-tooth" pattern, which occurs mostly on the expiratory component of the curve. However, if the situation is not corrected this pattern will also appear on the inspiratory curve.

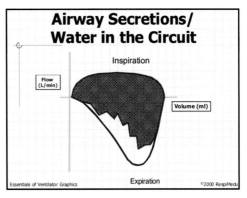

Recognition Of Different Modes of Ventilation

Spontaneous Modes	Modes of Mechanical Ventilation	
Spontaneous Breath	Volume-Targeted	Pressure-Targeted
CPAP	Controlled	Controlled
PSV	Assisted	Assisted
CPAP + PS	SIMV	SIMV
	SIMV + PS	SIMV + PS
	SIMV + PS + CPAP	SIMV + PS + CPAP

Spontaneous Modes

Spontaneous Breath

Observe the difference between the Flow vs. Time, the Pressure vs. Time and the Volume vs. Time scalars. Only the pressure curve shows a negative or below baseline tracing during inspiration; however, flow and volume are positive during inspiration.

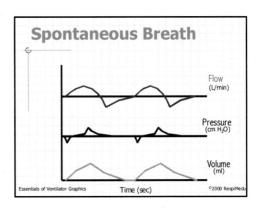

CPAP

A CPAP mode is identical to a spontaneous breath except that the baseline in the Pressure vs. Time curve is at a higher level. *CPAP can be verified from the P vs. T curve and P-V loop only.*

Pressure Support Ventilation

Pressure Support Ventilation is designed to augment spontaneous breath. It provides a higher volume with a lower inspiratory effort. Patients with Neuromuscular disorders, COPD, and post-operative patients benefit from PSV. It is also used during weaning from mechanical ventilation.

Observe the scalars: The key waveform for recognition of PSV is the Flow vs. Time curve. PSV terminates inspiration when the flow reaches a predetermined value (generally 25% of the peak flow). It is a flow-cycled mode. The Pressure vs. Time curve indicates a constant pressure tracing at the set pressure support level. Also notice the negative deflection on the Pressure vs. Time curve indicating that PSV is strictly an assist mode of ventilation. The delivered volume is dependent on the patient's lung compliance, airway resistance, patient's inspiratory effort and the pressure support level.

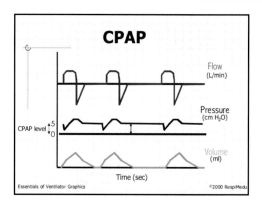

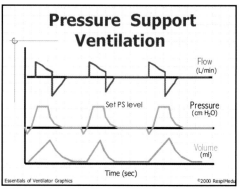

CPAP + PS

This mode is used to facilitate weaning from mechanical ventilation.

Observe the flow/time and pressure/time scalars confirm pressure support (PSV) mode. Also, the pressure/time scalar indicates that the baseline is at a higher level consistent with CPAP.

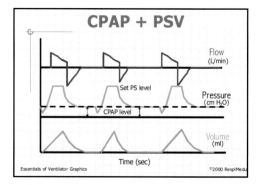

Modes of Mechanical Ventilation

Volume Targeted Ventilation

NOTE: A square flow pattern will be used to identify the inspiratory phase of the mechanical breaths in the Flow vs. Time curve.

Controlled Mode

In a controlled mode the ventilator provides the entire breathing. The ventilator exclusively performs the work of breathing. The ventilator initiates inspiration when a preset time elapses (Time-triggered).

It terminates inspiration when the preset tidal volume is delivered (volume cycled). Flow level is set by the clinician and remains constant throughout the inspiratory phase. Even in the event that the lung characteristics (resistance and compliance) change the flow rate remains constant. The flow parameter is termed as "limiting" parameter. Thus, volume controlled breath is classified as "Time triggered, flow limited, volume cycled".

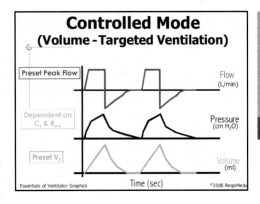

Assisted Mode

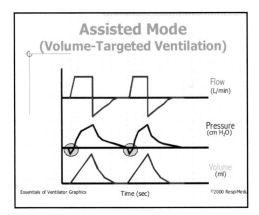

An assisted mode is identical to a controlled mode except that the Pressure vs. Time curve shows a negative deflection just prior to the mechanical breath. This negative deflection indicates patient triggering. An Assisted mode is termed as "Patient triggered, flow limited, volume cycled".

SIMV

This is the one of the common modes used in the clinical settings. It is primarily used to provide partial mechanical support. The patient's spontaneous breathing is supported with periodic assisted mechanical breaths. Observe small volume spontaneous breaths interposed between mechanical breaths.

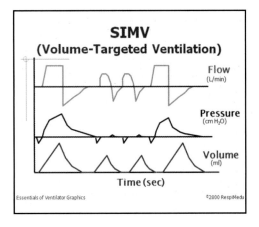

SIMV + PS

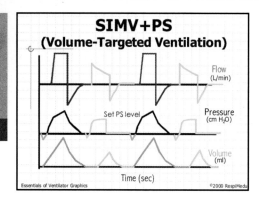

It is recommended that PS be added to SIMV to provide augmentation of unsupported spontaneous breath through the endotracheal tube. Each breath is a patient triggered breath. Volume delivered during mechanical breaths is preset. However, the volume delivered by the pressure supported breath is dependent on the level of pressure support, patient's lung compliance, airway resistance, and patient's inspiratory effort.

SIMV + PS + CPAP

The only difference in this waveform from the previous (SIMV + PSV) is that CPAP is added to the circuit as indicated on the Pressure/Time scalar.

Remember, the Pressure vs. Time curve and Pressure-Volume loop can be used to verify the use of CPAP. No other waveforms show CPAP.

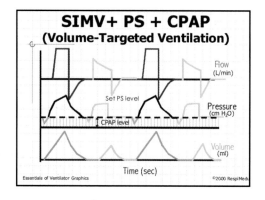

Pressure-Targeted Ventilation

Controlled Mode

A pressure targeted control breath is a pressure-limited (Preset pressure control level), time-cycled breath. The peak flow is a result of the set pressure level, the patient's lung characteristics and patient's inspiratory effort. Observe that the flow curve is decelerating and the flow decreases to zero at the end of preset inspiratory time.

In specific situations, such as decreased compliance (ARDS) the flow may return to

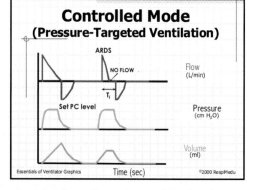

baseline prior to termination of inspiratory time and a state of zero flow exists until the inspiratory time elapses. The Pressure vs. Time curve exhibits a square pattern indicating that the pressure remains at the preset level throughout the inspiratory phase. The Volume vs. Time curve shows an initial sharp rise due to higher flow. However, the slope then tapers, indicating lesser amount of volume delivered as the lungs fill.

Essentials of Ventilator Waveforms

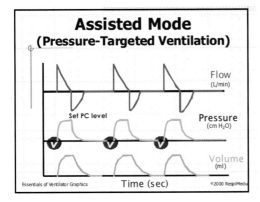

Assisted Mode

An assisted mode is identical to a controlled mode except that the Pressure vs. Time curve shows a negative deflection just prior to the mechanical breath. This negative deflection indicates patient triggering

SIMV

The patient's spontaneous breathing is supported with periodic assisted, pressure-targeted mechanical breaths.

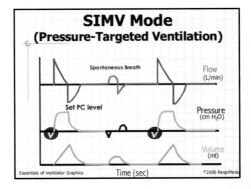

SIMV + PS

Exactly the same SIMV + PS mode as in volume-targeted ventilation, except the mechanical breaths are pressure-controlled breaths and PS augments the spontaneous breaths. The Pressure vs. Time curve is constant pressure curve since both the PCV and PS breaths are pressure limited and exhibit a square wave pressure pattern at their respective set levels. The Flow vs. Time curve shows the flow rate decaying to zero level for PC breaths; whereas PS breaths are flow cycled.

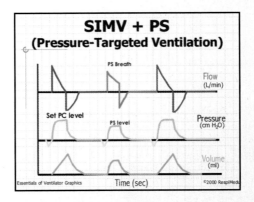

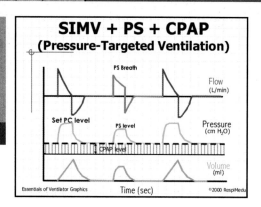

SIMV + PS + CPAP

Similar patterns as SIMV + PS with an addition of CPAP as shown on the Pressure vs. Time curve.

INITIATION OF MECHANICAL VENTILATION

Initiation of Gas Flow

Once a patient is diagnosed with Acute Respiratory Failure (ARF) mechanical ventilation should be instituted. Physiological definition of ventilation describes it as movement of gas in and out of the lungs. To ventilate the lungs, gas must flow from the airway opening to the alveoli. This requires a pressure gradient, meaning gas always flows from high pressure to low pressure area. Without a pressure gradient (ΔP), gas flow cannot be generated. The pressure gradient required to deliver gas to alveoli is referred to as Transairway Pressure ($\Delta P = P_{airway\ opening} - P_{alveolar}$). During spontaneous breathing, at end-inspiration and at end-exhalation the pressures in the alveoli and at the airway opening are equal and thus, there is no pressure gradient and no gas flow. A mechanical ventilator must generate either a negative intra-alveolar pressure or a positive airway opening pressure. The negative pressure ventilators such as Iron Lung and Curraise apply sub-atmospheric pressure to the chest wall. Consequently, the chest wall rises creating a negative intra-thoracic pressure ($< P_{atm}$). A Pressure gradient from atmospheric, at the airway opening, and negative pressure in the alveoli is generated resulting in gas flow. The Positive pressure ventilators are designed to deliver greater than atmospheric ($>P_{atm}$) pressure to the airways resulting in increased transairway pressure. The pressure gradient between the airway opening and alveoli produces gas flow. Figures 6.1 and 6.2 show anatomy of thorax and lung pressures. Figure 6.3 shows situation at end expiratory level with pressures at atmospheric (P_{atm}) with no gas flow, whereas, a delivery of positive pressure at the airway opening or generating a sub-atmospheric pressure in the alveoli results in a pressure gradient (ΔP) and gas flow to the alveoli.

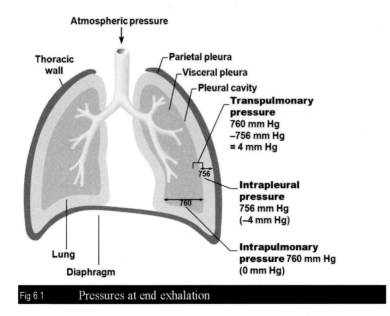

Fig 6.1   Pressures at end exhalation

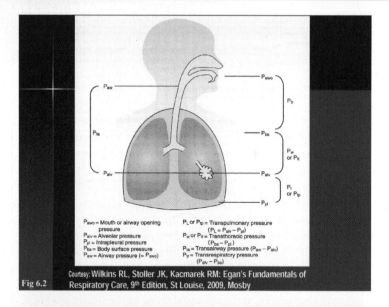

Fig 6.2 Courtesy: Wilkins RL, Stoller JK, Kacmarek RM: Egan's Fundamentals of Respiratory Care, 9th Edition, St Louise, 2009, Mosby

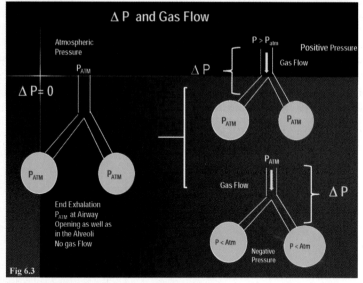

Fig 6.3

Phases of Ventilation and the Four (4) parameters

In clinical practice, the positive pressure ventilators are commonly used. From early mechanical ventilators with moving parts, advances in technology have progressed to the development of current microprocessor driven computerized ventilators. The positive pressure ventilators deliver pressure to the airway opening to ventilate the patient's lungs. Clinicians manipulate not only the pressure but other parameters such as volume delivered, inspiratory flow rate and termination of ventilatory cycle. The entire cyclic operation of the positive pressure ventilation involves four phases, beginning of inspiration with closed exhalation valve, inspiration, end of inspiration and beginning of expiratory phase by opening exhalation valve and finally, exhalation. The cycle repeats itself at a set frequency or on patient demand (Fig 6.4).

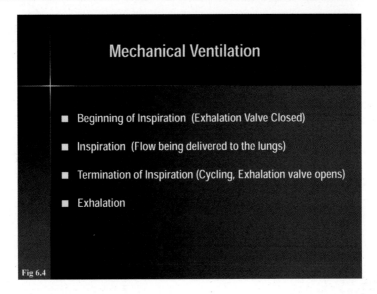
Fig 6.4

Mechanically ventilated breaths incorporate four parameters; pressure, flow, volume and time. The ventilator at any given point of time can only control the Volume (Flow × Time) or control the Pressure levels, but both these parameters cannot be controlled simultaneously. Manipulation can be done in these parameters to deliver breaths most suitable for the patient's need based on clinical judgment. There are parameters that trigger the ventilator to begin inspiration (pressure, time and flow). Some parameters or variables are limited and do not exceed their maximum (preset) value during inspiratory phase. It should be noted that reaching the limiting value does not terminate inspiration. In different modes of ventilation, as will be demonstrated in later chapters, specific variables are limited indicating a square pattern for that parameter on the scalar waveform. A mechanical breath that has started must be terminated at some point. Cycle variables terminate the inspiratory phase (pressure cycled, volume cycled, flow cycled and time cycled). Ventilator classification system describes triggering, limiting and cycling variables (Fig 6.5).

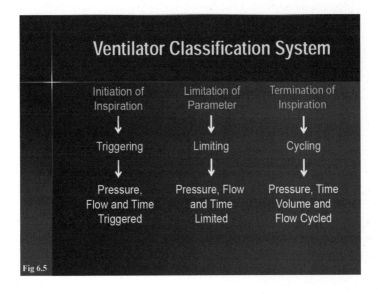
Fig 6.5

Triggering, Limiting and Cycling

Initiation of a mechanical breath (triggering) is provided when the patient makes an inspiratory effort, patient triggered, generally termed as "Assisted" breath or time triggered referred to as "Controlled" breath. The ventilator can be adjusted to provide triggering by any one of the two mechanisms, patient or time, whichever comes first (Assist/Control) – Fig 6.6. Patient triggering requires generation of a negative pressure from the patient. A sensitivity control is set to recognize this patient effort and initiate mechanical breath. A more sensitive flow triggering is introduced in most new ventilators. On the pressure-time scalar, a patient triggered breath shows a small negative deflection just before the breath is delivered, whereas a time triggered breath begins at the baseline (Fig 6.7).

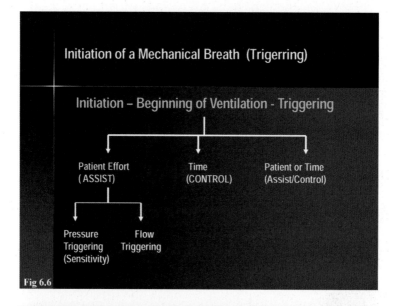

Fig 6.6

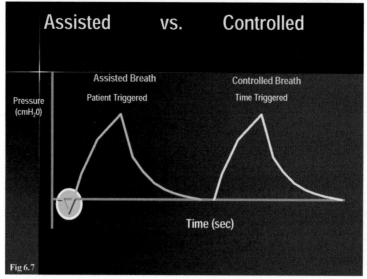

Fig 6.7

Initiation of Mechanical Ventilation

Termination of inspiration and beginning of exhalation, termed as cycling, can be accomplished by all four parameters. Figure 6.8 defines the cycling mechanisms by volume, time, flow and pressure parameters. As mentioned earlier in this chapter limiting a parameter does not allow it to exceed its preset value, even when the lung compliance and/or airway resistance deteriorate. Figure 6.9 identifies examples of limited variables and Fig 6.10 graphically shows square patterns of the parameters that are limited. In Pressure Control Ventilation the pressure and inspiratory time parameters are preset by clinician. The pressure-time scalar illustrates pressure and time are limited. In volume control ventilation the flow parameter is limited as indicated by the square pattern.

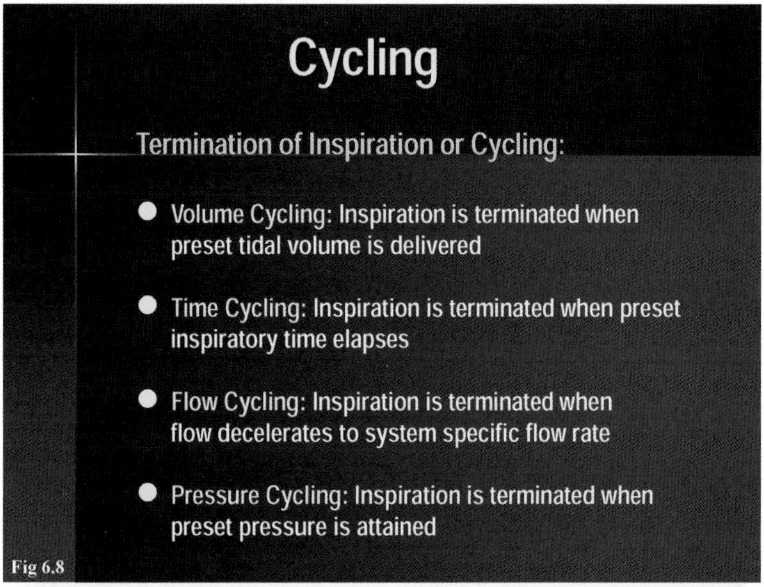

Cycling

Termination of Inspiration or Cycling:

- Volume Cycling: Inspiration is terminated when preset tidal volume is delivered

- Time Cycling: Inspiration is terminated when preset inspiratory time elapses

- Flow Cycling: Inspiration is terminated when flow decelerates to system specific flow rate

- Pressure Cycling: Inspiration is terminated when preset pressure is attained

Fig 6.8

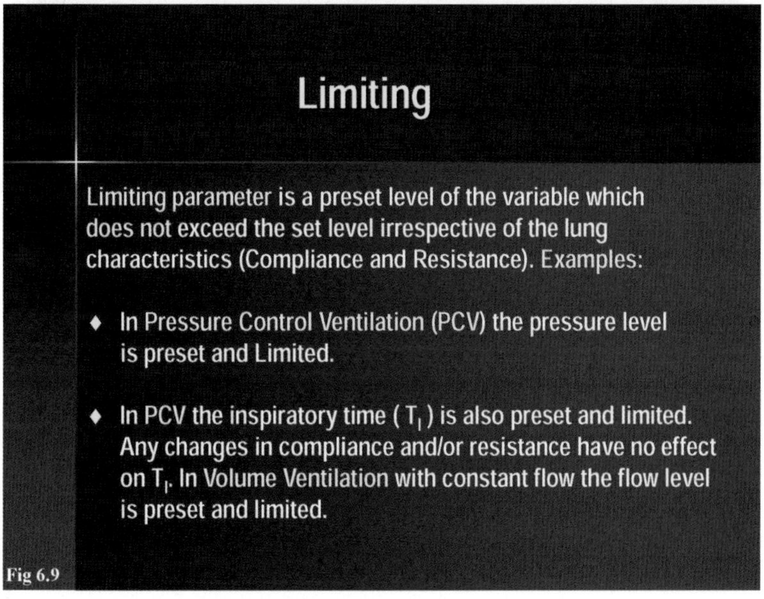

Limiting

Limiting parameter is a preset level of the variable which does not exceed the set level irrespective of the lung characteristics (Compliance and Resistance). Examples:

- In Pressure Control Ventilation (PCV) the pressure level is preset and Limited.

- In PCV the inspiratory time (T_I) is also preset and limited. Any changes in compliance and/or resistance have no effect on T_I. In Volume Ventilation with constant flow the flow level is preset and limited.

Fig 6.9

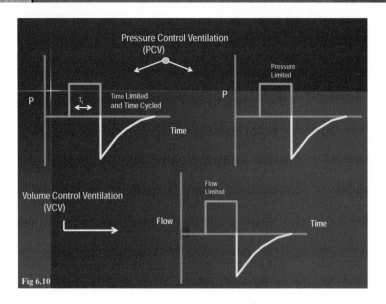

Fig 6.10

Volume Targeted Ventilation

When a decision is taken to initiate mechanical ventilation the clinician has to select the type of ventilation from three options- Volume Targeted Ventilation, Pressure Targeted Ventilation or Dual Mode (Fig 6.11).

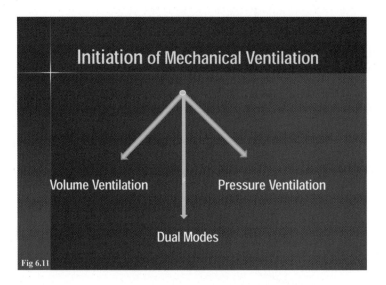

Fig 6.11

Volume targeted ventilation is commonly used in clinical practice. Typical features of volume ventilation are listed in Fig 6.12. Since the delivered tidal volume (V_T) is constant, it can be used to titrate $PaCO_2$ by adjusting V_T. It should be recognized that in volume targeted ventilation or commonly referred to as Volume Control Ventilation (VCV) with constant flow setting, not only the volume but also, flow and inspiratory time are constant, as long as the driving force is high. Clinicians can use a descending flow setting to improve gas distribution during inspiration.

Initiation of Mechanical Ventilation

The only variable parameter in volume ventilation is Pressure which is dependent on Airway Resistance (R_{aw}), Lung Compliance (C_L), inspiratory flow rate and the delivered tidal volume. In setting a volume ventilator the clinician sets desired tidal volume, respiratory frequency and inspiratory flow rate (Fig 6.13).

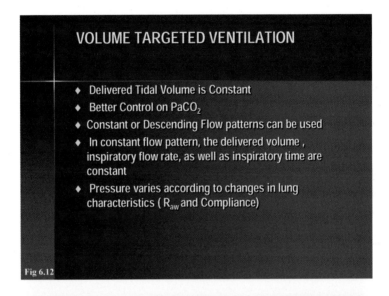

Fig 6.12

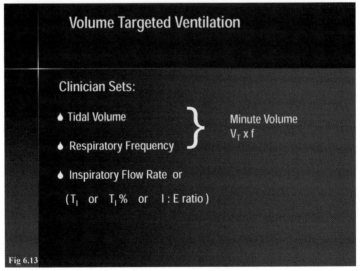

Fig 6.13

Setting Inspiratory Flow

In many current ventilators inspiratory flow rate is set indirectly and thus, do not have a flow rate control on the panel. Interrelationships between the time parameters allow a clinician to set inspiratory flow rate indirectly. If the ventilator has a "Flow Rate" setting, then it can be set directly. Some ventilators have an "Inspiratory Time" setting. Since inspiratory Flow Rate = Tidal Volume/Inspiratory Time, by adjusting inspiratory time at the given set tidal volume, flow rate can be obtained (flow rate = V_T / T_I) and adjusted as needed. Some ventilators adjust their inspiratory time by using $T_I\%$ control. $T_I\%$ is the percent (%) of cycle time (TCT) utilized for inspiration where the cycle time represents time required to complete one breathing cycle determined by the respiratory rate or frequency (f). Thus, TCT = 60 sec/F and $T_I\% = T_I/TCT \times 100$ (Fig 6.14).

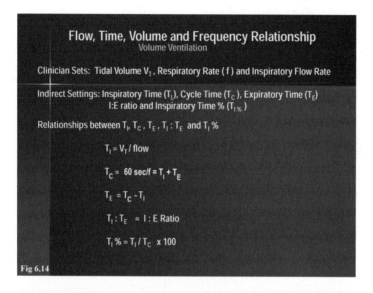

Fig 6.14

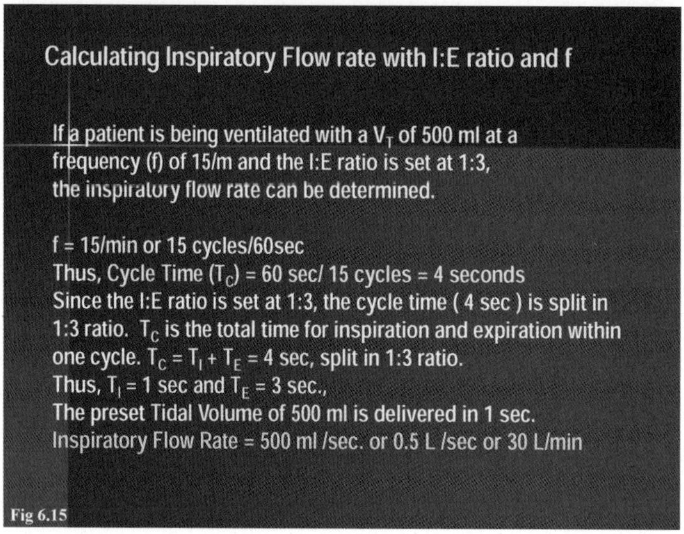

Fig 6.15

Some ventilators use the $T_I - T_E$ ratio, commonly known as I–E ratio, and respiratory frequency to calculate inspiratory time to deliver preset tidal volume. An example is given in Fig 6.15. Some ventilators have a $T_I\%$ setting to give the percent of T_I in relation to the total cycle time (TCT). The relationship between I:E ratio and $T_I\%$ is shown in Fig 6.16. In summary, in Volume Ventilation, Inspiratory Flow Rate can be set with controls on a given ventilator. The flow rate can be set directly, or indirectly via T_I, or $T_I\%$ or I–E ratio depending on the ventilator.

Initiation of Mechanical Ventilation

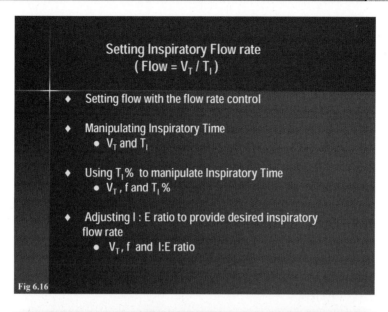

Fig 6.16

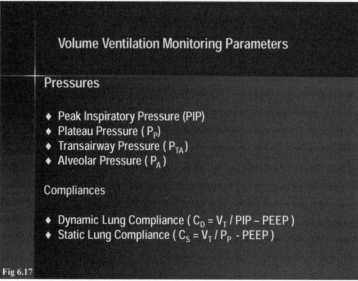

Fig 6.17

Monitoring Pressures during Volume Ventilation

During volume targeted ventilation a clinician monitors pressures and lung characteristics (Fig 6.17). PIP represents Peak Inspiratory Pressure (PIP) or the maximum pressure attained during the mechanical breath. P_P refers to Plateau Pressure which is the same as Alveolar Pressure (P_A). This pressure (P_P) is obtained by activating Inspiratory Pause or Inflation Hold control on the ventilator. The difference between PIP and P_P provides the Transairway Pressure (P_{TA}) or the pressure required to overcome airway resistance. From the measurement of Plateau Pressure (P_P) which is also termed as Static Pressure, we can determine Static Lung Compliance = V_T / P_P – PEEP. The value of PIP facilitates calculation of Dynamic Compliance = $V_T /$ PIP–PEEP.

Fig 6.18

Volume Targeted Ventilation

Key Alarms	Significance
▪ High Pressure Alarm	↑ Airway Resistance ↓ Compliance
▪ Low Pressure Alarm	Leak in the system
▪ Low Volume Alarm	Leak in the system

Fig 6.19

Figure 6.18 represents a tracing of pressure as the lung is inflated during inspiratory phase in volume ventilation. Upon initiation of inspiratory flow, the gas molecules experience frictional resistance during their transit through the airways all the way to terminal bronchioles. This generates trans-airway pressure, P_{TA}, (Fig 6.18). The tidal volume enters the alveolar zone against the recoiling force of the elastic fibers. Resulting pressure gradually increases until all the tidal volume is delivered. The pressure pattern depends on the compliance of the lung. At the end of tidal volume delivery the highest pressure, peak inspiratory pressure (PIP), is attained. The exhalation valve is supposed to open at this point to allow for exhalation. However, if the Inspiratory hold control is activated, the exhalation valve remains closed. Now the tidal volume is trapped in the lungs indicating alveolar pressure or plateau pressure (P_P). Since there is no gas flow the transairway pressure resulting from inspiratory flow is eliminated. Thus, P_P is always less than PIP in volume ventilation.

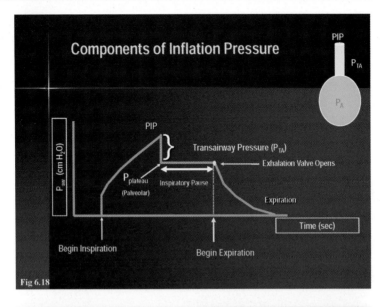

Initiation of Mechanical Ventilation

The exhalation valve opens when the inspiratory pause time elapses. Patient exhales the inspired tidal volume. The difference between PIP and PP provides the pressure required to overcome airway resistance (P_{TA}). During every ventilator check, the clinician is expected to monitor and record the above pressures. It is imperative that alarms should be set appropriately. In volume ventilation the two essential alarms are the High Pressure Alarm, indicating that the pressure has reached the set high pressure limit and the Low Pressure or Low Volume Alarm signifying that a leak in the circuit is causing the loss of pressure (Fig 6.19). As a rule of thumb, the high pressure alarm level is set at 5-10 cm H_2O higher than the ventilating pressure and the low pressure alarm level is set at 5-10 cm H_2O below the ventilating pressure (Fig 6.20).

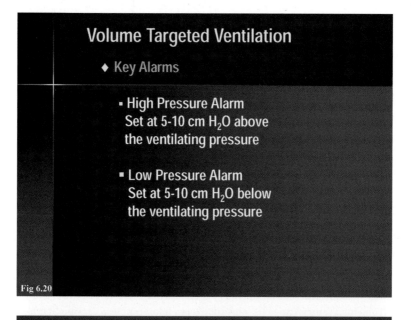

Fig 6.20

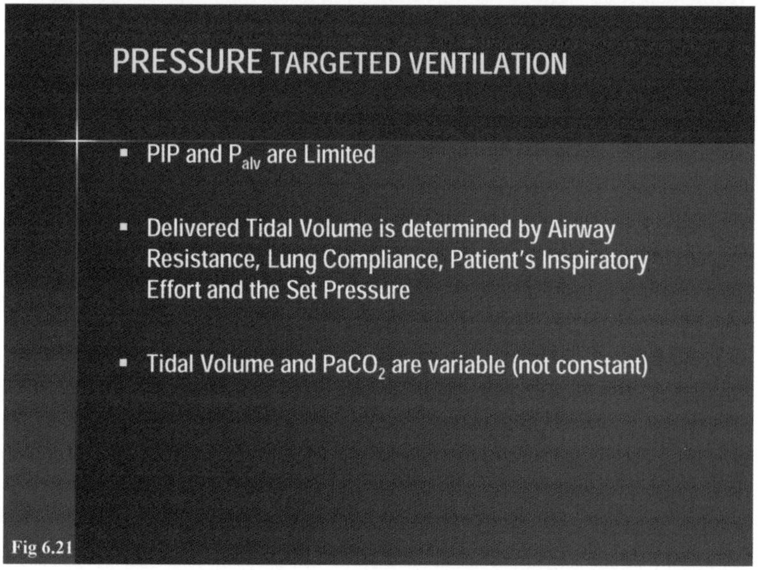

PRESSURE TARGETED VENTILATION

- PIP and P_{alv} are Limited

- Delivered Tidal Volume is determined by Airway Resistance, Lung Compliance, Patient's Inspiratory Effort and the Set Pressure

- Tidal Volume and $PaCO_2$ are variable (not constant)

Fig 6.21

In summary, during volume targeted ventilation the clinician sets V_T, respiratory rate (f) or Minute volume ($V_E = V_T \times f$). Actually, some ventilators do not have a tidal volume setting, instead it is set indirectly from V_E and frequency ($V_T = V_E /f$) as shown in Fig 6.13. The third parameter, Inspiratory Flow Rate, is derived from T_I or $T_I\%$ or I- E ratio.

Pressure Targeted Ventilation

Pressure Targeted Ventilation or Pressure Control Ventilation (PCV) provides preset pressure to the airways that does not exceed the set level irrespective of the changes in lung compliance and airway resistance (Pressure Limited). The volume delivered is dependent on Lung Compliance, R_{aw}, the Set Pressure and Patient effort during delivery of the pressure. Tidal volume is variable and so is $PaCO_2$ level (Figs 6.21 and 6.22).

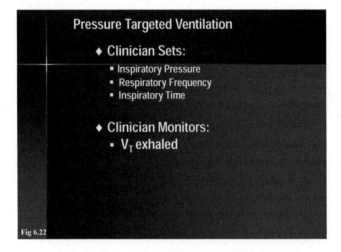
Fig 6.22

To initiate Pressure Control Ventilation (PCV) the clinician sets the Pressure level, Respiratory Frequency (f) and Inspiratory Time (T_I). Since delivered tidal volume is variable, it is monitored and a low volume alarm (or Low Minute Volume alarm) is set appropriately (Fig 6.23).

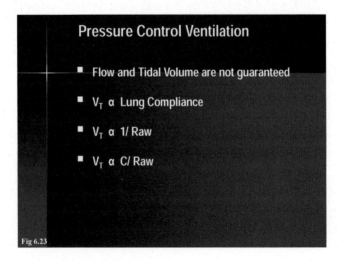
Fig 6.23

Initiation of Mechanical Ventilation

It is important to recognize that, unlike in volume ventilation, activation of Low Volume Alarm is not associated with a circuit leak but it indicates increased R_{aw} or decreased CL. In PCV, the volume delivered is directly proportional to the lung compliance. Lower the lung compliance lower the tidal volume delivered at the preset pressure control level. However, changes in R_{aw} inversely affect the delivered volume. As R_{aw} increases the delivered volume decreases during PCV. Thus, the delivered volume is proportional to the ratio of C/R_{aw} (Fig 6.23). The low volume alarm in PCV is identical to high pressure alarm in VCV, both alert the clinician that the lung characteristics have deteriorated (Decreased Compliance or Increased Airway Resistance, Figs 6.24 and 6.25).

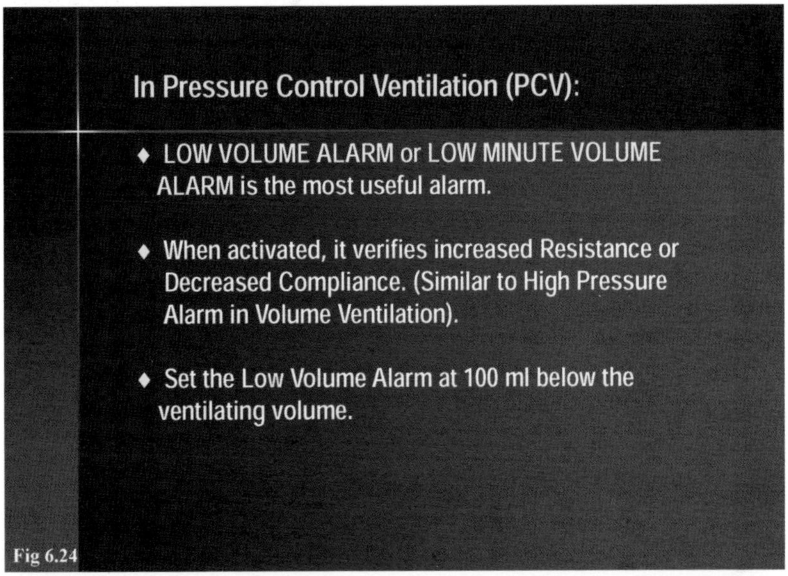

In Pressure Control Ventilation (PCV):

- LOW VOLUME ALARM or LOW MINUTE VOLUME ALARM is the most useful alarm.

- When activated, it verifies increased Resistance or Decreased Compliance. (Similar to High Pressure Alarm in Volume Ventilation).

- Set the Low Volume Alarm at 100 ml below the ventilating volume.

Fig 6.24

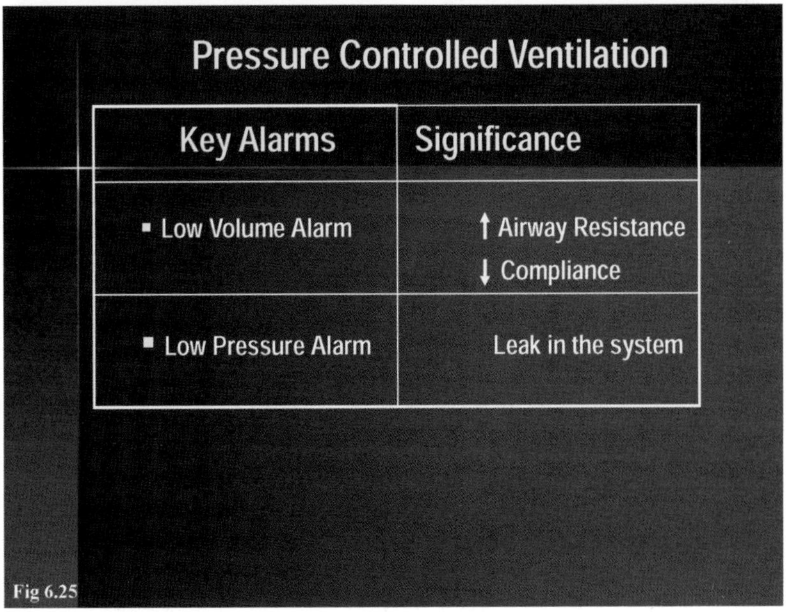

Pressure Controlled Ventilation

Key Alarms	Significance
■ Low Volume Alarm	↑ Airway Resistance ↓ Compliance
■ Low Pressure Alarm	Leak in the system

Fig 6.25

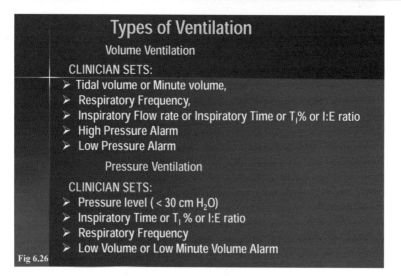

Fig 6.26

Figure 6.26 summarizes the role of a clinician in initiating volume or pressure ventilation.

Drawbacks in Volume and Pressure Ventilation

The clinicians had a choice of selecting either volume targeted ventilation or pressure targeted ventilation. Researchers recognized the limitations of both the volume and pressure ventilation causing dissynchrony between the patient and ventilator. Figure 6.27 identifies the drawbacks in Volume Ventilation.

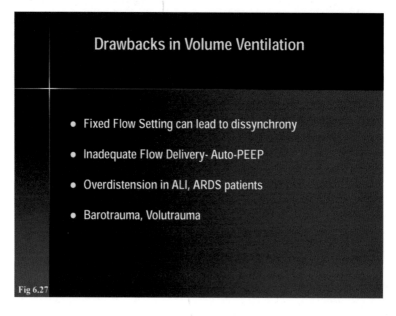

Fig 6.27

Since the inspiratory flow rate (or T_i) is set by the clinician, the patient cannot set their own flow demand. Consequently, the patient attempts to breathe spontaneously during the delivery of the mechanical breath resulting in dissynchrony. If the set flow rate is slower than the patient's demand it may increase inspiratory time leaving shorter expiratory time. This can result, in some cases, in air trapping or auto-PEEP. The pressure during volume ventilation is dependent on the lung characteristics (R_{aw} and C_L). In stiff lungs or emphasematous regions, delivery of positive pressure can cause barotraumas – trauma resulting from high intrathoracic pressures. Barotrauma is recognized from pneumothorax, pneumomediastinum, subcutaneous air when a patient is receiving positive pressure ventilation. Moreover, in situations like Acute Lung Injury (ALI) or Acute Respiratory Distress Syndrome (ARDS), where the lungs have regions of non-homogenously spread partially and completely collapsed alveoli. The open alveoli receive most of the delivered tidal volume resulting in overdistention which promotes release of chemical mediators and further damages the lung. Thus the use of volume ventilation has limitations.

The positive aspects of pressure ventilation are the adequacy of flow since the demand valve opens during inspiration allowing the patient to receive as much flow as needed and the pressure can be set at a safe level (< 30 cm H_2O). Pressure Ventilation has also, some disadvantages. The major problem with Pressure Ventilation is that the delivered pressure is fixed and the delivered volume depends on the set pressure, airway resistance, lung compliance and patient effort. If the lung characteristics deteriorate, the delivered volume decreases at the fixed set pressure. This can promote hypoventilation and hypercapnia (increased $PaCO_2$). If the set pressure is high it may lead to barotrauma (Fig 6.28)

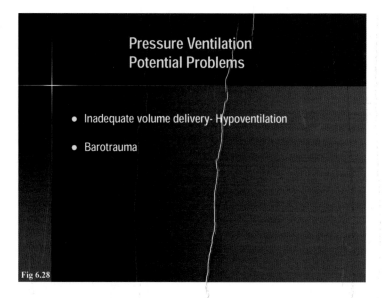

Fig 6.28

Dual Modes of Ventilation

Recognizing the limitations of volume and pressure ventilation, manufacturers introduced dual ventilation system. Essentially, Dual Ventilation uses the beneficial aspects of both volume ventilation and pressure ventilation. In most cases, it delivers pressure ventilation with volume target. Thus the patient is protected from high pressure levels and yet, receives desired tidal volume. The ventilator adjusts pressure (< 30 cm H_2O) based on calculated dynamic compliance and delivers desired volume (Fig 6.29). Currently, different ventilators employ dual modes. Figure 6.30 lists the names of commonly use Dual Modes. Subsequent chapters will discuss these modes in details.

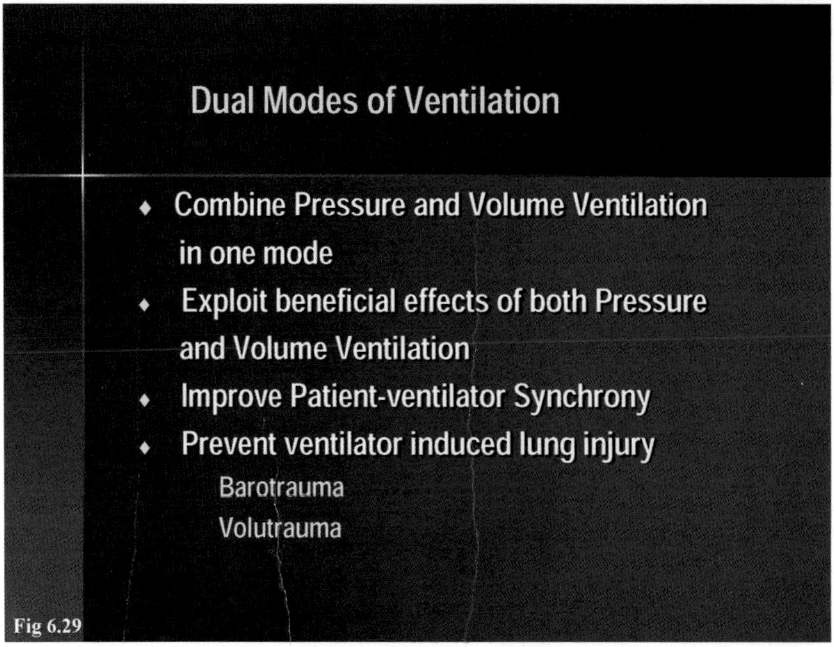

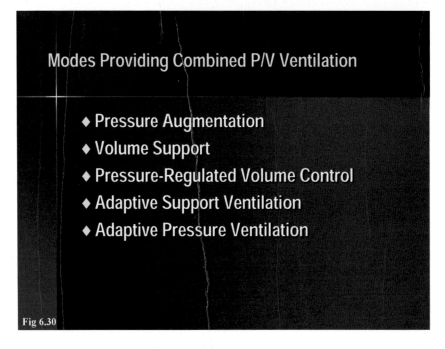

Fig 6.29

Fig 6.30

After taking into consideration all aspects of the types of mechanical ventilation discussed in this chapter, the clinician should also consider the patient's underlying cause for respiratory failure before initiating mechanical ventilation.

★★★

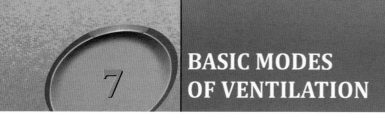

BASIC MODES OF VENTILATION

A mode of ventilation can be described as a predefined pattern of interaction between the patient and ventilator.

According to the Equation of motion, the pressure required to inflate the lungs and chest wall during spontaneous breathing comes from the muscles (diaphragm, accessory muscles of respiration). This pressure overcomes the elastic and resistive forces in delivering the volume to the lungs. Since elastic recoil depends on the elastance ($E = 1/\text{Compliance}$) and frictional resistance depends on the caliber of the airways (patency) and the gas flow, the pressure required to deliver gas to alveoli is expressed by the Equation of Motion:

$$P_{mus} = (E \times V_T) + (R_{aw} \times \text{Flow})$$

When a patient requires mechanical support the pressure is shared by the respiratory muscles and the ventilator

$$P_{mus} + P_{vent} = (E \times V_T) + (R_{aw} \times \text{Flow})$$

Elastance or reciprocal of compliance (1/Compliance) and Tidal Volume represent the pressure required to overcome the recoiling force of the lungs against which the volume is being delivered. Whereas, the resistive component involves overcoming the frictional resistance to gas flow and is dependent on the airway resistance and flow (Fig 7.1).

Pressure required to Inflate the Lung

$$PIP = P_{TA} + P_{alv}$$

$$= (R_{aw} \times \text{Flow}) + \frac{\text{Tidal Volume}}{C_L}$$

Equation of Motion

$$P_{mus} + P_{vent} = (R_{aw} \times \text{Flow}) + (V_T \times 1/C_L)$$

Fig 7.1

By convention, control variable is either volume or pressure. Volume control mode is also known as Volume Targeted Ventilation. In volume targeted ventilation the ventilator delivers desired tidal volume and the lung characteristics, compliance and resistance, do not affect the delivery of the volume. Whereas, in Pressure Control Ventilation or Pressure Targeted Ventilation the set pressure is delivered irrespective of respiratory system mechanics (compliance, resistance or patient effort).

Thus, when a decision is made to ventilate a patient the clinician has to decide the control variable, volume or pressure and then select a mode of ventilation. The clinician can also select Dual Mode which delivers clinician's set tidal volume at a minimal pressure keeping alveolar (plateau) pressure < 30 cm H_2O (Fig 7.2).

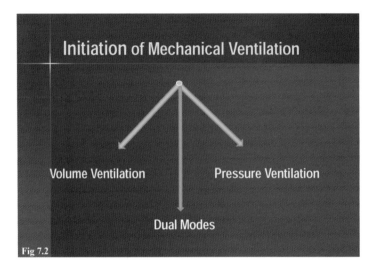

Fig 7.2

Upon selecting volume ventilation or pressure ventilation option the clinician selects certain parameters to instruct the ventilator to deliver specific types of breaths. In volume ventilation the desired volume (Tidal Volume or Minute volume), respiratory rate (f) and inspiratory flow rate (set by T_I, T_I%, or I–E ratio) are set to establish the character of every mandatory breath (Fig 7.3A). In

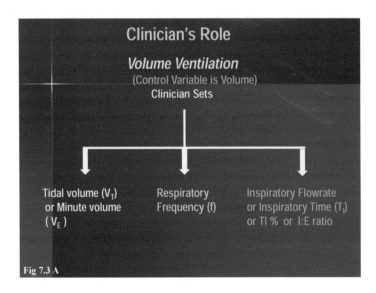

Fig 7.3 A

Pressure Ventilation the clinician sets the target pressure (below 30 cm H_2O), respiratory rate (f) and Inspiratory Time (T_I or T_I% or I–E ratio) (Fig 7.3 B).

Basic Modes of Ventilation

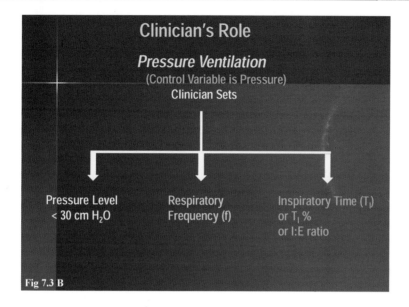

Fig 7.3 B

Over the past 40 years, technology has advanced significantly. New modes of ventilation were introduced to rectify drawbacks identified by researchers about the earlier ways of ventilating patients. Figure 7.4 identifies technological advancement in modes of ventilation from Assist/Control to currently introduced Closed Loop Ventilation. Under Volume Control and Pressure Control

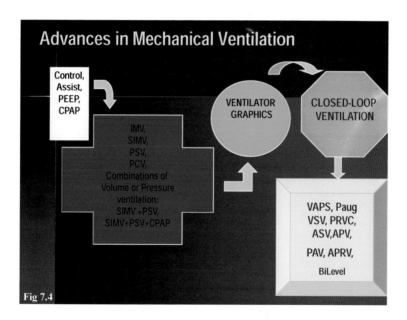

Fig 7.4

ventilation a clinician can utilize Control Mode, Assist Mode, synchronized intermittent mandatory ventilation (SIMV), SIMV with Pressure Support as well as combination of SIMV with Pressure Support (PSV) and continuous positive airway pressure (CPAP) (Fig 7.5). Each of the mode associated with a mandatory breath are described below with graphics. These graphs are repeated in many chapters in this book to maintain continuity. These graphs are also described in chapter 5.

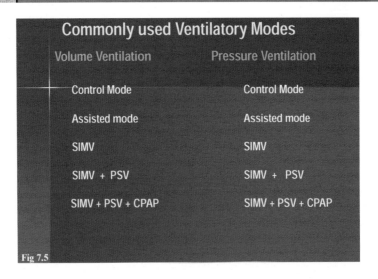

Fig 7.5

CONTROL VENTILATION

When a breath is triggered by the patient, it is termed as an Assisted Breath, whereas, a time triggered breath is known as a Controlled breath. Figure 7.6 shows scalars-Flow/Time, Pressure/Time and Volume/Time-for Controlled Ventilation (Time Triggered, Flow Limited and Volume Cycled) in Volume Targeted or Volume Controlled or simply Volume Ventilation. Recognize that the characteristics of volume ventilation are flow limited (constant), variable pressure and set, constant tidal volume. The ventilator terminates the mechanical breath when the set tidal volume is delivered (Volume Cycled).

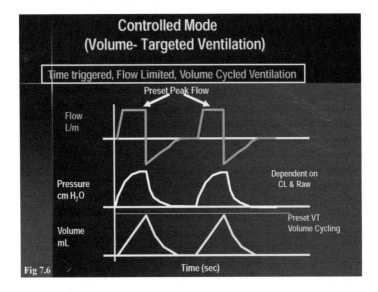

Fig 7.6

Controlled breath implies that the entire breathing process is controlled by the ventilator and the patient has no participation. Generally, patients receiving controlled ventilation are incapable of initiating spontaneous breath. Fig 7.7 lists typical patients that require controlled ventilation. There are obvious hazards of controlled ventilation. If the patient desires to take a spontaneous breath the

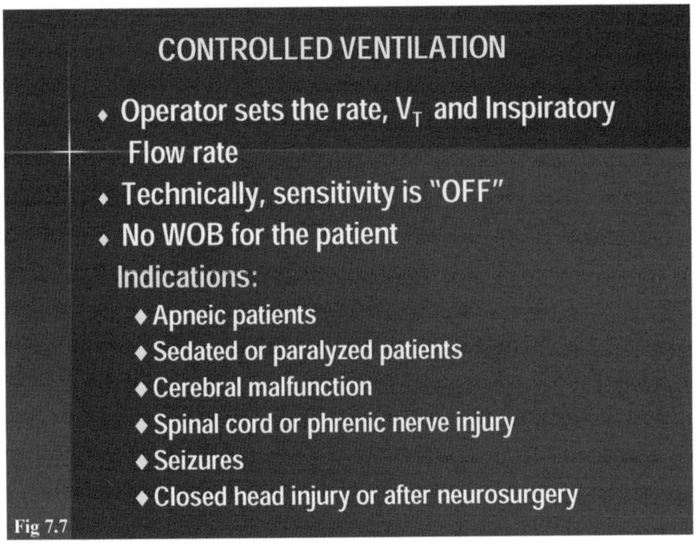

Basic Modes of Ventilation

CONTROLLED VENTILATION
- Operator sets the rate, V_T and Inspiratory Flow rate
- Technically, sensitivity is "OFF"
- No WOB for the patient

Indications:
- Apneic patients
- Sedated or paralyzed patients
- Cerebral malfunction
- Spinal cord or phrenic nerve injury
- Seizures
- Closed head injury or after neurosurgery

Fig 7.7

ventilator will not allow since every breath is time triggered. This causes anxiety in patient and he gets in dissynchrony with the ventilator. The pressure alarm goes off and the patient is considered to be "fighting" the ventilator. Moreover, the patient is stuck with clinician set tidal volume and flow which may be inadequate (Fig 7.8). In clinical practice the patient is always placed on assisted

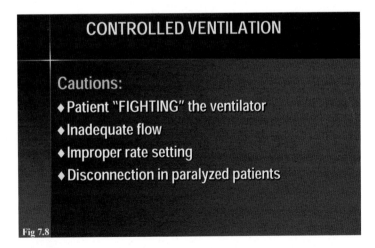

CONTROLLED VENTILATION

Cautions:
- Patient "FIGHTING" the ventilator
- Inadequate flow
- Improper rate setting
- Disconnection in paralyzed patients

Fig 7.8

ventilation with backup frequency adjusted to give adequate ventilation. Sensitivity should never be "off" (difficult for patient to trigger the ventilator).

ASSISTED VENTILATION

Most common initial mode used is volume ventilation in assisted breath. Switching from controlled mode to assisted mode involves simply activating "sensitivity" control.

In assisted ventilation every breath is mandatory, delivering clinician-set tidal volume. Clinician sets only the back-up frequency to ascertain ventilation in unforeseen situation such as apnea. The patient determines the total frequency. Figure 7.9 shows scalars for assisted ventilation.

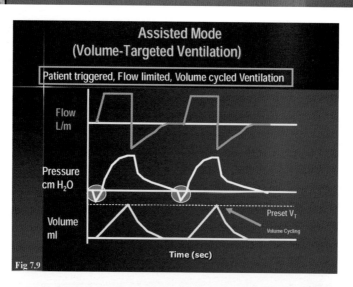
Fig 7.9

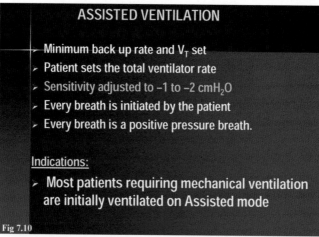
Fig 7.10

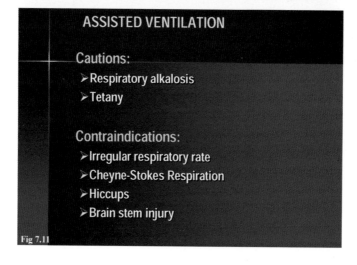
Fig 7.11

Basic Modes of Ventilation

Observed, the only difference between the controlled breath and assisted breath is that every breath in assisted ventilation is initiated by the patient as seen by the small negative deflection on Pressure-Time scalar. Key points, indications, cautions and hazards of assisted ventilation are listed in Figs 7.10 and 7.11.

ALARMS IN VOLUME VENTILATION

Besides setting the parameters in the given mode of ventilation the clinician must set alarms to ensure proper functioning and preserve patient safety. The key alarms that must be routinely set during Volume Ventilation are the High Pressure Alarm and the Low Pressure Alarm. The high

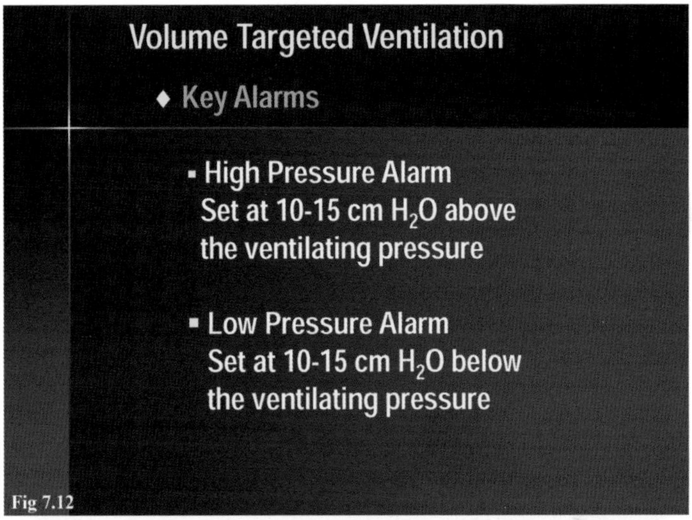

Volume Targeted Ventilation

♦ Key Alarms

- High Pressure Alarm
  Set at 10-15 cm H_2O above the ventilating pressure

- Low Pressure Alarm
  Set at 10-15 cm H_2O below the ventilating pressure

Fig 7.12

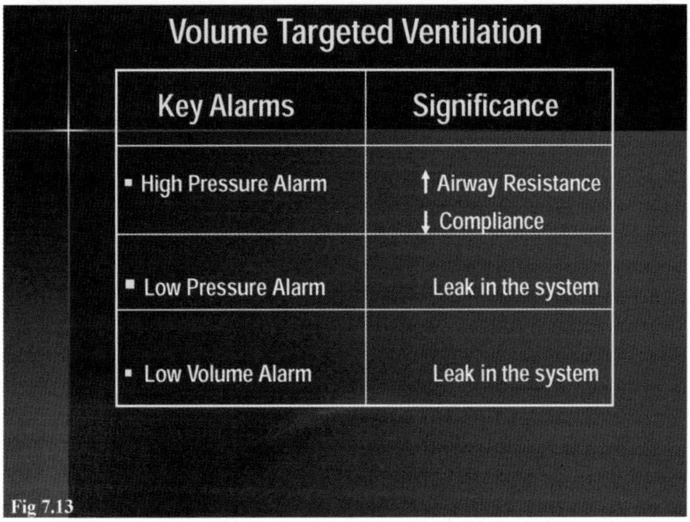

Volume Targeted Ventilation

Key Alarms	Significance
High Pressure Alarm	↑ Airway Resistance ↓ Compliance
Low Pressure Alarm	Leak in the system
Low Volume Alarm	Leak in the system

Fig 7.13

pressure alarm, an audible as well as visible alarm, on all mechanical ventilators makes the clinicians aware of increased airway pressure. The alarm is set at 10–15 cm H_2O above the Peak Inspiratory Pressure (PIP). Similarly, to detect leaks in the system or ventilator, disconnection of Low

Pressure Alarms are incorporated in all ventilators. Low Volume Alarm is also activated when a leak in the system is present. Generally, low pressure alarm is set at 10–15 cm H_2O below the PIP (Fig 7.12). Figure 7.13 identifies the underlying causes of activation of these alarms. Thus, when high pressure alarm sounds, the clinician interprets it as increase in airway pressure above the PIP. This generally occurs as a result of increased airways resistance (most common cause) or decreased compliance. Based on patient assessment the clinician corrects the problem by tracheal suctioning or bronchodilator therapy to decrease R_{aw}.

MODES IN PRESSURE VENTILATION

Similar to volume ventilation all basic modes are available during Pressure Ventilation. The ventilator is instructed to deliver set pressure and not the volume. The character of the breath is set as controlled breath or Assisted breath. Figure 7.14 shows scalars in Pressure Control mode.

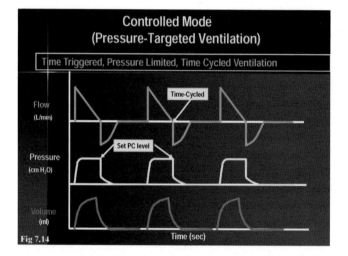
Fig 7.14

Observe the flow-time scalar indicating a decelerating flow throughout the inspiratory phase. This pattern is seen in all pressure ventilation modes that will be discussed later. Since flow is generated

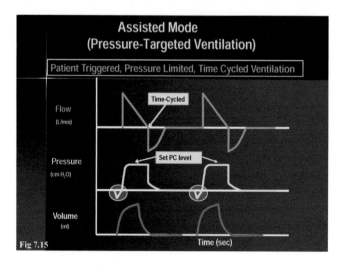
Fig 7.15

Basic Modes of Ventilation

from pressure gradient, in Pressure ventilation the clinician applies desired positive pressure at the airway opening at which time the alveolar pressure is the same as atmospheric. The pressure gradient between airway opening pressure and alveolar pressure produces flow. As the lungs start filling, the pressure gradient from airway opening (preset pressure) and alveoli begins to decrease. Consequently, the flow starts decreasing. This decrease in flow is seen until the termination of inspiration. In pressure ventilation the pressure is constant and so is inspiratory time. The only variable is delivered volume. Figure 7.15 shows pressure control ventilation in assist mode as indicated by the negative deflection on the pressure-time scalar.

ALARMS IN PRESSURE VENTILATION

Unlike volume ventilation, changes in R_{aw}, and lung compliance affect delivered volume in pressure ventilation. Since the pressure to be delivered is set by the clinician, under no circumstances

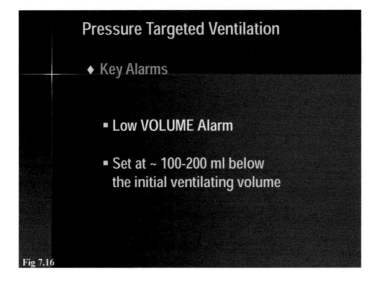
Fig 7.16

pressure will exceed this set value (pressure limited). This pressure ceiling makes high pressure alarm useless. The most essential alarm in Pressure Ventilation is LOW VOLUME (OR LOW MINUTE VOLUME) ALARM. In volume ventilation low volume alarm indicates a leak in the circuit. However, activation of low volume alarm during Pressure Ventilation indicates delivery of lower volume due to loss of pressure available for lung inflation. Increased airway resistance uses some of the applied pressure to negotiate flow of gas molecules to the lungs. Thus, lesser pressure is available to deliver tidal volume. Decreasing lung compliance delivers lower volume for the set pressure. Once again it is imperative that the clinician activates Low Volume (or Low Minute Volume) alarm when using pressure ventilation (Fig 7.16).

SYNCHRONIZED INTERMITTENT MANDATORY VENTILATION (SIMV)

In 1973 John Downs and colleagues published their research findings in Pediatric patients with a new approach to ventilation called intermittent mandatory ventilation (IMV). This new mode incorporated mandatory breaths with preset tidal volume at specified intervals while allowing the patient to take spontaneous breaths between the controlled mandatory mechanical breaths. This article revolutionized ventilator management. It was a controversial approach and opposing articles flooded the literature. Both sides, pros and cons, for the IMV justified their arguments. IMV was further improved to SIMV where the spontaneous breathing was allowed between Assisted

Breaths avoiding breath stacking (Fig 7.17). Today, patients are ventilated on both Assisted Ventilation and synchronized intermittent mandatory ventilation (SIMV). Scalars for SIMV in Volume and Pressure Ventilation are shown in Figs 7.18 and 7.19. Observe small volume spontaneous breaths between mechanical breaths. One major drawback of SIMV is that the patient, sick enough to have tracheal intubation, is permitted to take spontaneous breaths through the tracheal tube.

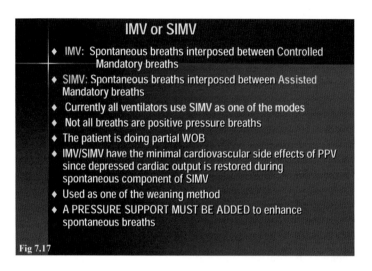

Fig 7.17

This unsupported ventilation offers significantly increased resistance and thus, increases work of breathing. As indicated in Fig 7.20, the pressure at the airway opening is higher than at Carina. Currently, Pressure Support is added to all patients on SIMV to offset increased work of breathing imposed by the tracheal tube. The level of pressure required to overcome the imposed resistance by the tracheal tube can be estimated as transairway pressure, or pressure difference between PIP and Plateau pressure (alveolar pressure). Thus, a clinician can add pressure support equivalent to PIP − P_{Plat} as the initial level and then adjust according to the patient's clinical condition. Generally, 5 cm

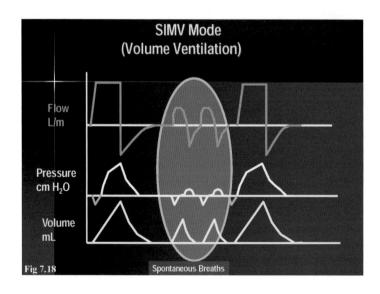

Fig 7.18

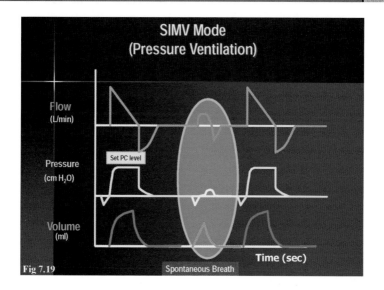
Fig 7.19

H₂O of pressure support (PS) is used in all SIMV patients as the beginning point. Figure 7.21 represents SIMV + PSV scalars. Compared to Fig 7.19, it is obvious that added PS increases spontaneous volume.

Since SIMV involves two types of breaths, in manipulating minute ventilation the clinician must be cognizant of mandatory and spontaneous breaths.

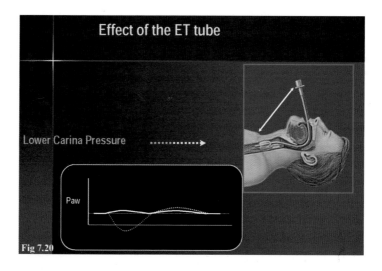
Fig 7.20

In Assisted ventilation,

Minute Ventilation = Tidal Volume × Respiratory Rate

$$= V_T \times f$$

In SIMV,

Minute Ventilation = Mandatory Minute Ventilation + Spontaneous Minute Ventilation

$$= (V_T \times f)_{mandatory} + (VT \times f)_{spontaneous}$$

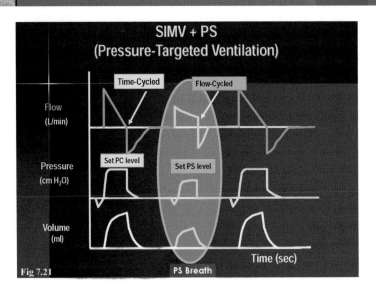
Fig 7.21

PRESSURE SUPPORT VENTILATION

Pressure support ventilation (PSV) has become an integral part of mechanical ventilation. PSV provides inspiratory flow in response to patient's inspiratory effort. The flow increases airway pressure to the preset level. The flow continues to decelerate to a system specific level (~ 25 % of the peak flow). All this time the exhalation valve is closed until the threshold flow level is reached and

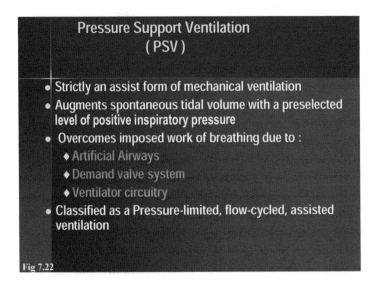
Fig 7.22

the breath is terminated (flow cycled). PS augments spontaneous tidal volume. PS delivers higher tidal volume with lower patient effort. PSV is an assisted form of ventilation where it only enhances patient triggered spontaneous breaths. PSV is inoperative during mandatory ventilation. Only spontaneous breaths are augmented. PSV overcomes the imposed work of breathing due to tracheal tube, and ventilator circuitry (Fig 7.22). The mechanism of delivery of PSV is explained in Figs 7.23 and 7.24.

Basic Modes of Ventilation

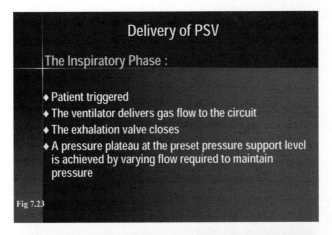

Fig 7.23

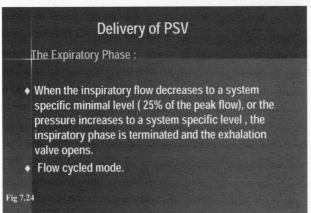

Fig 7.24

Observe scalars for Pressure Support breaths (Fig 7.25). The flow decelerates from its peak level throughout the inspiratory phase. Pressure plateau is attained at the set pressure.

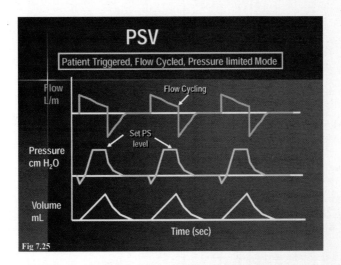

Fig 7.25

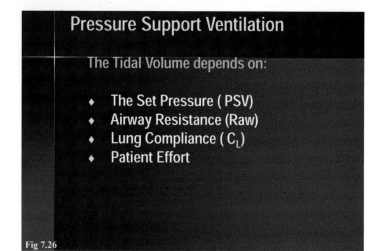
Fig 7.26

Delivered volume is a function of Pressure Support Level, patient's inspiratory effort, airway resistance and lung compliance (Fig 7.26). Any changes in these factors affect the delivered volume. Thus, tidal volume is not constant during application of preset pressure support. PSV is indicated to support feeble patient efforts in neuromuscular diseases, and augment volume in spontaneous phase of SIMV. It is one of the major technique used to assist COPD patients in exacerbation and during weaning a patient off mechanical ventilation (Fig 7.27). PSV can also be used as a stand-alone mode of ventilation for spontaneously breathing patients which can be delivered via tracheal tube or nasal or face mask (non-invasive ventilation).

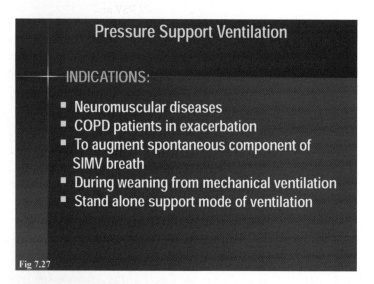
Fig 7.27

Continuous Positive Airway Pressure (CPAP)

CPAP does not provide ventilation. It simply maintains clinician-set positive pressure throughout the ventilatory cycle. The baseline is elevated for every breath, spontaneous or SIMV. CPAP increases functional residual capacity (FRC). Two terms are generally used in mechanical ventilation that refer to higher baseline- PEEP and CPAP. Positive end expiratory pressure (PEEP) is

Basic Modes of Ventilation

recognized when the baseline is higher during mechanical breath whereas elevated baseline during spontaneous breath is termed as CPAP. Basically, CPAP is spontaneous PEEP and PEEP is mechanical CPAP. More discussion on PEEP and CPAP can be found in later chapters. Figure 7.28 shows scalars for a CPAP breath. Observe that the baseline is elevated only in Pressure–Time scalar.

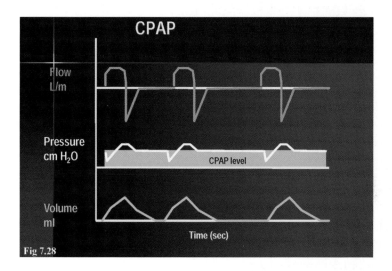
Fig 7.28

COMBINATION MODES

It is very common to use combination of these basic modes to provide support to the patient.

Figure 7.29 shows a typical combination of modes- SIMV, PSV and CPAP in pressure ventilation. Observe mechanical breaths are pressure controlled breaths delivered at fixed intervals during SIMV. The spontaneous component of SIMV is supported by Pressure Support and the entire ventilation is carried out at higher baseline (CPAP). Figure 7.30 demonstrates SIMV + PSV + CPAP in Volume control ventilation. Most patients recovering from acute ventilatory problems benefit from the combination of modes.

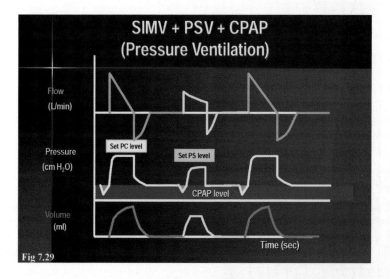
Fig 7.29

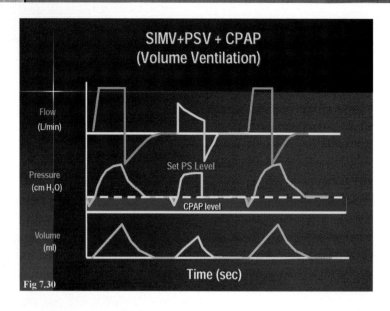
Fig 7.30

BiPAP

Most common non-invasive positive pressure ventilation is known as BiPAP, incorporating PSV and CPAP (Fig 7.31). The dedicated version of BiPAP uses slightly different terminology for pressures. The maximum pressure set is termed as inspiratory positive airway pressure (IPAP), the traditional CPAP level is termed as expiratory positive airway pressure (EPAP) and the difference between IPAP and EPAP is the Pressure Support.

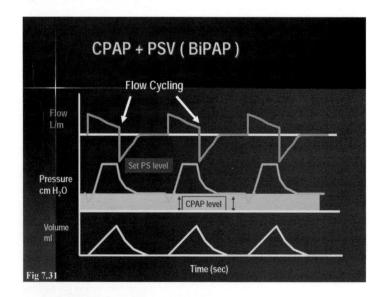
Fig 7.31

★ ★ ★

VOLUME vs. PRESSURE VENTILATION

In the previous chapter basic modes of ventilation under volume and pressure control were discussed. Figure 8.1 compares scalars for assisted mode in Volume and Pressure ventilation. The variables in different modes are shown in a tabular form in Fig 8.2. Most clinicians are familiar with volume ventilation, and find it user friendly since it delivers precise clinician-set tidal volume and is useful in titrating $PaCO_2$ to the normal level.

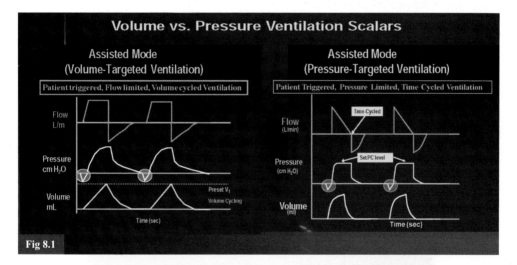

Fig 8.1

Mode	Variables	Trigger Variable	Limiting Variable	Cycling Variable
Volume Targeted A/C		Pressure, Flow, or Time	Flow	Set Tidal Volume
Pressure Targeted A/C		Pressure, Flow, or Time	Pressure	Set Inspiratory Time
Pressure Support		Pressure or Flow	Pressure	System-Specific Flow

Fig 8.2

Drawback of Volume Ventilation

There are specific drawbacks of volume ventilation. Since the flow is set by the clinician, it can be inadequate for some patients.

This flow starving may lead to flow dissynchrony and also, promote auto-PEEP. Similarly, clinician-set improper sensitivity may increase work of breathing (Fig 8.3).

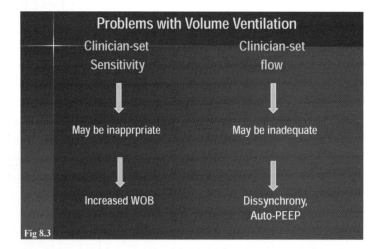

Fig 8.3

As the volume delivered in Volume ventilation is constant and preset, changes in compliance and resistance affect the airway pressure. As demonstrated in the pressure-volume loops (Fig 8.4), at fixed volume the PIP varies as compliance changes.

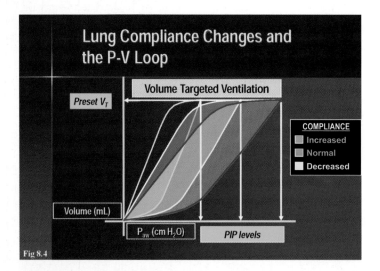

Fig 8.4

In acute cases persistent use of volume ventilation in presence of increased resistance or decreased compliance can develop barotrauma. It has been argued that volume ventilation may be detrimental when ventilating acute lung injury (ALI) and ARDS patients. Volume delivered can result in volutauma, patient-ventilator dissynchrony and ventilator induced lung injury (discussed in later chapters) (Fig 8.5). ALI and ARDS posed a major problem for ventilation. In early years the mortality rate was very high. Figure 8.6 shows the definitions and criteria established at the European-American Consensus Conference differentiating ALI and ARDS.

Potential Hazards of Volume Ventilation

- In the presence of increased R_{aw} or decreased Lung Compliance the airway pressure rises and may promote Barotrauma

- Potential for local Alveolar Over-distention that may result in Volutrauma

- May promote patient-ventilator dyssynchrony and increased WOB

- Higher risk of Ventilator-induced Lung Injury

Fig 8.5

American - European Consensus Conference Criteria For ALI And ARDS

Clinical Variable	Criteria for ALI	Criteria for ARDS
Onset	Acute	Acute
Hypoxemia	$PaO_2/FiO_2 \leq 300$ mmHg	$PaO_2/FiO_2 \leq 200$ mmHg
Chest Radiograph	Bilateral infiltrates consistent with pulmonary edema	Bilateral infiltrates consistent with pulmonary edema
Noncardiac cause	No clinical evidence of left atrial hypertension or, if measured, pulmonary artery occlusion pressure ≤ 18 mmHg	No clinical evidence of left atrial hypertension or, if measured, pulmonary artery occlusion pressure ≤ 18 mmHg

Fig 8.6

Dilemma in Ventilating ALI and ARDS patients with Volume Ventilation

To appreciate the dilemma in ventilating these patients it must be recognized that even in severe cases of ALI and ARDS approximately 1/3 lung is normal, whereas, other parts of the lung are either collapsed or partially collapsed (Fig 8.7).

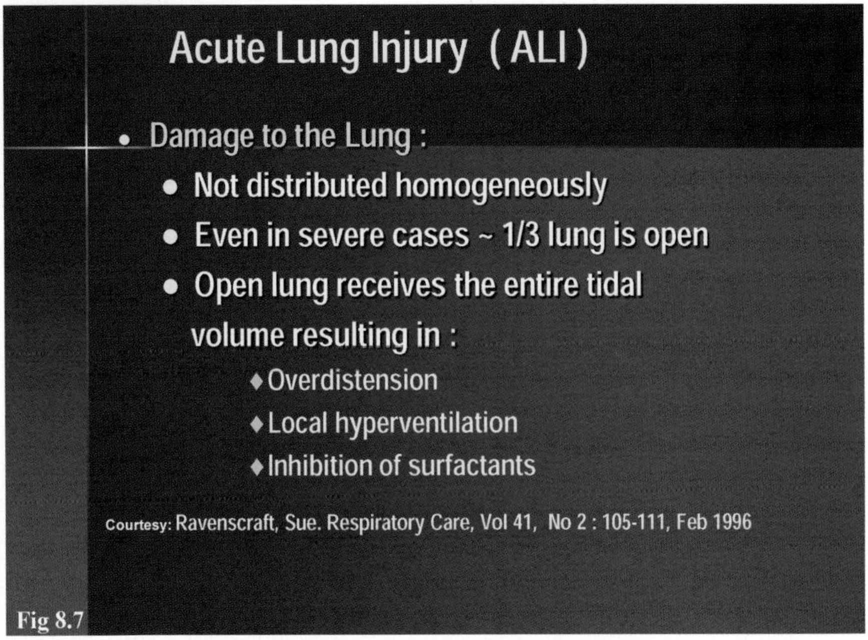

Acute Lung Injury (ALI)
• Damage to the Lung :
• Not distributed homogeneously
• Even in severe cases ~ 1/3 lung is open
• Open lung receives the entire tidal volume resulting in :
♦ Overdistension
♦ Local hyperventilation
♦ Inhibition of surfactants
Courtesy: Ravenscraft, Sue. Respiratory Care, Vol 41, No 2 : 105-111, Feb 1996

Fig 8.7

This non-homogeneity is the major problem in ventilating ALI and ARDS patients. During volume breath the entire tidal volume finds the path of least resistance and enters the normal lung units. Thus the normal lung over-distends and shearing forces damage the normal parts of the lung (Figs 8.8 and 8.9).

ALI and ARDS
Non-Homogeneous Lung Units
Collapsed
Recruitable
Normal
Lung Units

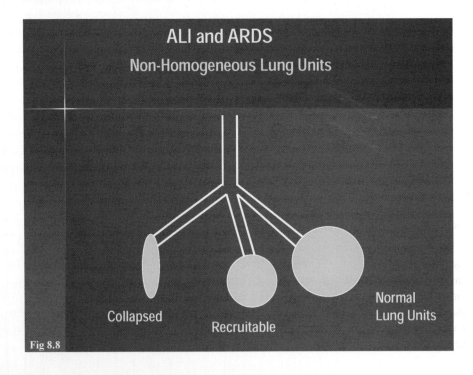

Fig 8.8

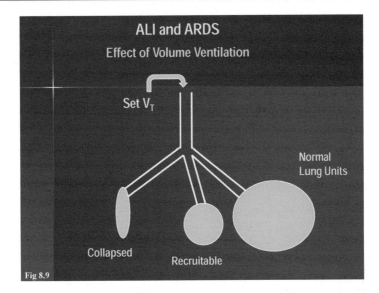
Fig 8.9

On a pressure-volume loop a clinician can observe the over-distension tracing indicating a "beak-like" appearance associated with increase in pressure without any appreciable volume delivery (Fig 8.10).

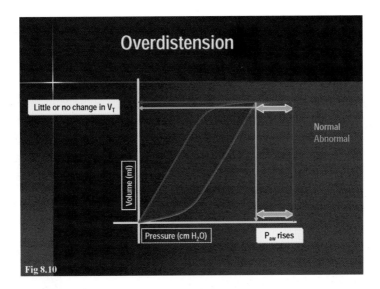
Fig 8.10

Management of ARDS will be discussed in a separate chapter later in this book.

Pressure Ventilation

To protect healthy lung in ARDS it was recognized that Pressure ventilation may be a viable option since delivering pressure to the non-homogeneous lung does not over-distend it. When fixed amount of pressure is delivered to non-homogeneous lung the healthy lung receives volume until the pressure in the lungs and in the airways is equal, no more gas is delivered further in the healthy lung units preventing over-distension. Pressure ventilation is time cycled, the remaining time is used to inflate re-cruitable alveoli (Fig 8.11).

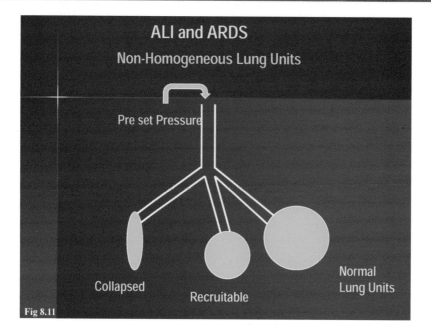
Fig 8.11

There are other advantages of pressure ventilation. Pressure is the driving force and flow is not preset. The patient is not limited to receive clinician-set flow. Potential flow dissynchrony is avoided. Pressure is kept at a safer level <30 cm H_2O. The clinician has the flexibility to manipulate inspiratory time to recruit partially collapsed alveoli (discussed later as Inverse Ratio Ventilation)

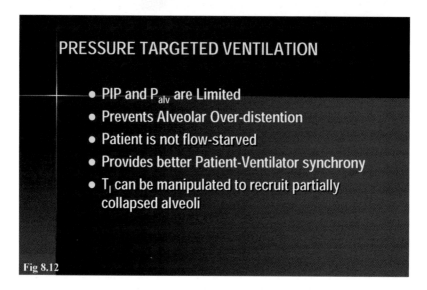
Fig 8.12

(Fig 8.12). Just like Volume ventilation, Pressure ventilation also has drawbacks. Although Pressure and Inspiratory time are constant (Pressure Limited and Time cycled), delivered tidal volume is variable. In face of increased R_{aw} and decreased C_L tidal volume decreases. A care should be taken to monitor exhaled tidal volume and a Low Volume Alarm should be set appropriately (Fig 8.13).

Volume vs. Pressure Ventilation

Limitation of Pressure Control Ventilation

- Pressure and Inspiratory Time are constant
- Flow and Tidal Volume are not guaranteed
- Increased R_{aw} and Decreased C_L decrease delivered Tidal Volume and may increase $PaCO_2$
- Low Volume alarm should be properly set

Fig 8.13

The delivered tidal volume is directly proportional to lung compliance as exhibited in Fig 8.14. As compliance increases so does delivered tidal volume and decreasing compliance results in delivering lesser tidal volume at fixed airway opening pressure.

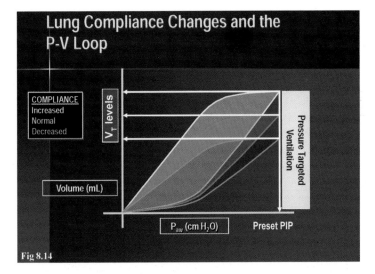

Fig 8.14

Types of Pressure Ventilation

Technically, pressure ventilation implies delivery of pressure. There are three types of Pressure Ventilation utilized in mechanical ventilation. In late 1960 till mid 1980s, pressure ventilation was used to deliver short term hyperinflation therapy called intermittent positive pressure breathing or IPPB. It also served to deliver bronchodilators to the lungs. IPPB lost it's popularity when other less labor intensive ways to deliver medication to the lung were introduced. The ventilators that delivered IPPB were Pressure Cycled units. When the set pressure reached, inspiration was terminated. In Pressure Support Ventilation inspiration is terminated when the flow reaches system-specific flow level or Flow Cycled, and the Pressure Control Ventilation is designed to be

Time cycled where inspiration is terminated when preset inspiratory time elapses. Figure 8.15 identifies the three types of Pressure Ventilation with Pressure/Time and Flow/Time scalars for each.

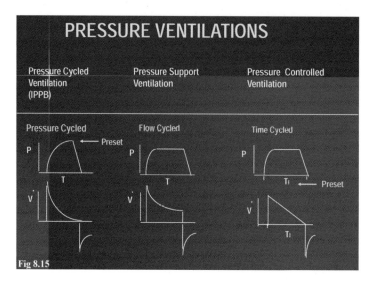

Fig 8.15

Flow-Time Scalar in Pressure Ventilation

In pressure ventilation as the pressure is kept constant the flow is always descending. At the end of inspiration the flow may return to the baseline depending on the set inspiratory time and lung characteristics (R_{aw} and C_L). Figure 8.16 represents a typical flow-time scalar for a pressure control breath. The Pressure and Inspiratory Time are preset by the clinician. Observe, in this case, the flow returns to the baseline at the same time as inspiratory time elapses and the exhalation valve opens. However, if the clinician sets long inspiratory time the flow may decrease all the way to the baseline before the inspiratory time has completed. This implies that the flow has decreased to zero and yet, the exhalation valve has not opened. This causes a period of NO FLOW situation as shown in Fig 8.17 and

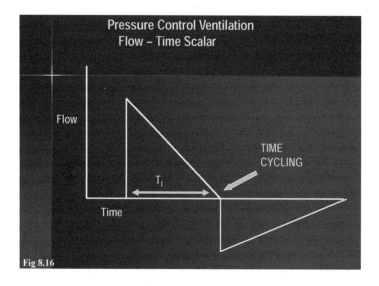

Fig 8.16

Volume vs. Pressure Ventilation

the flow stays at the baseline until the exhalation valve opens. Similar situation occurs when the lung compliance is decreased. Opposite also can occur. If the set T_I is shorter than the time required for the flow to descend to the baseline, the pattern looks like in Fig 8.18 where inspiration is terminated before the flow returns to the baseline. This pattern is also observed in Pressure Support Ventilation (Flow Cycling) (Fig 8.18).

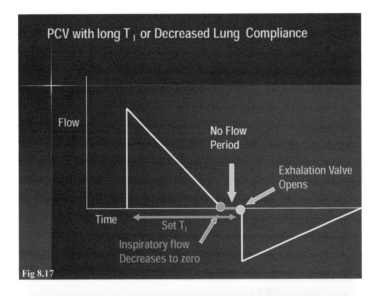

Fig 8.17

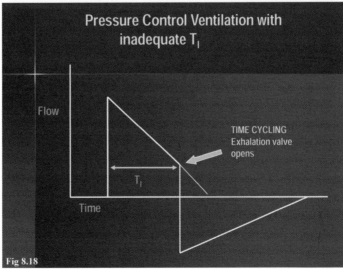

Fig 8.18

Figure 8.19 demonstrates the effect on flow patterns associated with varying clinical conditions during pressure control ventilation. Recognize that the exhalation valve opens at point "B". The yellow descending line descends to the baseline at the normal T_I, the red line depicts effect of severe decrease in compliance as it descends to the baseline much faster (Point "A") and in case of increased dynamic compliance the inspiration is terminated before the flow returns to the baseline (Point "C").

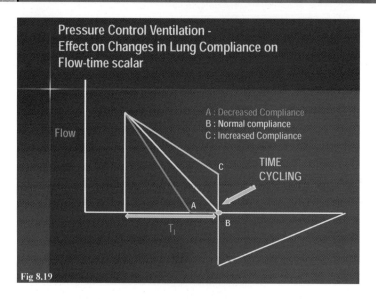

Fig 8.19

Key aspects of Pressure Control Ventilation are listed in Fig 8.20.

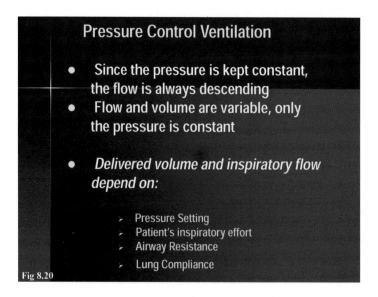

Fig 8.20

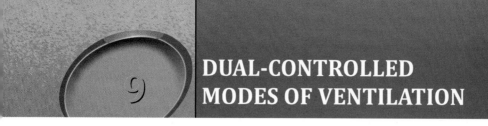

DUAL-CONTROLLED MODES OF VENTILATION

The mortality in ARDS patients was alarming and researchers were engaged in collecting data to determine the best way to open the collapsed and recruitable alveoli. Various modes were tried. In 2000, New England Journal of Medicine published their findings on the multicenter study on using 6 ml/kg vs. 12 ml/kg tidal volumes (Fig 9.1). The study showed that high tidal volumes were detrimental to patients in ALI and ARDS. Subsequent articles related to high tidal volumes, resulting in volutrauma, overdistension, upper inflection point etc. were published in literature. ARDS Net's findings were the best tool for the clinicians at the bedside.

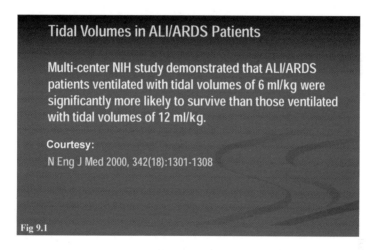

Fig 9.1

Lower tidal volumes reduced mortality in ALI/ARDS patients; however, this promotes decreased minute ventilation and could affect CO_2 removal. To compensate for low minute ventilation, the

ARDSnet Findings

- Lower Tidal Volumes
- Use of rapid rates avoiding auto-PEEP (< 35/min)
- P_{PLAT} < 30 cm H_2O reduces mortality
- Lower P_{PLAT} showed better outcome

ARDSnet: 6ml/kg reduces mortality vs. 12 ml/kg

Fig 9.2

respiratory rate can be increased but not too high to result in Auto-PEEP. Ventilating stiff lung as in ALI/ARDS requires higher pressure. ARDS net determined that a plateau pressure of <30 cm H_2O was the safe level and lower the plateau pressure better the outcome (Fig 9.2).

As seen in previous chapters, volume ventilation in ALI/ARDS patients leads to overdistension and volutrauma (Fig 8.8). Whereas, pressure ventilation delivers variable volumes and may not be sufficient to open the lungs at pressures < 30 cm H_2O. Recognizing that high Volumes and high Pressures cause lung injury and dissynchrony, a safer way to ventilate using a combined volume and pressure modes (Dual-Controlled Mode) were developed (Fig 9.3).

Dual-Controlled Mode

- Exploits beneficial effects of both Pressure and Volume Ventilation
- Operates with Pressure Support or Pressure Control modes to attain and maintain clinician-set tidal volume
- Improves Patient-ventilator Synchrony
- Prevents ventilator induced lung injury

Fig 9.3

Dual-controlled modes combine beneficial features of pressure and volume ventilation to provide desired V_T at minimal pressure. These modes can be triggered by patient (Volume Support) or time triggered (PRVC), the flow delivered is variable and cycling occurs as time cycled (e.g. Pressure Control breaths in PRVC) or flow cycled (e.g. PSV breaths in Volume Support). Currently most ventilators

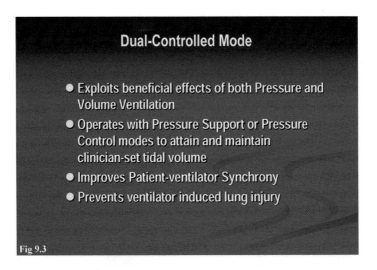

Combined Pressure and Volume Ventilation

- Pressure Augmentation
- Volume Assured Pressure Support (VAPS)
- Volume Support
- Pressure-Regulated Volume Control
- Auto Mode
- VC+
- Auto Flow
- Adaptive Support Ventilation

Fig 9.4

Dual-Controlled Modes of Ventilation

have incorporated some variation of dual modes. Figure 9.4 lists some of the dual modes available on various mechanical ventilators.

In later chapters on closed-loop ventilation these modes will be discussed in more details.

Dual-controlled breaths are delivered in two ways, as "Within a Breath" where the ventilator switches from Pressure Ventilation to Volume Ventilation to fine tune the volume delivery to preset level (VAPS and P_{aug}) (Fig 9.5) or "Breath-to-Breath" where the ventilator delivers either Pressure Support or Pressure Control ventilation and adjusts pressure level until the clinician-set tidal volume is attained (VS, PRVC, VC+, Auto Flow). Pressure Augmentation (P_{aug}) and volume assured pressure support (VAPS) provide "Within-a-Breath" version of Dual-controlled Ventilation (Fig 9.6).

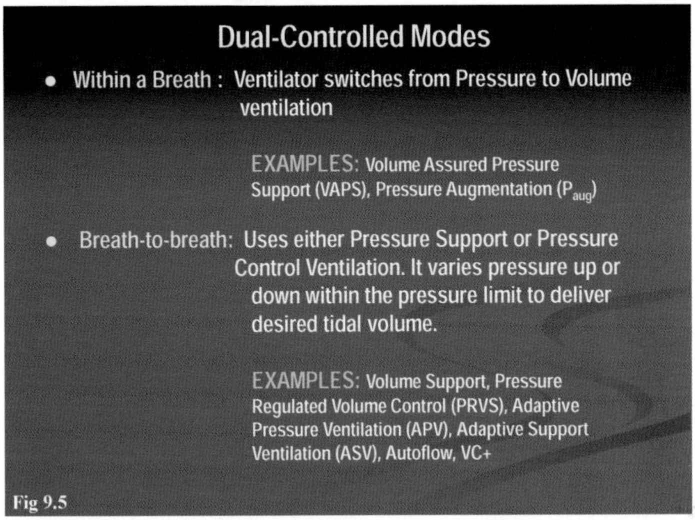

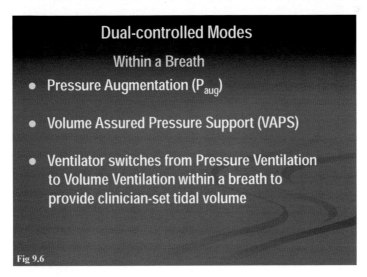

Fig 9.5

Fig 9.6

Dual Control "Within-a-Breath"

In P_{aug} and VAPS, the ventilator delivers a PSV or PCV breath triggered by the patient or time, rapidly attains the set pressure level with descending flow and monitors delivered volume. If the volume delivered is same as set volume, the ventilator continues ventilation in Pressure Support mode. If the delivered volume is less than the clinician-set tidal volume, the ventilator switches from pressure ventilation to volume ventilation within the breath. As shown in Fig 9.7, the switch in modes provides constant flow (VCV) as against decelerating flow in PCV resulting in increased volume delivery during this phase. This allows the ventilator to fine tune potential deficit in delivered volume.

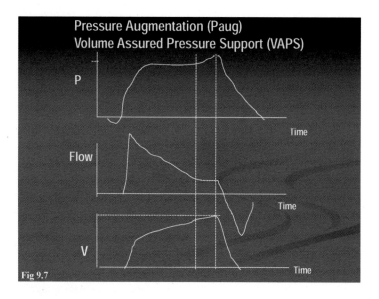

Fig 9.7

Dual Control "Breath-to-Breath" (Fig 9.8)

This version of dual-controlled ventilation is the most common since it is incorporated in most currently used ventilators. Volume support (VS) mode delivers Pressure support breaths to achieve clinician-set tidal volume. When activated, it delivers a trial breath; measures delivered tidal volume and calculates compliance.

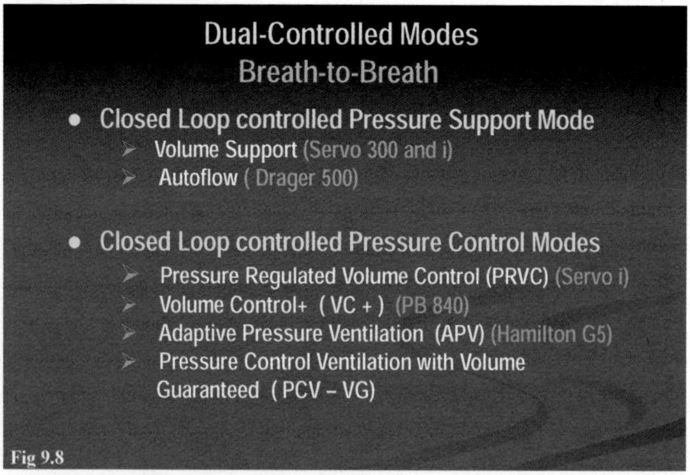

Dual-Controlled Modes
Breath-to-Breath

- **Closed Loop controlled Pressure Support Mode**
  - Volume Support (Servo 300 and i)
  - Autoflow (Drager 500)

- **Closed Loop controlled Pressure Control Modes**
  - Pressure Regulated Volume Control (PRVC) (Servo i)
  - Volume Control+ (VC +) (PB 840)
  - Adaptive Pressure Ventilation (APV) (Hamilton G5)
  - Pressure Control Ventilation with Volume Guaranteed (PCV – VG)

Fig 9.8

Dual-Controlled Modes of Ventilation

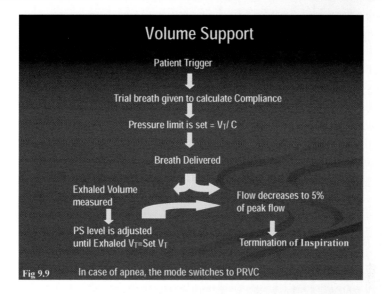

Fig 9.9   In case of apnea, the mode switches to PRVC

The pressure is increased step-wise over several breaths until the desired tidal volume is attained. The clinician sets desired V_T and upper pressure limit (Fig 9.9). Since it is purely a spontaneous breath, sensitivity should be at normal level (–1 to –2 cm H_2O). In some cases the desired volume is not achieved. The decelerating flow can decrease upto 5% of the peak flow and then the inspiration is terminated. The clinician should assess the patient and make further decision about the mode of ventilation. In case the patient becomes apneic the ventilator switches to PRVC.

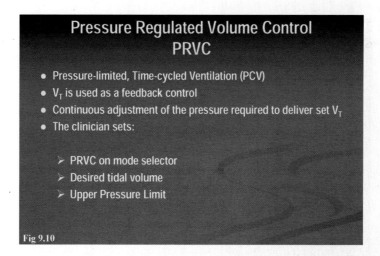

Fig 9.10

PRVC is a pressure control - pressure limited, time cycled mode. It is incorporated on most ventilators with different names (Fig 9.8). Basically, it functions just like Volume Support mode (pressure limited, flow cycled) except PRVC which is a control mode (Pressure limited, time cycled) with volume target. The clinician simply sets the mode; desired V_T and upper pressure limit (Fig 9.10). Upon initiation of PRVC it gives a Volume Control breath and measures the plateau pressure. Using the plateau pressure static compliance is calculated. The pressure is gradually increased for

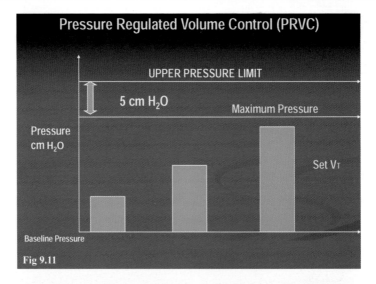

Fig 9.11

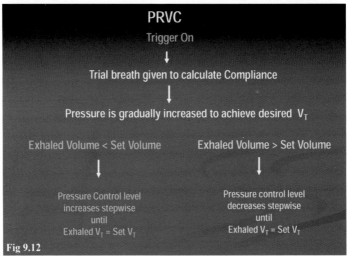

Fig 9.12

several breaths (Fig 9.11) until it reaches the set tidal volume. The pressure adjusts every time the compliance increases or decreases to deliver set volume (Fig 9.12).

A new control, automode, was introduced on Servo I ventilator. Automode allows the ventilator to switch from control mode to support mode and vice versa. Thus the patient can be switched, using closed-loop, from mandatory breathing to spontaneous breathing and vice versa. Automode couples pressure control with pressure support mode, volume control with volume support mode and PRVC with volume support mode. In PRVC the every breath is a control breath until the patient takes two consecutive spontaneous breaths at each time, if the Automode is activated, the ventilator switches to the spontaneous Volume Support mode. In both situations the ventilator adjusts the pressure up or down, to maintain the set volume. If the patient becomes apneic for 12 seconds, the Automode switches back to PRVC (Fig 9.13).

Adaptive Support Ventilation is the sophisticated version of Dual-Controlled Ventilation. The ventilator is designed to deliver precise tidal volume and respiratory frequency in varying clinical situations.

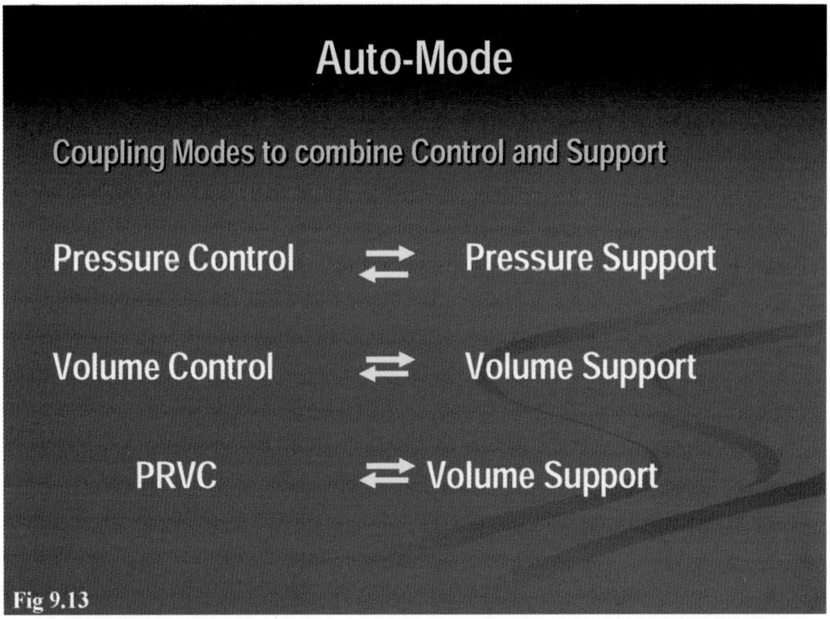

Dual-Controlled Modes of Ventilation

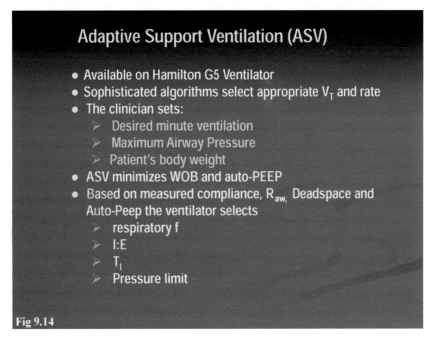

Fig 9.13

Fig 9.14

Figure 9.14 identifies the parameters that the clinician feeds in and the ventilator measures. From this data the ventilator selects specific parameters and limits to deliver required minute ventilation. ASV delivers a blend of spontaneous and mandatory breaths to maintain desired minute ventilation. If the patient improves and increases his spontaneous rate, the ventilator decreases mandatory rate. In case the patient deteriorates the ventilator increases mandatory rate. The patient is protected from apnea and Auto-PEEP (Fig 9.15).

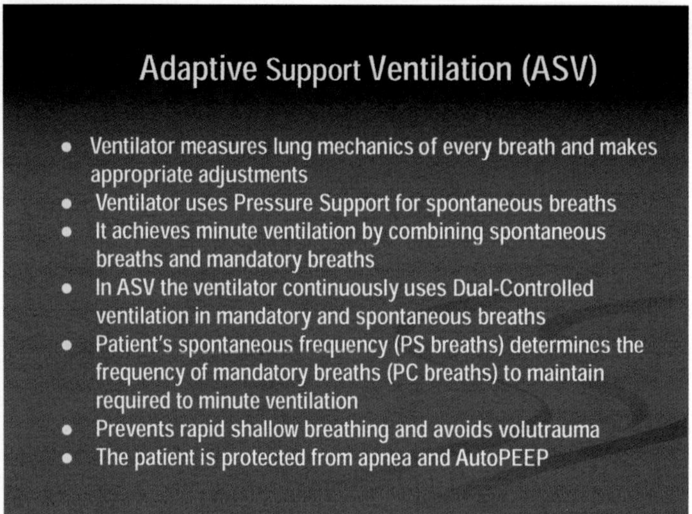

Adaptive Support Ventilation (ASV)

- Ventilator measures lung mechanics of every breath and makes appropriate adjustments
- Ventilator uses Pressure Support for spontaneous breaths
- It achieves minute ventilation by combining spontaneous breaths and mandatory breaths
- In ASV the ventilator continuously uses Dual-Controlled ventilation in mandatory and spontaneous breaths
- Patient's spontaneous frequency (PS breaths) determines the frequency of mandatory breaths (PC breaths) to maintain required to minute ventilation
- Prevents rapid shallow breathing and avoids volutrauma
- The patient is protected from apnea and AutoPEEP

Fig 9.15

In future chapters some of this material will be repeated to maintain continuity of closeloop ventilation or advanced modes of ventilation.

INITIAL SETTINGS

In earlier chapters, criteria for mechanical ventilation, initiation of ventilation, modes of ventilations and ventilator graphics are discussed. However, when the clinician is faced with initiating mechanical ventilation, it is important to go through the sequence of parameter settings before the ventilator is turned on. When a patient meets the criteria for mechanical ventilation the clinician assesses the patient for proper ventilator settings. It is imperative that the clinician identifies the underlying disorder that has caused inability to achieve effective gas exchange. Pulmonary mechanics associated with the underlying cause must be taken into consideration when setting the ventilator parameters. A patient in COPD exacerbation is not ventilated with the same parameters as a neuromuscular disease patient (Fig 10.1).

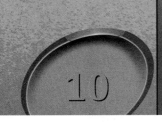

Instituting Mechanical Ventilation

Initial Considerations
- Objective evaluation of Acute Respiratory Failure (ARF)
- Underlying Disorder
- Pulmonary Status:
  - Normal Lung Mechanics
  - Obstructive Lung Disease
  - Restrictive Lung Disorder

Fig 10.1

When instituting mechanical ventilation, the first decision the clinician takes is the control variable, Volume or Pressure. It is a common practice to provide full ventilatory support using Volume A/C or Pressure A/C mode. An unstable patient is generally sedated to ensure that the patient is in synchrony with the ventilator. The backup rate on the Assist Control (A/C) mode is kept high enough to ascertain that the work of breathing is done entirely by the ventilator (Fig 10.2).

The initial parameters in Volume Ventilation depend on patient's lung characteristics, underlying pathophysiology and the type of ventilator. Most current ventilators are designed to compensate for tubing compliance or compressible volume and deliver set volume; on the other hand, ventilators that do not compensate for tubing compliance must be set to deliver higher volume to account for volume lost to the tubing compliance. In pediatric and neonatal patients requiring mechanical ventilation with small tidal volumes, compressible volume loss can have profound effect on the actual volume delivered to the patient.

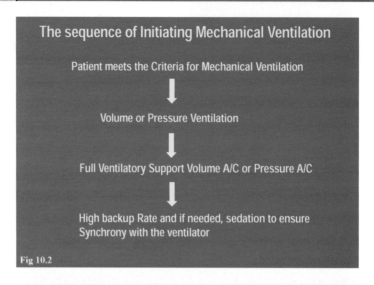

Fig 10.2

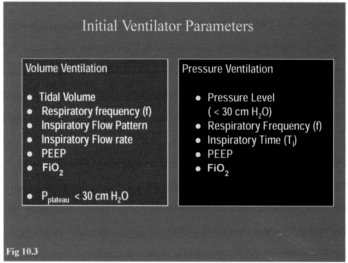

Fig 10.3

The parameters that must be set on the ventilators before it is connected to the patient are listed in (Fig 10.3).

Tidal Volume in Volume Ventilation

In volume ventilation tidal volume (V_T) is calculated on the basis of ideal body weight (IBW). Figure 10.4 shows the formulae for Ideal Body Weight calculation with typical example IBW should always be used to calculate tidal volume especially in overweight patients. The other consideration when V_T is set is patient's underlying pulmonary condition. If the pulmonary mechanics is normal such as in Drug Overdose, Organophosphate Ingestion, and Neuromuscular diseases, a tidal volume up to 6-8 ml/kg ideal body weight (IBW) at a rate of 8 to 12 breaths per minute can be set, keeping a watch on P_{Plat} not to exceed 30 cm H_2O. In patients with obstructive diseases where the lungs may be very compliant a tidal volume of 8 to 10 ml/kg at a rate of 8–12/min is used. Potential for auto-PEEP must be recognized and the rate and V_T should be adjusted to eliminate any Auto-PEEP and high pressure

Initial Settings

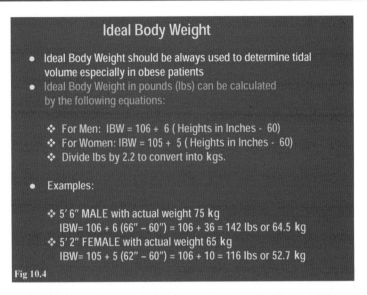

Fig 10.4

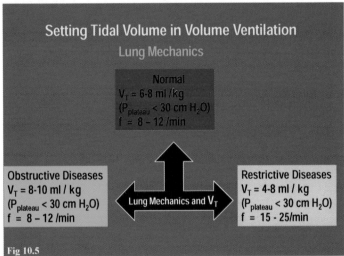

Fig 10.5

(keep it < 30 cm H_2O). More attention has been paid to restrictive disorders especially ALI/ARDS in setting low tidal volumes due to increased mortality in patients receiving high tidal volumes. In restrictive disorders recommended V_T is 5–7 ml/kg at a rate of 15–25/min to account for low tidal volumes. High respiratory rates can result in Auto-PEEP and it should be avoided (Fig 10.5).

Tidal Volume in Pressure Ventilation

There are two ways to set tidal volume in Pressure Control ventilation. Since tidal volume is not directly set during pressure ventilation, (except when Dual-Controlled mode is used) a volume breath is given with desired V_T and the plateau pressure is measured. Now, pressure can be set to the level of Plateau Pressure from volume breath at the same inspiratory time, the resulting tidal volume should be approximately the same as during volume targeted breath. The delivered volume in pressure ventilation varies with changes in lung compliance and RAW and should be frequently monitored (Fig 10.6).

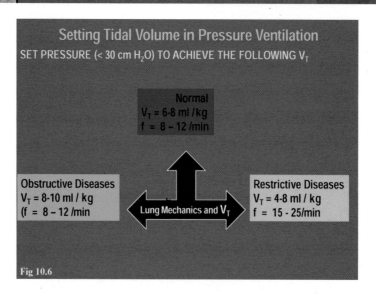

Fig 10.6

Another way is to start pressure targeted ventilation at a lower pressure (~ 15 cm H_2O) and check the delivered volume. Adjust pressure until the desired tidal volume is attained. The tidal volume range is the same as for volume ventilation, 6-8 ml/kg for normal lungs, 5-7 ml/kg in restrictive disorders and 8-10 ml/kg for obstructive patients.

Respiratory Frequency (*f*)

Respiratory rate is set to deliver sufficient minute ventilation ($V_T \times f$) to support patient's metabolic demand. High set frequency may result in auto-PEEP and excessive ventilation. The rate can be adjusted after the initial setting to titrate patient's ABGs to normal level. Figures 10.5 and 10.6 show the initial settings for respiratory rate to deliver adequate minute volume at the set tidal volume in normal, obstructive and restrictive lung mechanics.

Inspiratory Flow Pattern

In pressure ventilation the flow is always decelerating and the clinician cannot change the flow pattern.

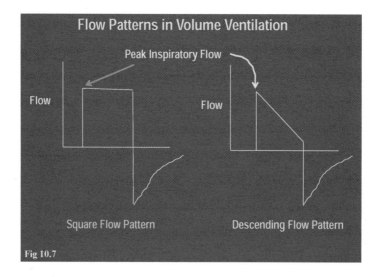

Fig 10.7

Initial Settings

However, in volume ventilation two flow patterns are available - constant or square flow and descending flow. Although descending flow pattern improves gas distribution, square flow is commonly used while initiating mechanical ventilation. Changing from square flow pattern to descending pattern does not change peak flow setting, however, Inspiratory time and I–E ratio change. The clinician should adjust the peak flow to deliver set tidal volume at an improved I–E ratio. For normal lung mechanics both flow patterns are acceptable. In restrictive disorders (ALI/ARDS) descending flow pattern maintains low peak pressure and high mean airway pressure as well as improves gas distribution. In obstructive diseases descending flow pattern is desirable for better gas distribution (Fig 10.7).

As indicated in Fig 10.8 high inspiratory flow rates shorten inspiratory time, have higher peak inspiratory pressure and the gas distribution is poor in obstructed airways. On the other hand descending flow pattern improves gas exchange at low PIP and high mean airway pressure.

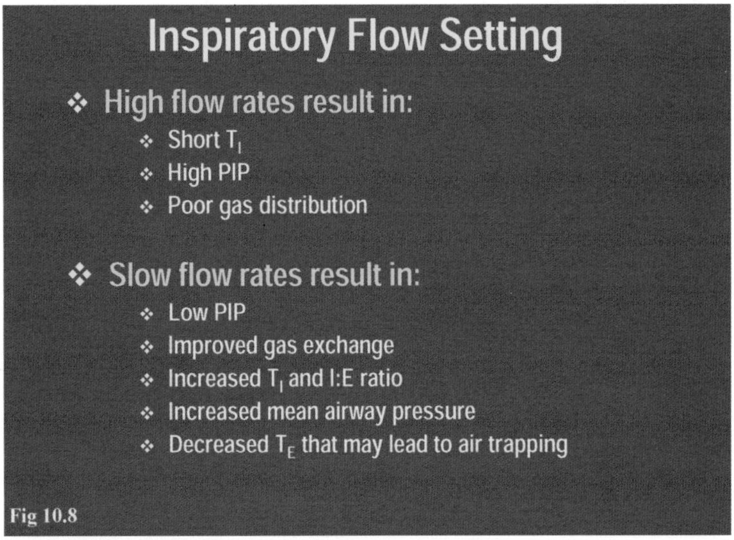

Inspiratory Flow Setting

- **High flow rates result in:**
  - Short T_I
  - High PIP
  - Poor gas distribution

- **Slow flow rates result in:**
  - Low PIP
  - Improved gas exchange
  - Increased T_I and I:E ratio
  - Increased mean airway pressure
  - Decreased T_E that may lead to air trapping

Fig 10.8

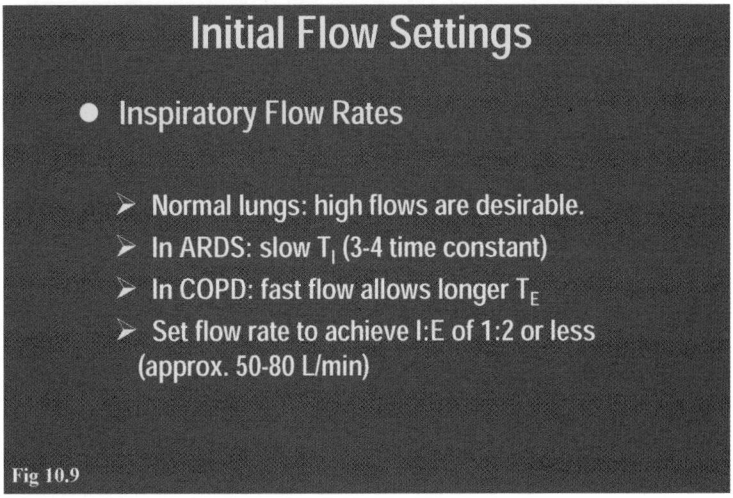

Initial Flow Settings

- **Inspiratory Flow Rates**
  - Normal lungs: high flows are desirable.
  - In ARDS: slow T_I (3-4 time constant)
  - In COPD: fast flow allows longer T_E
  - Set flow rate to achieve I:E of 1:2 or less (approx. 50-80 L/min)

Fig 10.9

It also increases inspiratory time and decreases expiratory time which can promote air trapping or auto-PEEP. In normal lungs the flow is set high (50-60 l/min), in restrictive disorders slow flows are desirable to increase inspiratory and mean airway pressure and in COPD patients high flows are used to eliminate or prevent air trapping (Fig 10.9). In Pressure Ventilation the ventilator opens a demand valve and allows the patient to take as much flow as desired, however the flow pattern is always decelerating and termination occurs when inspiratory time elapses.

PEEP and FIO_2

Generally a low level of PEEP is recommended to maintain functional residual capacity (FRC). The FiO_2 set at 1.0 (100%) to eliminate V/Q mismatch situations to prevent hypoxemic hyperventilation. Subsequently the FiO_2 is reduced to safe level using SpO_2 as a guide.

Upon initiating mechanical ventilation with appropriate settings the clinician monitors the patient's physiological parameters, and ventilator graphics to make suitable changes in ventilator settings to eventually, wean the patient off the ventilator.

Later Chapters include more detailed information.

★ ★ ★

PATIENT MONITORING AND ABNORMAL VENTILATOR WAVEFORMS

Once the patient is connected to mechanical ventilator the clinician records initial ventilator parameters. The first assessment of the patient after connecting to the mechanical ventilator is very thorough and crucial. It gives a baseline record to compare with similar assessments later during ICU stay.

Initial Assessments for the "Ventilator Records Document"

Figure 11.1 identifies the three major areas of parameter monitoring, typically done on all mechanically ventilated patients. The parameters, Mode of Ventilation, Tidal Volume, Respiratory frequency, Minute Volume, PIP, P_{plat}, FiO_2, PEEP/CPAP and alarm settings, must be recorded on a "Ventilator

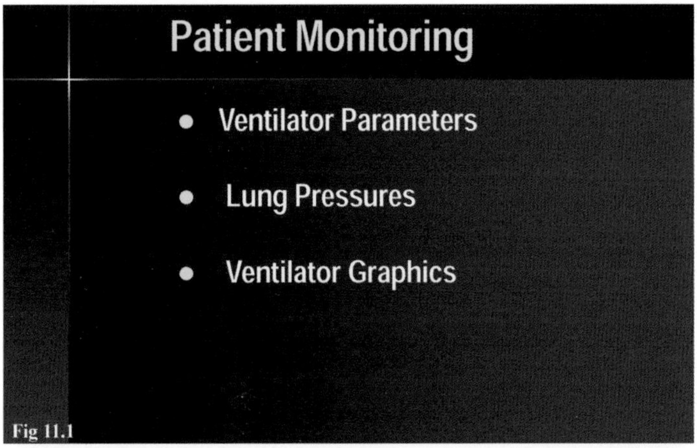

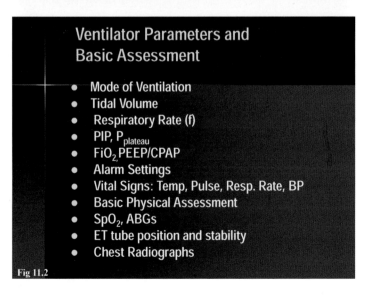

Fig 11.1

Fig 11.2

Record Sheet" designed by the ICU clinicians. While recording the ventilator parameters, the clinicians should also record the basic patient evaluation findings such as vital Signs, initial chest physical examination including inspection of chest wall expansion, absence of uneven expansion, auscultation, SpO_2 and ABG and if needed a chest radiogram. It is imperative that the clinician inspects the ET tube position and stability (Fig 11.2).

Since Volume Ventilation is used most often, especially in short term mechanical support as well as in other situations except ALI/ARDS, it is vital that the clinicians understand all aspects of

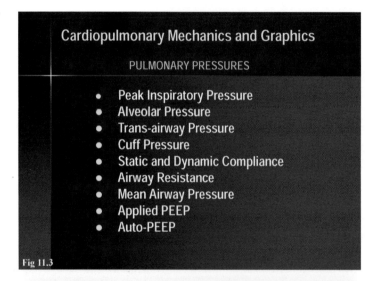

Fig 11.3

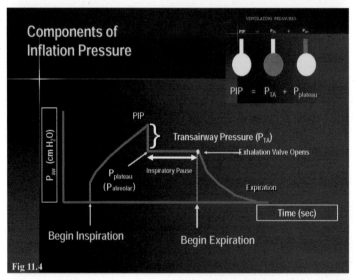

Fig 11.4

associated pressures and significance of changes in these pressures. Figure 11.3 identifies these pressures. The waveform of inflation pressure (Fig 11.4) traced when inspiratory pause control is activated, identifying PIP, P_{plat} and transairway pressure (P_{TA}), was discussed previously (Chapter 5).

Peak Inspiratory Pressure and Alarms

PIP is the total pressure measured by the ventilator and incorporates resistive and elastic pressures (Fig 11.5). PIP is always recorded as a yardstick to compare later during management of the ventilated patient. It gives a quick view of dynamic compliance. It should be noted that PIP includes P_{TA} and P_{alv}. The High Pressure Alarm is set at a 5-10 cm H_2O above the PIP level. During mechanical ventilation when the high pressure alarm is activated, an audio sound and a visual display on the ventilator screen, the clinician should quickly identify the cause of the increased PIP.

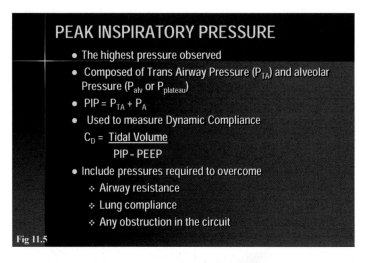

Fig 11.5

Generally, increased airway secretions, bronchospasm, kinking of the ET tube or any obstruction in the inspiratory limb results in high pressure and alarm sounds (Fig 11.6). It is important to address the situation immediately to prevent barotrauma. In case the clinician cannot identify the underlying cause, the patient should be disconnected and hand ventilated with a resuscitation bag until the reason for high pressure is ascertained. Setting the Low Pressure Alarm is equally

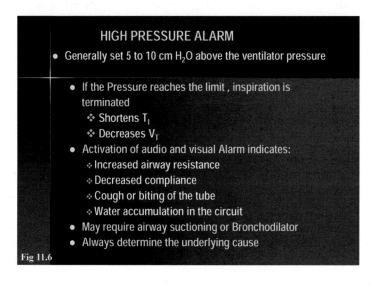

Fig 11.6

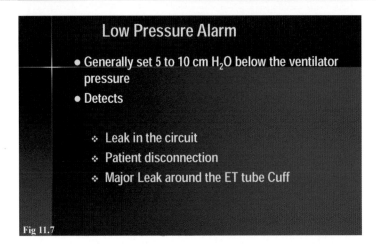
Fig 11.7

important to detect disconnection, leaks in the system or occasionally, leak around the ET tube cuff (Fig 11.7).

Plateau Pressure (P_{plat})

During volume breath when the Inflation Hold or Inspiratory Pause is activated, at the end of inspiration, inspiratory flow stops and the ventilator keeps the exhalation valve closed for the duration of the pause time set by the clinician. Plateau pressure should be measured during each ventilator check. It is the pressure generated by the recoil of the lung in the closed system.

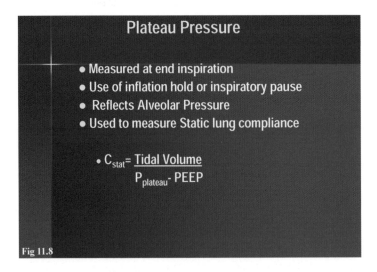
Fig 11.8

Plateau Pressure is generally considered as equivalent to Alveolar Pressure (P_{Alv}). It gives the direct measure of Static Lung Compliance. Increase in Plateau pressure is indicative of decreased lung compliance (Fig 11.8).

Transairway Pressure (P_{TA})

Frictional resistance to gas flow during its transit through the airways results in transairway pressure. This pressure exists only in the airways during gas flow. In absence of gas flow there is no PTA.

When gas flows from the mouth to alveoli, the pressure at the mouth cascades down the airways influenced by airway caliber and gas flow.

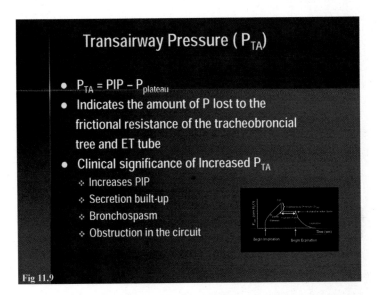

Transairway Pressure (P_{TA})
• P_{TA} = PIP – $P_{plateau}$
• Indicates the amount of P lost to the frictional resistance of the tracheobroncial tree and ET tube
• Clinical significance of Increased P_{TA}
❖ Increases PIP
❖ Secretion built-up
❖ Bronchospasm
❖ Obstruction in the circuit
Time (sec)
Begin Inspiration
Begin Expiration

Fig 11.9

At the terminal bronchioles the remaining pressure is delivered to the alveoli (to deliver Tidal volume). Changes in airway caliber secondary to increased secretions, bronchospasm and any obstruction in the circuit increases P_{TA} and thus PIP. It is vital that the patient should be protected from high airway pressures by setting the high pressure alarm (Fig 11.9).

Dynamic and Static Lung Compliance

Compliance is defined as ease of distensibility and in pulmonary medicine it is simply measured as volume delivered per unit pressure or ∇V/∇P. In Mechanical ventilation ∇V is the tidal volume and ∇P is either PIP or P_{plat}. Dynamic compliance, as the term reflects, includes pressure generated by gas flow.

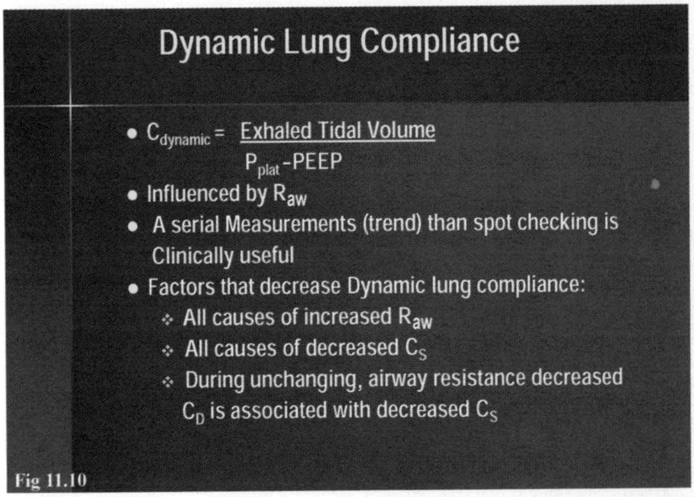

Dynamic Lung Compliance
• $C_{dynamic}$ = Exhaled Tidal Volume / P_{plat}-PEEP
• Influenced by R_{aw}
• A serial Measurements (trend) than spot checking is Clinically useful
• Factors that decrease Dynamic lung compliance:
❖ All causes of increased R_{aw}
❖ All causes of decreased C_S
❖ During unchanging, airway resistance decreased C_D is associated with decreased C_S

Fig 11.10

It also includes pressure resulting from volume delivery against recoiling force of the alveoli. Dynamic compliance is calculated as:

$$C_D = \frac{\text{Exhaled Tidal Volume}}{\text{PIP} - \text{PEEP}}$$

Clinically dynamic compliance reflects Static Compliance provided RAW is constant (Fig 11.10). Static Compliance is the amount of volume delivered to alveoli per unit of alveolar pressure.

$$C_S = \frac{\text{Exhaled Tidal Volume}}{P_{Plat} - \text{PEEP}}$$

PEEP being a constant pressure applied during inspiration and expiration is subtracted from PIP and Plateau pressures. A spontaneously breathing individual has a Static Compliance of ~ 100 mL/cm H$_2$O. Compliance value of 50–60 ml/cm H$_2$O is considered as normal for intubated patients. Thus, when a patient on mechanical ventilation with severe decrease in compliance (20-25 mL/cm H$_2$O)

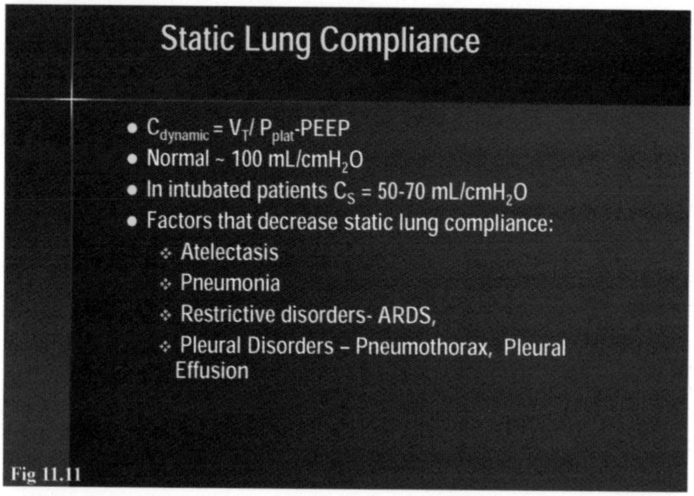

Static Lung Compliance

- $C_{dynamic} = V_T / P_{plat} - PEEP$
- Normal ~ 100 mL/cmH$_2$O
- In intubated patients C_S = 50-70 mL/cmH$_2$O
- Factors that decrease static lung compliance:
  - Atelectasis
  - Pneumonia
  - Restrictive disorders- ARDS,
  - Pleural Disorders – Pneumothorax, Pleural Effusion

Fig 11.11

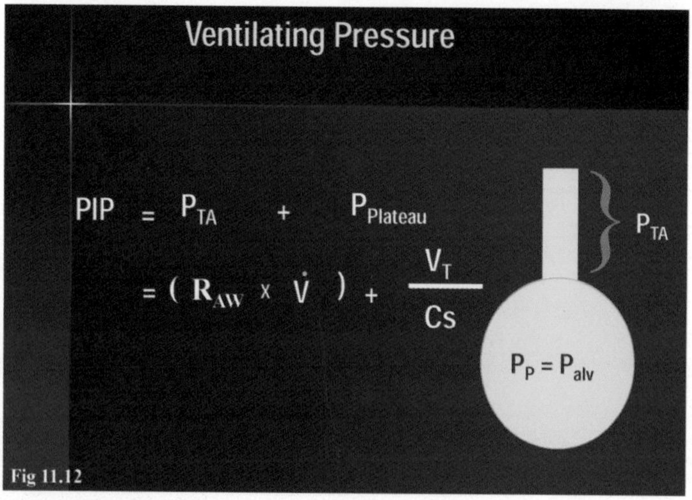

Ventilating Pressure

$$PIP = P_{TA} + P_{Plateau}$$
$$= (R_{AW} \times \dot{V}) + \frac{V_T}{C_S}$$

$P_P = P_{alv}$

Fig 11.12

improves to a compliance of 50 mL/cm H_2O, weaning should be strongly considered. All restrictive disorders have low lung compliance. Incidentally, Emphysema is the only disease where Static Lung Compliance is increased due to loss of recoiling force (Fig 11.11).

Interrelationship Between PIP, P_{TA}, P_{plat} and Lung Compliances

The total ventilating pressure during a mechanical breath depends on transairway pressure and alveolar pressure. P_{TA} results from airway resistance and the gas flow, whereas, Alveolar pressure is dependent on tidal volume and lung compliance (Fig 11.12). Increased R_{aw} and gas flow result in increased P_{TA} (Fig 11.13).

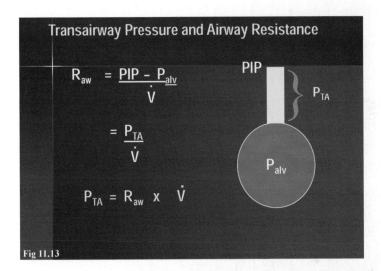

Fig 11.13

The relationship between Tidal Volume, Static Compliance and Plateau Pressure (Alveolar Pressure) is demonstrated in Fig 11.14. During mechanical ventilation situations occur where the R_{aw} increases suddenly as a consequence of Mucus Plug in large bronchi or severe asthmatic episode.

The PIP increases (Fig 11.15). Notice that there is no change in plateau pressure indicating that the lung compliance is not affected, only the airways are experiencing partial occlusion (increased P_{TA} and PIP).

The PIP can also increase when the lung compliance decreases. Figure 11.16 demon-strates the effect of decreased lung compliance (increased P_{plat} and PIP). P_{TA} is unchanged indicating that the problem originated in the lungs and did not affect airways.

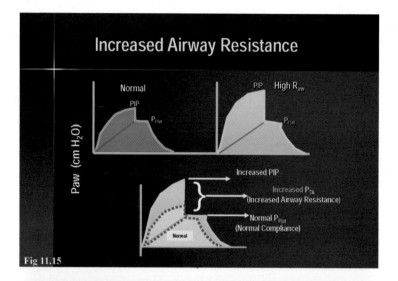

Fig 11.15

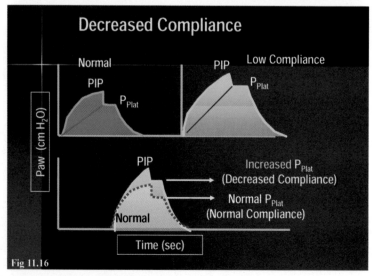

Fig 11.16

Cuff Pressure

During initial evaluation the clinician is expected to check the position and security of the ET tube as well as the cuff pressure. It is argued by some clinicians that high cuff pressures result in damage to tracheal wall due to tracheal necrosis, mucosal edema and ischemia.

The cuff pressure is recommended not to exceed 25 mm Hg. Figure 11.17 shows the effect of increased cuff pressures on the blood flow and lymphatic flow to tracheal mucosa. Cuff pressure-measuring devices, cuffalators, also allow the clinician to add or remove air from the cuff. To protect the airways from high cuff pressures, the Minimal Leak Techniques is recommended.

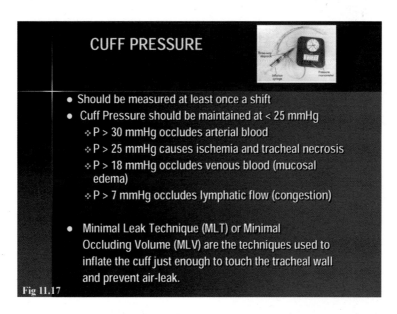

Fig 11.17

Mean Airway Pressure

Finally, it is desirable to monitor Mean Airway Pressure which the clinicians manipulates to open recruitable lung in ALI and ARDS. Fig 11.18 shows the basic formula for estimating Mean Airway Pressure. Since the pressure is applied only during inspiratory phase the first equation indicates Mean airway pressure = ½ PIP × T_I / TCT, where, T_I is the inspiratory time and TCT is the total cycle time. If PEEP is added, then the equation incorporates PEEP recognizing that it is applied throughout

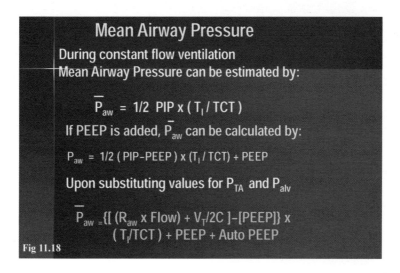

Fig 11.18

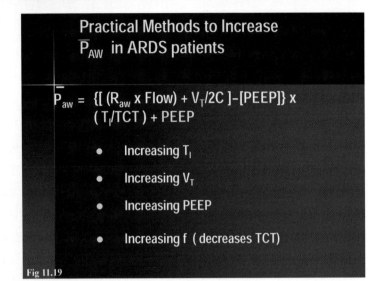

Fig 11.19

the respiratory cycle, PEEP is subtracted from PIP and added at the end of the equation. Getting a little more academic the equation expands to the final version where values for P_{TA} and P_{Alv}, the two components of PIP, are substituted. This equation provides all the factors that can be manipulated by the clinician to increase or decrease Mean Airway Pressure. Figure 11.19 identifies parameters, V_T, T_I, TCT and PEEP that are readily available for changing mean airway pressure whereas R_{aw} and C are lung characteristics and cannot be manipulated.

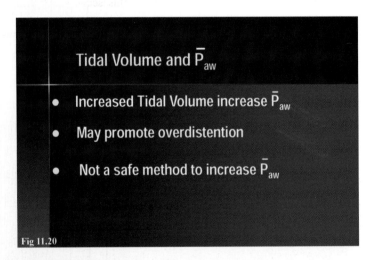

Fig 11.20

In ALI/ARDS patients increasing Mean Airway Pressure by increasing tidal volume may be detrimental for the patient as it can promote overdistention and volutrauma (Fig 11.20). However, in clinical practice, mean airway pressure is increased by manipulating T_I (inverse ratio ventilation- IRV) and by decreasing total cycle time (TCT) via increased frequency. Application of PEEP has been a cornerstone in managing ALI/ARDS patients. PEEP, not only increases Mean Airway Pressure but it also prevents decruitment. Increased Mean Airway pressure increases alveolar

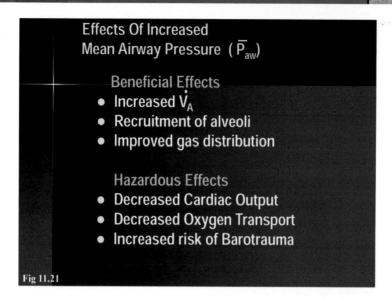

Fig 11.21

ventilation by opening recruitable alveoli and improves gas exchange (Fig 11.21). It must be recognized that in lungs that are not stiff, increased Mean Airway Pressure may decrease cardiac output and can also promote Barotrauma.

Commonly Encountered Abnormal Ventilator Waveforms

Ventilator waveforms have opened the door for evaluating clinical situations by observing changes in ventilator graphics. Nuances in abnormal waveforms are published in literatures identifying waveforms indicating different types of dissynchrony. This section will identify only three commonly observed abnormal waveforms–Auto-PEEP, Air Leak and Inadequate Inspiratory Flow (Fig 11.22). These abnormalities are very common in most ICUs and can be fixed easily. Identification of Auto-PEEP, small leak and especially inadequate inspiratory flow is missed in most cases. Ventilator waveforms are the best tool to verify these correctable situations.

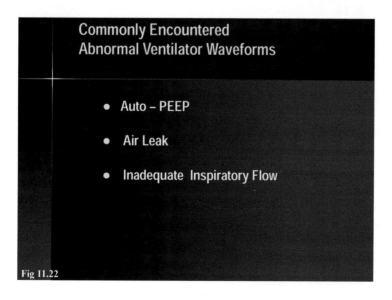

Fig 11.22

Auto-PEEP or Air Trapping

PEEP set on the ventilator by the clinician is termed as Extrinsic PEEP. Auto-PEEP is referred to as Intrinsic PEEP, since it occurs from altered intrinsic function of the lung leading to inadequate expiratory time. Technically, at end exhalation the pressure in the lungs should be at atmospheric. In situations such as premature bronchiolar collapse (COPD), high minute ventilation and expiratory flow limitation due to increased airway resistance (Asthma) or decreased recoiling force (Emphysema),

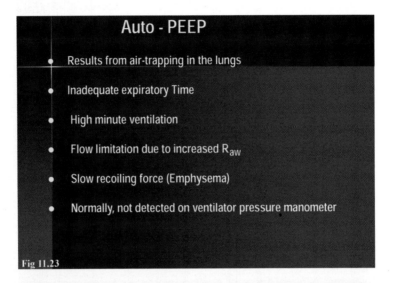
Fig 11.23

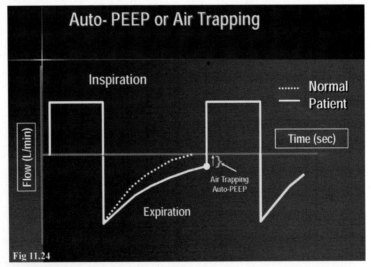
Fig 11.24

the lung pressure does not return to the baseline (atmospheric). The pressure remaining in the lung is called Auto-PEEP. Unfortunately, in normal circumstances, Auto-PEEP is not indicated on ventilator pressure manometer (Fig 11.23). Current ventilators are able to close inspiratory and expiratory ports and not only identify presence of auto-PEEP but also quantify the magnitude of Auto-PEEP.

Patient Monitoring

Ventilator graphics provide an avenue to detect Auto-PEEP. Figure 11.24 shows that the expiratory flow for the ventilator cycle does not have adequate time to complete exhalation and the next breath is delivered before the expiratory flow returns to the baseline. The dotted line on expiratory limb represents normal expiratory time returning to the baseline. Auto-PEEP can also be detected on a Flow-Volume loop (Chapter 5). Another way to detect Auto-PEEP is to add extrinsic PEEP on the ventilator until the PIP begins to increase. The PIP does not increase until the applied PEEP has exceeded auto-PEEP level.

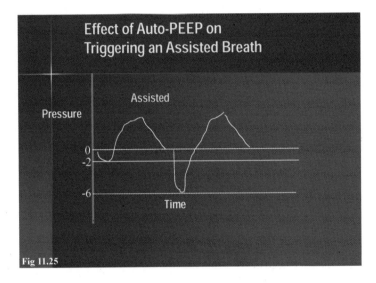
Fig 11.25

Auto-PEEP is undesirable in ventilated patients, since it can increase work of breathing, hyperinflate the lung and most importantly, auto-PEEP can interfere with triggering the ventilator breath (Fig 11.25). Missed breaths in assisted ventilation are commonly seen in patients with auto-PEEP. In presence of Auto-PEEP, the patient on A/C mode has to make an inspiratory effort greater than the auto-PEEP level, to trigger the ventilator and in many cases the patient is incapable of creating negative pressure of that magnitude, missing the breath (Fig 11.25).

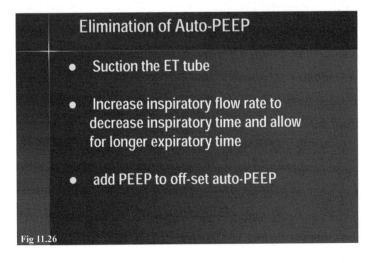
Fig 11.26

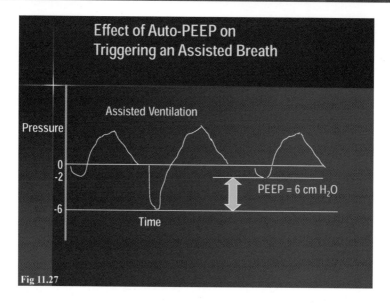

Fig 11.27

Elimination of auto-PEEP is essential in managing ventilated patients. This can be accomplished by suctioning the airways, increasing expiratory time by decreasing inspiratory time or add extrinsic PEEP (Fig 11.26). In spontaneously breathing patients such as COPD and those unable to trigger the ventilator, auto-PEEP can be reduced by applying extrinsic PEEP. Up to 80% of auto-PEEP can be nullified by extrinsic PEEP decreasing effort needed to trigger ventilator breath (Fig 11.27).

Air Leak

Volume vs. Time Scalar detects leaks in the ventilator circuit. Normally, the volume tracing descends to the baseline at end exhalation. In presence of air leak the tracing does not return to the baseline. It stagnates at the level of leaked volume and for the next breath abruptly drops to the baseline and proceeds with the next inspiratory tracing (Fig 11.28). Occasionally the patient makes an extra expiratory effort and the exhaled volume tracing goes below the baseline (Fig 11.29).

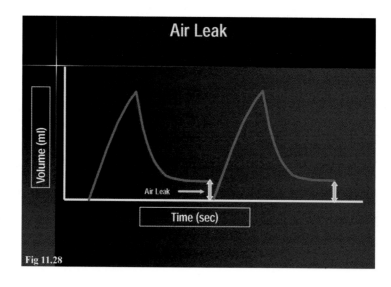

Fig 11.28

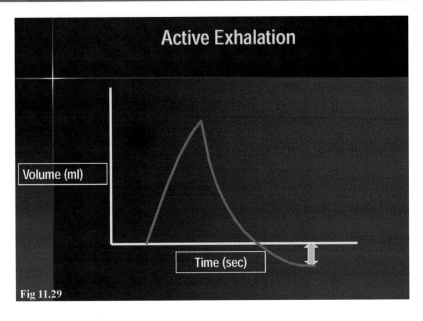

Fig 11.29

Inadequate Inspiratory Flow

It is claimed that inadequate inspiratory time is most commonly observed in ICUs. Clinicians are reluctant to give high flows to patients. A most standard setting is 30L/min flow for all patients. This can promote flow dissynchrony demonstrated on Flow/Time, Pressure/Time, and most profoundly on Pressure/Volume loop. On Flow/Time scalar an uneven pattern is observed in place of square flow (Volume Ventilation) indicating patient's effort to add more flow (Fig 11.30). On pressure/Time scalar the smooth contour of the pressure waveform shows concavity (Fig 11.31) caused by patient's inspiratory effort.

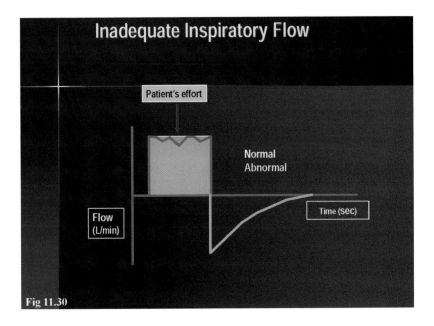

Fig 11.30

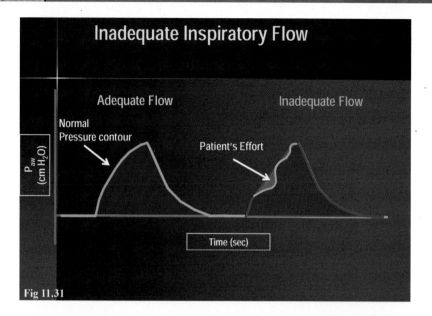

Fig 11.31

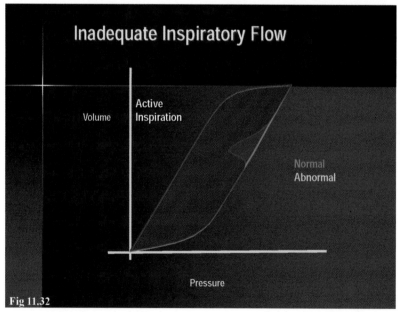

Fig 11.32

Pressure-Volume loop shows a sudden depression in the inspiratory tracing signifying patient's inspiratory activity while the ventilator breath is in progress (Fig 11.32). Upon encountering these waveforms the clinician, simply increases inspiratory flow (decreased T_I, or T_I % or manipulating I–E ratio).

In later chapters more complex ventilator graphics are discussed.

★ ★ ★

WEANING FROM MECHANICAL VENTILATOR

When the underlying disease process overwhelms the ability of the patient to support ventilatory demand by the metabolism, mechanical ventilation is instituted. Once the underlying cause has reversed, mechanical ventilation can be discontinued. Weaning is defined as gradually decreasing mechanical ventilatory support and transfer ventilation process from mechanical support to patient's spontaneous breathing apparatus. About 80% of the patients requiring temporary mechanical support do not need intricate, slow process to wean from mechanical support. They are disconnected within hours. Figure 12.1 shows the balance between the demands and capabilities. When demands overweigh capabilities, then the balance shifts to the left indicating the need for

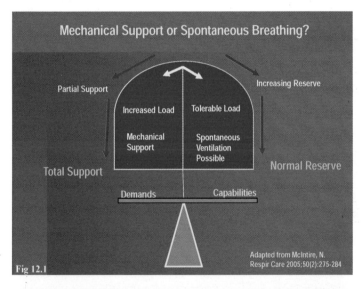

Fig 12.1

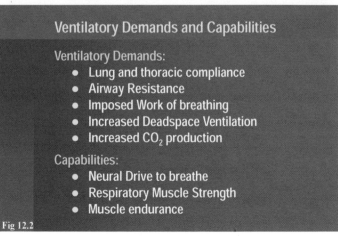

Fig 12.2

more ventilatory support. Upon reversal of the underlying problem the patient's capability increases and the balance shifts to the right in the direction of regaining the normal reserves.

Figure 12.2 identifies factors increasing demands and capabilities. Ventilatory demand increases with deterioration in lung characteristics (compliance and resistance), increased deadspace ventilation as well as increased imposed work by the tracheal tube and ventilator circuitry.

The capabilities of the patient to provide adequate spontaneous ventilation can be judged by evaluating neural drive, muscle strength and endurance.

Discontinuation of mechanical support is the ultimate goal of mechanical ventilation.

Successful weaning is defined as effective spontaneous breathing for more than 24 hours, whereas weaning attempt is considered failed when the patient demonstrates signs of worsening clinical condition such as; increased use of accessory muscles of breathing, diaphoresis, arrhythmias and abnormal blood gases, requiring return to mechanical ventilation (Fig 12.3).

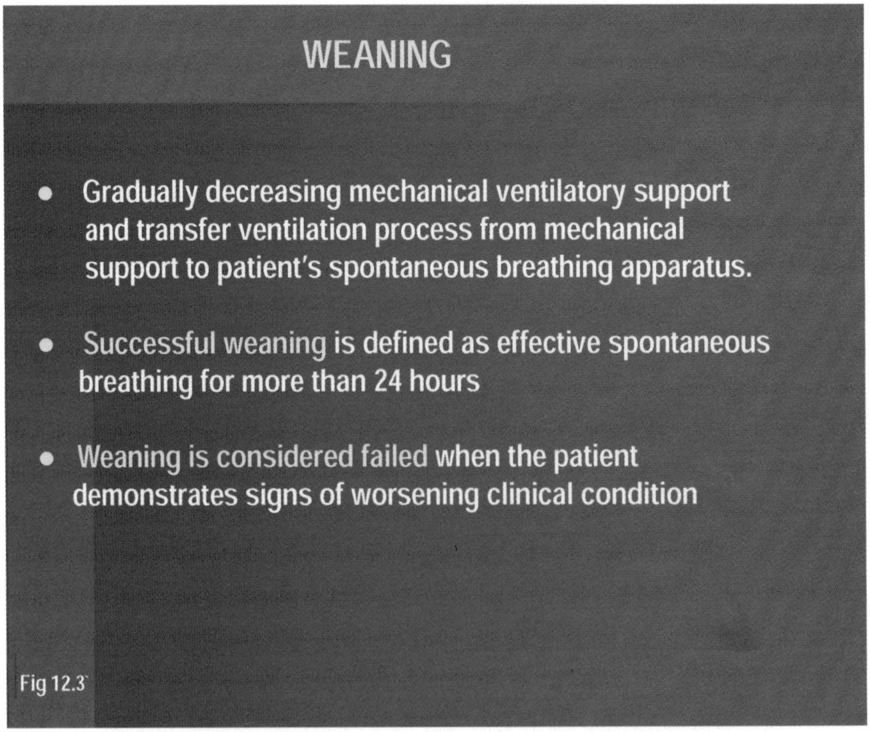

WEANING

- Gradually decreasing mechanical ventilatory support and transfer ventilation process from mechanical support to patient's spontaneous breathing apparatus.

- Successful weaning is defined as effective spontaneous breathing for more than 24 hours

- Weaning is considered failed when the patient demonstrates signs of worsening clinical condition

Fig 12.3

In most patients weaning is feasible when the underlying physiologic cause of respiratory failure is reversed. A small percent of patients do not completely return to condition suitable for weaning. Brochard and coworkers classified patients from their weanability (Fig 12.4).

They used spontaneous breathing trials (SBT) as the yardstick to identify patients in three categories: Simple Weaning, Difficult Weaning and Prolonged Weaning. The patients requiring prolonged weaning may require long term mechanical support and perhaps Home Mechanical Ventilation.

Weaning from Mechanical Ventilator

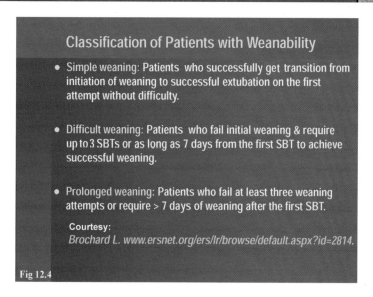

Fig 12.4

Weaning should be initiated as soon as possible to avoid potential hazards of mechanical ventilation and yet, should not be discontinued prematurely. Figure 12.5 lists the hazards associated with mechanical ventilation as well as adverse effects of premature discontinuation of mechanical support.

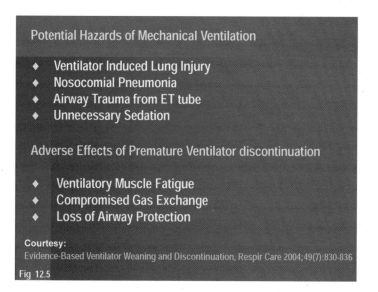

Fig 12.5

Patient's Readiness to Wean

Weaning is a major transition from transferring the WOB from the ventilator to the patient.

Patient's ability to perform the work of breathing must be evaluated. Not only the acute phase of underlying disorder should be resolved, but also, the patient must have adequate cough to maintaining patency of airways and ability to clear any secretions (Fig 12.6). Other objective parameters should be measured to ascertain that the patient is ready to be weaned (Fig 12.7).

Assessing readiness to wean

Clinical Evaluation

- Adequate cough.

- Absence of excessive tracheobronchial secretions.

- Resolution of acute phase of disease process for which the patient was intubated.

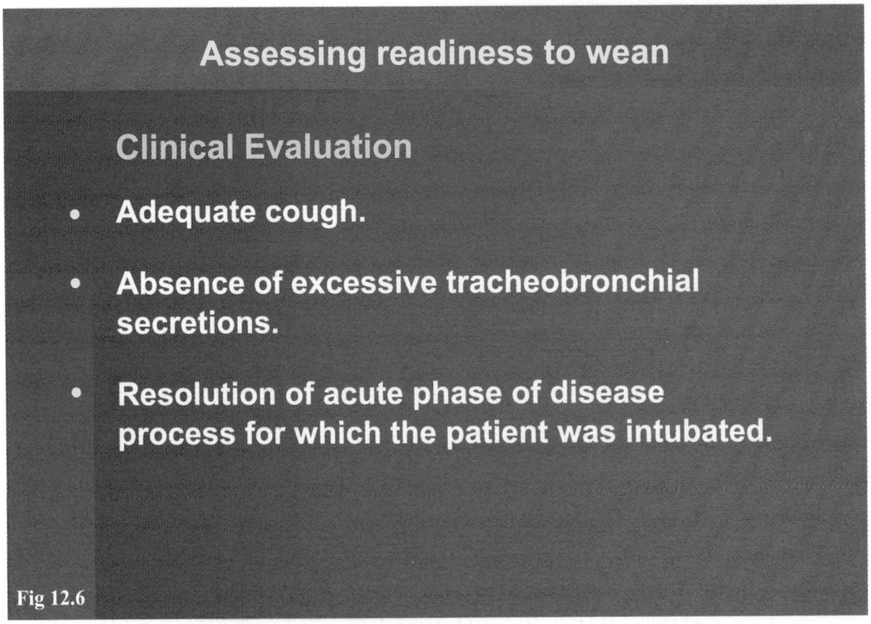

Fig 12.6

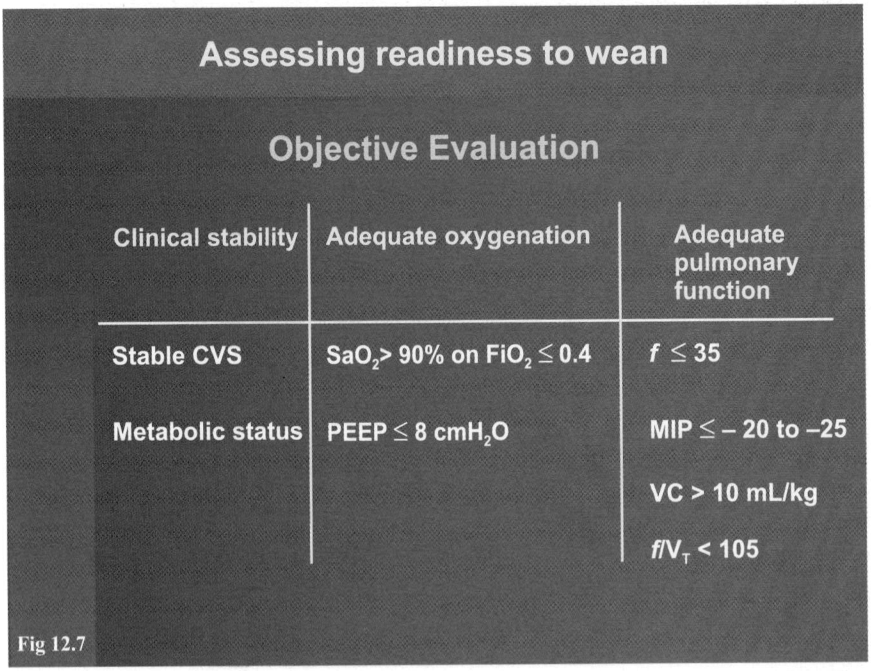

Assessing readiness to wean

Objective Evaluation

Clinical stability	Adequate oxygenation	Adequate pulmonary function
Stable CVS	$SaO_2 > 90\%$ on $FiO_2 \leq 0.4$	$f \leq 35$
Metabolic status	$PEEP \leq 8$ cmH_2O	$MIP \leq -20$ to -25
		$VC > 10$ mL/kg
		$f/V_T < 105$

Fig 12.7

Stable cardiovascular system, adequate oxygenation and reliable pulmonary mechanics are essential for successful weaning. Many parameters which are routinely measured during mechanical ventilation can be used to verify weanability of the patient. A detailed list of commonly measured physiological parameters to determine adequacy in oxygenation and ventilation with their acceptable values are shown in Fig 12.8 (Oxygenation) and Fig 12.9 (Ventilation).

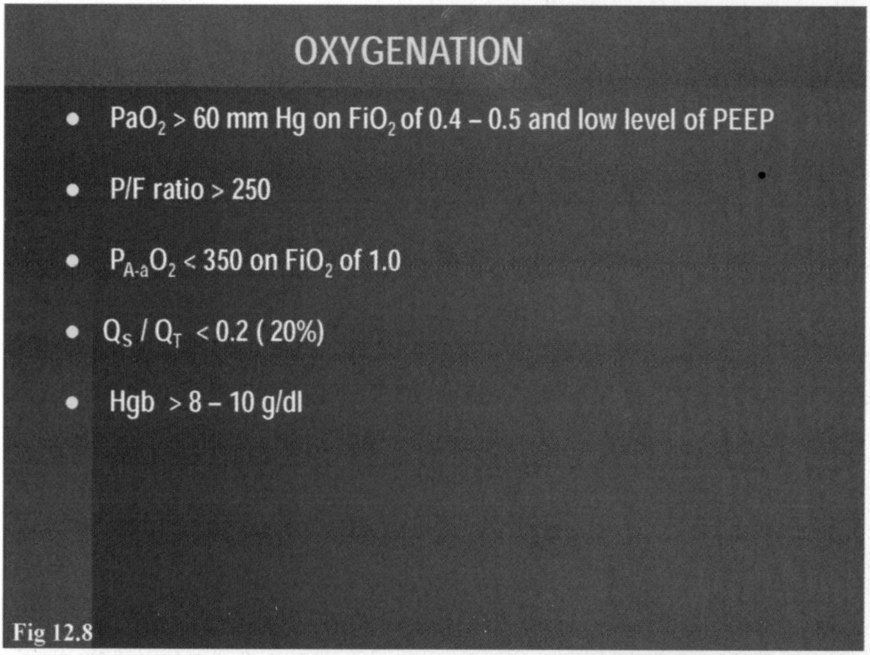

OXYGENATION

- $PaO_2 > 60$ mm Hg on FiO_2 of 0.4 – 0.5 and low level of PEEP
- P/F ratio > 250
- $P_{A-a}O_2 < 350$ on FiO_2 of 1.0
- $Q_S / Q_T < 0.2$ (20%)
- Hgb > 8 – 10 g/dl

Fig 12.8

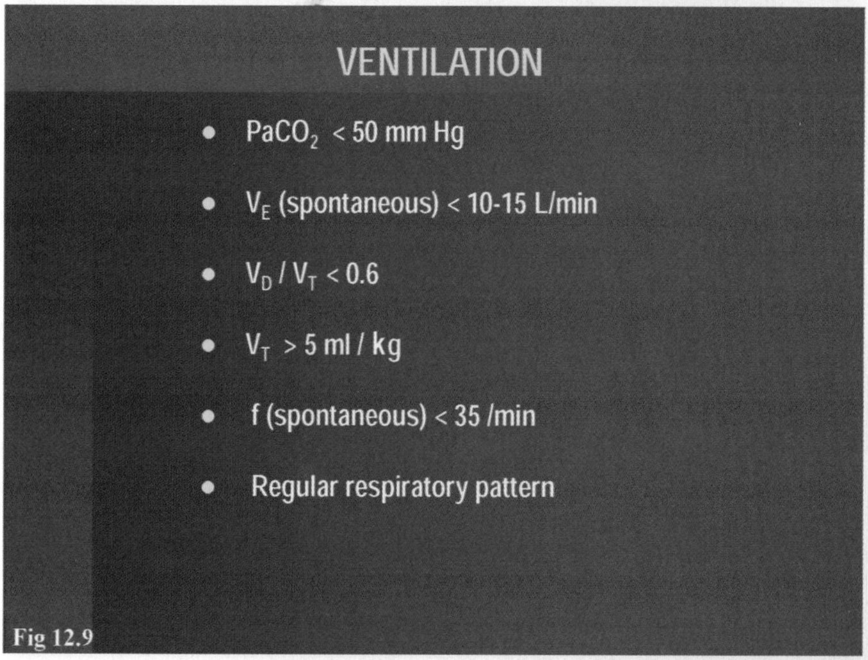

VENTILATION

- $PaCO_2 < 50$ mm Hg
- V_E (spontaneous) < 10-15 L/min
- $V_D / V_T < 0.6$
- $V_T > 5$ ml / kg
- f (spontaneous) < 35 /min
- Regular respiratory pattern

Fig 12.9

It is expected that these values are within the normal ranges and a regular respiratory pattern to predict successful weaning. Along the same line, measurement of pulmonary mechanics is essential. The value for static lung compliance (C_L), can be obtained during a mechanical breath from the ventilator ($C_L = V_T / PP$). A value of > 30 mL/cm H_2O is desirable (Fig 12.10).

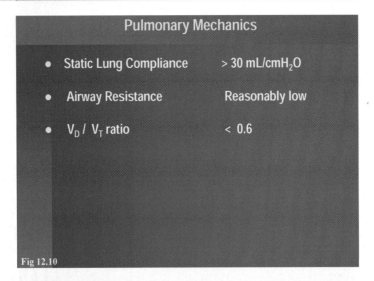

Fig 12.10

Pulmonary Mechanics

- Static Lung Compliance   > 30 mL/cmH$_2$O
- Airway Resistance   Reasonably low
- V_D / V_T ratio   < 0.6

Parameters Predicting Success or Failure of Weaning

- Rapid Shallow Breathing Index (RSBI)
- Ventilatory Drive
- Ventilatory Muscle Strength
- Work of Breathing
- Spontaneous Breathing Trials (SBT)

Fig 12.11

Parameters Predicting Success or Failure of Weaning

Researchers identified some tests that could predict the success or failure of weaning. The most successful predictor of weaning is rapid-shallow breathing index (RSBI). Other commonly used predictors of weaning listed in Fig 12.11, include Ventilatory Drive, Ventilatory Muscle strength, Work of Breathing and spontaneous breathing trials (SBT).

Rapid Shallow Breathing Index (RSBI)

The success rate of weaning depends on the number of these criteria met by the patient. Rapid Shallow Breathing Index has been identified as a yardstick to verify weanability. RSBI (f / V_T) less than 100 is associated high probability of success and RSBI greater than 100 indicates a greater probability of failure. The tidal volume is measured in Liters. Statistically RSBI has 97% sensitivity and 65% specificity (12.12). The physiological parameters associated with potential successful weaning are as shown in Fig 12.13. Measurement of RSBI is also described. Volumes are measured by a respirometer or directly from the ventilator in liters.

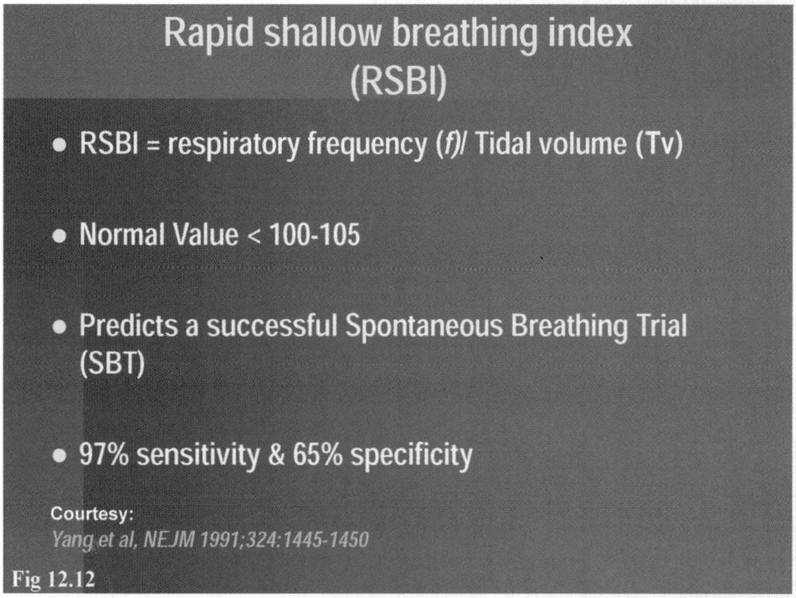

Rapid shallow breathing index (RSBI)

- RSBI = respiratory frequency (f)/ Tidal volume (Tv)

- Normal Value < 100-105

- Predicts a successful Spontaneous Breathing Trial (SBT)

- 97% sensitivity & 65% specificity

Courtesy:
Yang et al, NEJM 1991;324:1445-1450

Fig 12.12

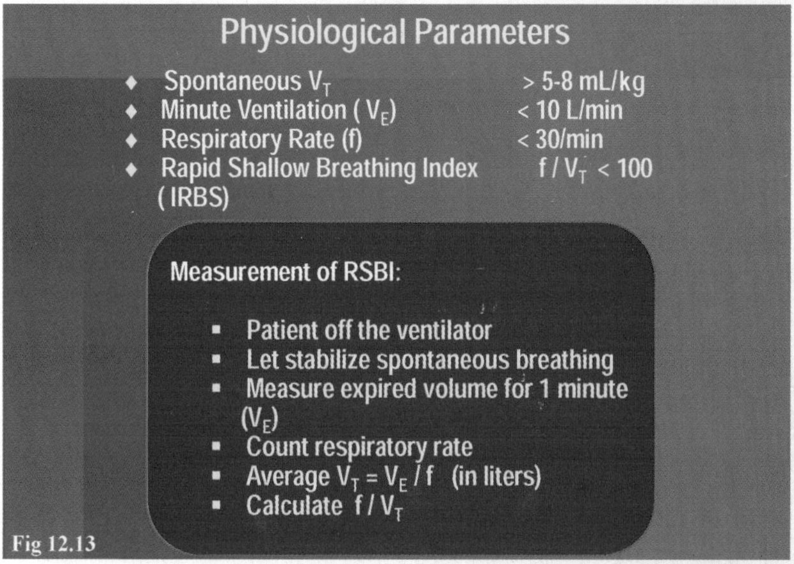

Physiological Parameters

- Spontaneous V_T — > 5-8 mL/kg
- Minute Ventilation (V_E) — < 10 L/min
- Respiratory Rate (f) — < 30/min
- Rapid Shallow Breathing Index (IRBS) — $f/V_T < 100$

Measurement of RSBI:

- Patient off the ventilator
- Let stabilize spontaneous breathing
- Measure expired volume for 1 minute (V_E)
- Count respiratory rate
- Average $V_T = V_E / f$ (in liters)
- Calculate f / V_T

Fig 12.13

Ventilatory Muscle Strength

Ventilator muscles must be strong enough to sustain spontaneous breathing. Assessment of patient effort dependent tests such as, Vital Capacity, Maximal Inspiratory Pressure (PI_{max}) or Negative Inspiratory Force (NIF) and MVV verify muscle strength (Fig 12.14). PI_{max} is measured from residual volume with an occluded airway, keeping a watch on oxygen desaturation and arrhythmia. PI_{max} is the best predictor of weaning failure. A value of $PI_{max} >/= -15$ cm H_2O indicates inadequate muscle strength for weaning. Vital Capacity (VC) is completely dependent on patient cooperation and thus is not very useful in predicting weaning outcome. Mandatory minute ventilation (MMV) is not commonly used as it can lead to muscle fatigue.

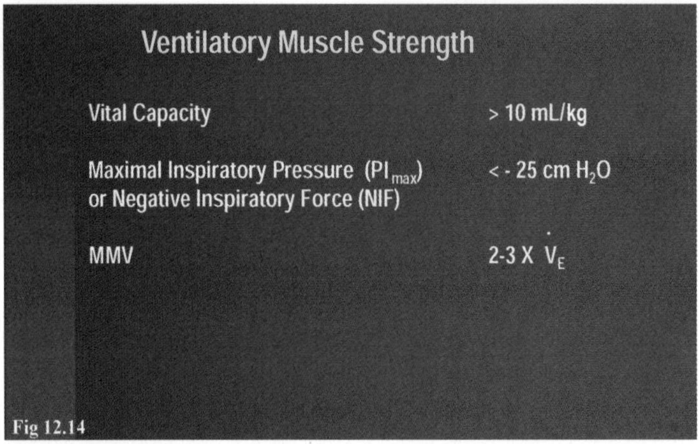

Ventilatory Muscle Strength

Vital Capacity	> 10 mL/kg
Maximal Inspiratory Pressure (PI_{max}) or Negative Inspiratory Force (NIF)	< -25 cm H_2O
MMV	2-3 X $\dot{V}_E$

Fig 12.14

Ventilatory Drive

The primary index of ventilator drive is P_{100} or $P_{0.1}$ which reflects on patient's drive to breath and muscle strength. Normal value for $P_{0.1}$ is 0 to -2 cm H_2O. Value below normal indicates weak muscles inadequate strength for weaning. Whereas value less negative than -6 cm H_2O is associated with a high drive to breathe and may promote exhaustion during weaning (Fig 12.15)

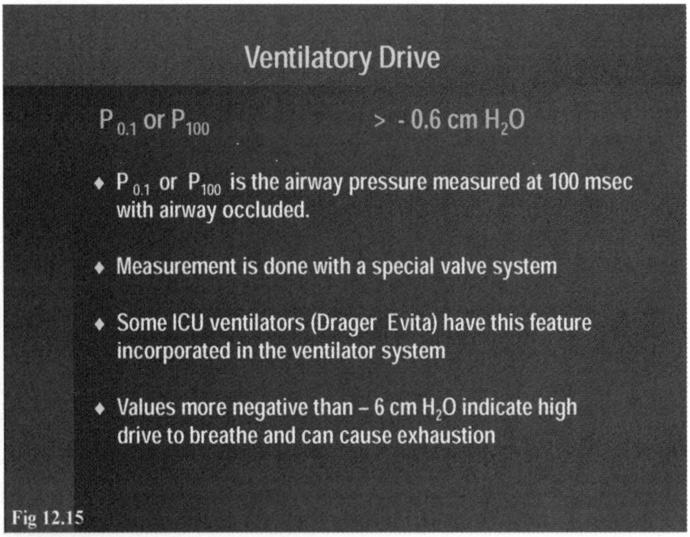

Ventilatory Drive

$P_{0.1}$ or P_{100} > -0.6 cm H_2O

- $P_{0.1}$ or P_{100} is the airway pressure measured at 100 msec with airway occluded.
- Measurement is done with a special valve system
- Some ICU ventilators (Drager Evita) have this feature incorporated in the ventilator system
- Values more negative than -6 cm H_2O indicate high drive to breathe and can cause exhaustion

Fig 12.15

Patient's spontaneous work of breathing (WOB) plays an important role in success of weaning. To begin with, tracheal intubation increases resistive component of WOB, reducing dynamic compliance. A dynamic compliance ($C_D = V_T / PIP - PEEP$) greater than 25 mL/cm H_2O is desirable to initiate weaning. Similarly, presence of increased deadspace precipitates increased respiratory rate and WOB. A V_D / V_T value below 0.6 is considered acceptable (Fig 12.16). Increased WOB and ventilatory muscle fatigue lead to ventilator dependency. During mechanical ventilation all efforts should be made to minimize WOB. Selecting appropriate level of sensitivity, use of flow sensitivity over pressure sensitivity and eliminating auto-PEEP, if any, reduce triggering work of breathing.

Selecting appropriate mode of ventilation and providing adequate inspiratory flow avoids dissynchrony. In situations of increased airway resistance, tracheal suctioning and giving bronchodilators decrease WOB, use of accessory muscles of breathing and asynchronous breathing confirm increased work of breathing.

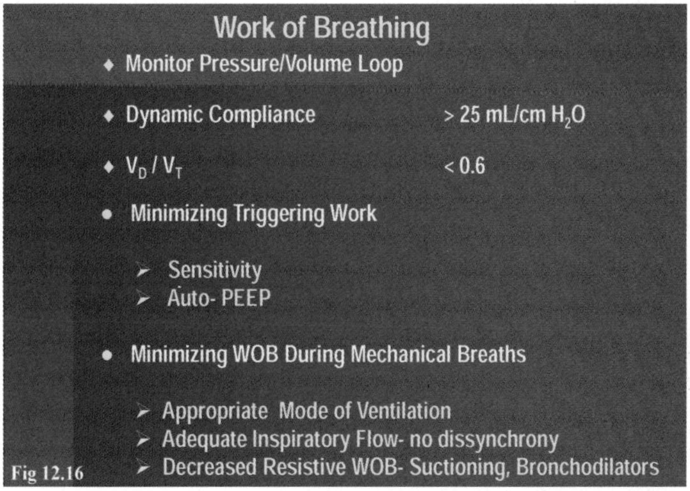

Work of Breathing
- Monitor Pressure/Volume Loop
- Dynamic Compliance   > 25 mL/cm H_2O
- V_D / V_T < 0.6
- Minimizing Triggering Work
  - Sensitivity
  - Auto- PEEP
- Minimizing WOB During Mechanical Breaths
  - Appropriate Mode of Ventilation
  - Adequate Inspiratory Flow- no dissynchrony
  - Decreased Resistive WOB- Suctioning, Bronchodilators

Fig 12.16

After evaluating all the essential parameters a final confirmation of readiness for weaning is determined from spontaneous breathing trial (SBT). A patient demonstrates weanability when he/she sustains spontaneous breathing on a T-piece, without any ventilatory support, for more than 30 minutes provided adequate flow is available. In case the trial is done on a ventilator, a continuous flow is added to the circuit with or without a low level of CPAP or PSV (Fig 20.17).

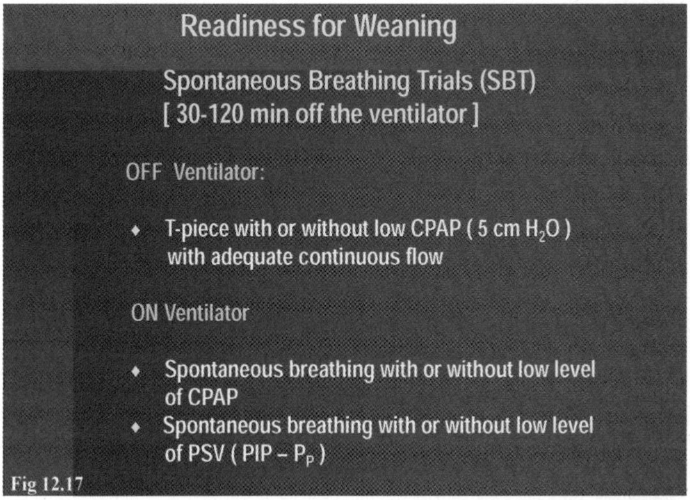

Readiness for Weaning
Spontaneous Breathing Trials (SBT)
[30-120 min off the ventilator]

OFF Ventilator:
- T-piece with or without low CPAP (5 cm H_2O) with adequate continuous flow

ON Ventilator
- Spontaneous breathing with or without low level of CPAP
- Spontaneous breathing with or without low level of PSV (PIP – P_P)

Fig 12.17

It is demonstrated that patients successfully passing the SBT have a 77-85% probability to wean off the mechanical support (Fig 20.18). SBT involves alternating spontaneous breathing and complete

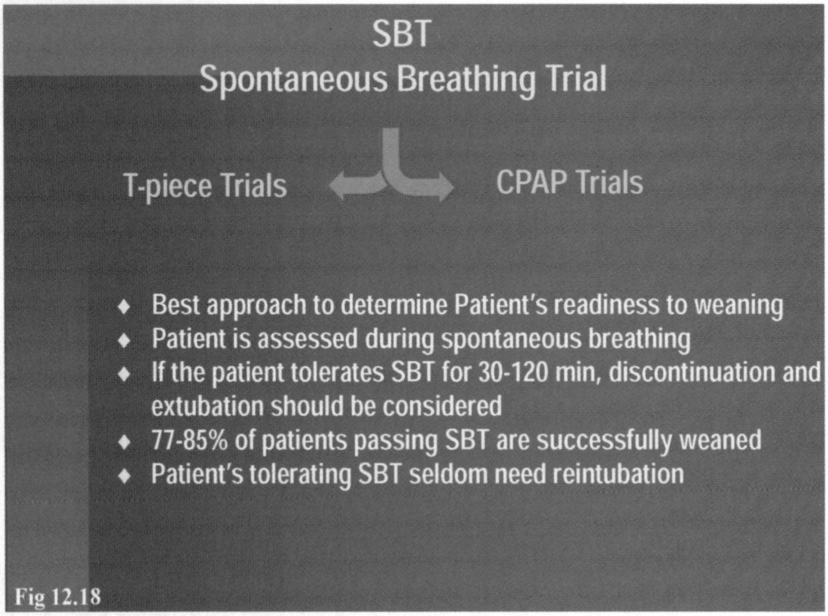

SBT
Spontaneous Breathing Trial

T-piece Trials ⟷ CPAP Trials

- Best approach to determine Patient's readiness to weaning
- Patient is assessed during spontaneous breathing
- If the patient tolerates SBT for 30-120 min, discontinuation and extubation should be considered
- 77-85% of patients passing SBT are successfully weaned
- Patient's tolerating SBT seldom need reintubation

Fig 12.18

mechanical support. As tolerated by the patient, time "off" the ventilator is increased. Low levels (~ 5 cm H_2O) of CPAP may benefit COPD patients who potentially experience Auto-PEEP. Patients with Asthma or neuromuscular disease benefit from low levels PSV during spontaneous breathing (Fig 20.19). SBT trials are viewed as most acceptable method of weaning by gradually transferring work of breathing from the ventilator to the patient.

Vallverdu *et al* have identified clinically useful objective and subjective indices associated with SBT failure (Fig 12.20).

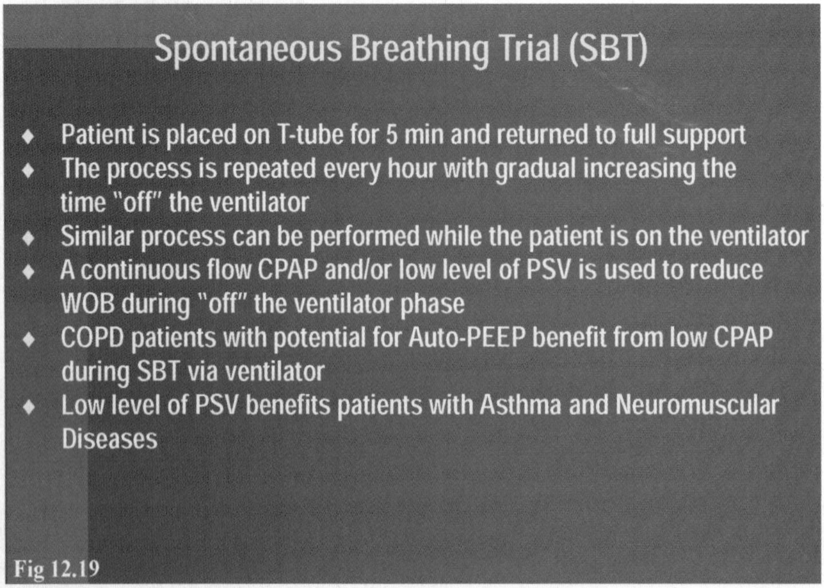

Spontaneous Breathing Trial (SBT)

- Patient is placed on T-tube for 5 min and returned to full support
- The process is repeated every hour with gradual increasing the time "off" the ventilator
- Similar process can be performed while the patient is on the ventilator
- A continuous flow CPAP and/or low level of PSV is used to reduce WOB during "off" the ventilator phase
- COPD patients with potential for Auto-PEEP benefit from low CPAP during SBT via ventilator
- Low level of PSV benefits patients with Asthma and Neuromuscular Diseases

Fig 12.19

Failure of SBT

Objective Indices	Subjective indices
Tachypnea,	Agitation or distress
Tachycardia,	Depressed mental status
Hyper or hypotension,	Diaphoresis
Hypoxemia or acidosis,	Evidence of increased WOB
Arrthythmias.	

Courtesy: Vallverdu et al, Am J Respir Crit Care Med 1998;158:1855-1862

Fig 12.20

Some patients may not pass the SBT. They can be weaned by employing other methods such as PSV, SIMV, SIMV+PSV, NPPV and closed loop weaning (Fig 12.21). Weaning attempts with stand-alone PSV are also reported. One group decided to increase PSV level until the desired VT, was delivered on spontaneous trigger (PSV_{max}). The other group increased PSV until the desired respiratory frequency was achieved. In either case, if the patient tolerated the procedure, PSV level was gradually decreased to the minimal level of 5 cm H_2O. Vital signs and other essential clinical parameters (ABG, ECG, use of accessary muscles etc.) need to be continually monitored during PSV weaning process (Fig 12.22).

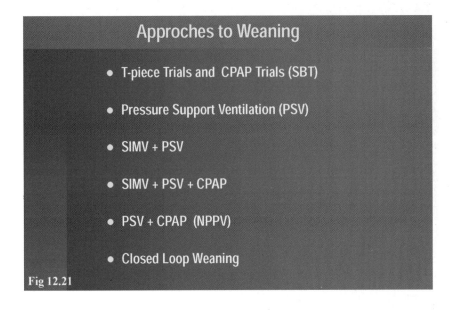

Approches to Weaning

- T-piece Trials and CPAP Trials (SBT)
- Pressure Support Ventilation (PSV)
- SIMV + PSV
- SIMV + PSV + CPAP
- PSV + CPAP (NPPV)
- Closed Loop Weaning

Fig 12.21

PSV Weaning

- PSV can be used as stand-alone mode for weaning

- PSV level can be increased to achieve desired V_T (~ 5-7 ml/kg)

- PSV level can be increased until desired spontaneous frequency is achieved (< 35/min)

- Gradually PSV level is decreased (3-5 cm H_2O increments) to the minimal level of 5 cm H_2O

- If the patient tolerates this reduction in PSV extubation can be considered

- Periodic assessment is crucial (ABG, ECG, Vital Signs, WOB)

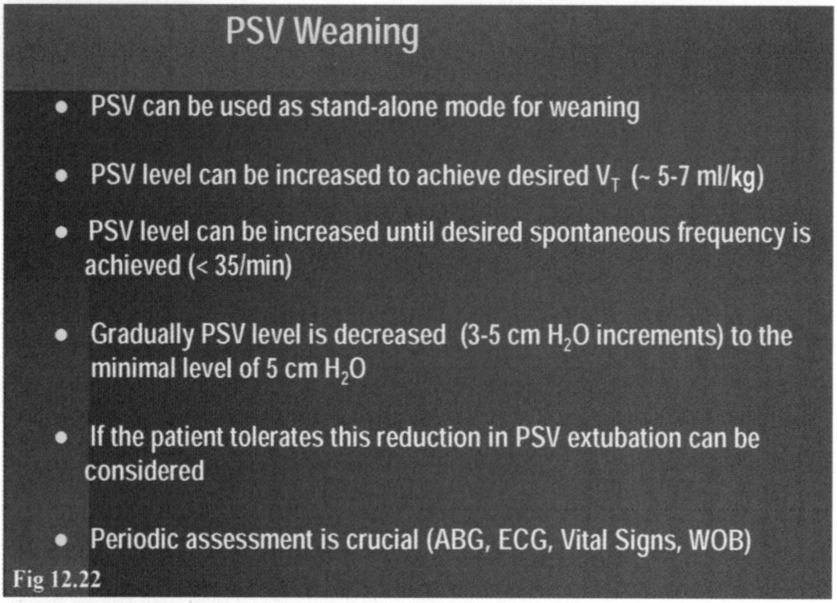

Fig 12.22

Synchronized intermittent mandatory ventilation (SIMV) was primarily used as a weaning tool for several years. It was practical and convenient to ventilate patients using high SIMV rate (12–15/min). As the patient stabilized, the SIMV rate was gradually reduced. Since SIMV involves assisted ventilation interposed by unsupported spontaneous breathing, use of PSV to overcome imposed WOB was employed during spontaneous component of SIMV. Esteban and Tobin published their findings indicating SIMV method of weaning had the worst outcome. Currently, unsupported SIMV is not recommended for weaning (Fig 12.23).

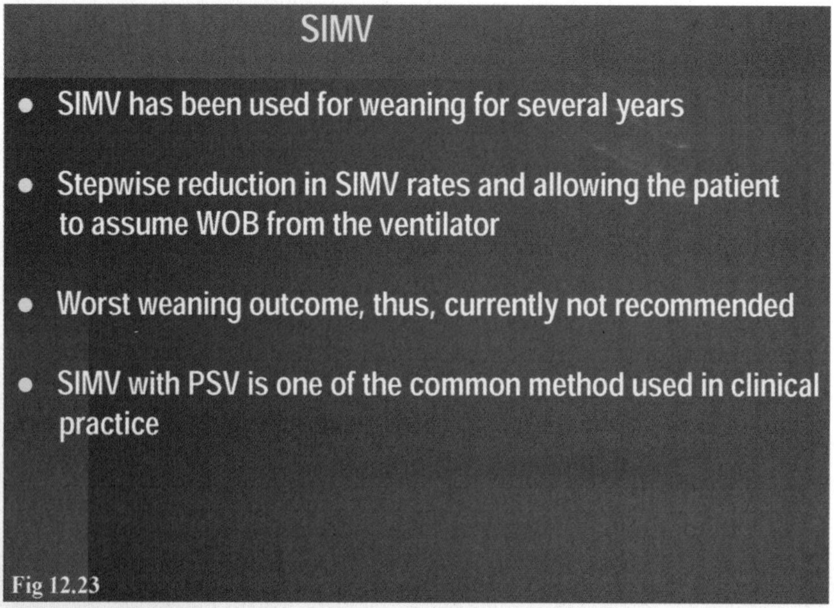

SIMV

- SIMV has been used for weaning for several years

- Stepwise reduction in SIMV rates and allowing the patient to assume WOB from the ventilator

- Worst weaning outcome, thus, currently not recommended

- SIMV with PSV is one of the common method used in clinical practice

Fig 12.23

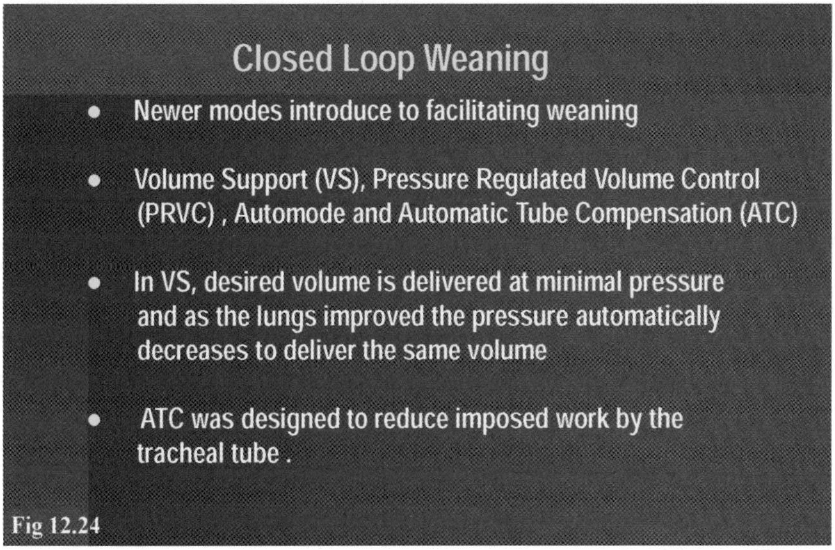

Closed Loop Weaning

- Newer modes introduce to facilitating weaning

- Volume Support (VS), Pressure Regulated Volume Control (PRVC), Automode and Automatic Tube Compensation (ATC)

- In VS, desired volume is delivered at minimal pressure and as the lungs improved the pressure automatically decreases to deliver the same volume

- ATC was designed to reduce imposed work by the tracheal tube.

Fig 12.24

Technological advances introduced newer approaches to weaning with closed-loop mechanism. Volume Support, Automode and automatic tube compensation (ATC) were added to the alphabet soup of ventilator modes. Volume support allows the clinician to set a desired tidal volume. The ventilator delivers this volume at a lowest possible pressure support. As the patient improves the delivered PS is decreased to provide desired pre-set volume. Automode monitors patients who need mechanical support for some periods of time (post-anesthesia). As the patient makes a spontaneous effort, the ventilator switches to volume support (VS). If the patient becomes apneic, the ventilator switches to control mode. ATC activation uses data such as the tracheal tube size and type to provide adequate pressure at the airways to overcome imposed WOB due to ET tube (Fig 12.24). Adaptive support ventilation (ASV) is designed to accomplish weaning using Servo Controlled closed-loop ventilation, gradually decreasing support (Fig 12.25).

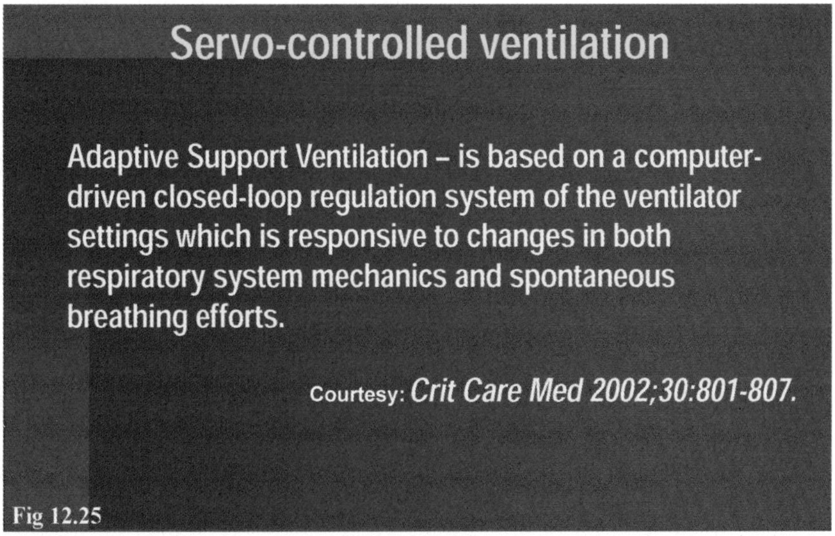

Servo-controlled ventilation

Adaptive Support Ventilation – is based on a computer-driven closed-loop regulation system of the ventilator settings which is responsive to changes in both respiratory system mechanics and spontaneous breathing efforts.

Courtesy: *Crit Care Med 2002;30:801-807.*

Fig 12.25

REFERENCES

1. Brochard L et al. Comparison of three methods of gradual withdrawal from ventilatory support during weaning from mechanical ventilation. Am J Respir Crit Care Med 1994; 150:896-903
2. Esteban A, Tobin MJ et al. A comparison of four methods of weaning Patients from mechanical ventilation. New Engl J Med 1995; 332:345-350
3. ACCP, AARC, SCCM Task Force. Evidence based guidelines for weaning and discontinuing mechanical ventilatory support. CHEST 2001;120 Suppl 6:375S-484S.
4. Respir Care 47(1); 69-90.
5. Kollef MH, Shapiro SD et al. A Randomized, controlled trial of protocol-directed versus physician-directed weaning from mechanical ventilation. Crit Care Med 1997;25(4):567-574
6. MacIntire, Neil and Branson, Richard in Mechanical Ventilation; W.B. Saunders Company, Philadelphia, 2001
7. Pilbeam, Susan and Cairo, J.M. in Mechanical Ventilation-Physiologica and Clinical applications, Mosby-Elsevier, Saint Louise, Missouri, Fourth Edition, 1998
8. Chang, David in Clinical Application of Mechanical Ventilation, Delmar Learning, Third Edition, 2006
9. Hess, Dean and Kacmarek, Robert in Essentials of Mechanical Ventilation, The McGraw Hill, Second Edition, 2002

References for Chapters 1-11

10. Intermittent mandatory ventilation: a new approach to weaning patients from mechanical ventilators. Downs JB, Klein EF, Desautels D, et al. Chest 1973; 64:331-335.
11. Intermittent Mandatory Ventilation, John M. Luce, M.D.; David I. Pierson, M.D., F.C.C.P.; and Leonard D. Hudson, M.D., F.C.C.P. ,CHEST, 79: 6, JUNE, 1981
12. Essentials of Mechanical Ventilation, Dean Hess and Robert Kacmarek, McGraw Hill Companies 2002, Second Edition.
13. Pilbeam's Mechanical Ventilation- Physiological and Clinical Applications, J.M.Cairo, Mosby Inc. 2006 Fifth Edition.
14. Clinical Application of Mechanical Ventilation, David W. Chang, Delmar Learning 2006, Third Edition.
15. Yang, K.L, et al. (1991), A prospective study if indices predicting the outcome of trials of weaning from mechanical ventilation. N Eng J Med, 324, 1445-1450
16. Evidence-Based Ventilator Weaning and Discontinuation, Respir Care 2004;49(7):830-836
17. Vallverdu et al, Am J Respir Crit Care Med 1998;158:1855-1862
18. Brochard L et al. Comparison of three methods of gradual ventilatory support during weaning from mechanical ventilation. Am J Respir Crit Care Med 1994; 150:896-903
19. Esteban A, Tobin MJ et al. A comparison of four methods of weaning Patients from mechanical ventilation. New Eng J Med 1995; 332:345-350
20. Hess DR: Managing the artificial Airway, Respir Care 44: 759, 1999.
21. Rapid Interpretation of Ventilator Waveforms, Jonathan Waugh, Vijay Deshpande, Robert Harwood, Melissa Brown, Paerson Education Inc, New Jersey, 2007, Second Edition.

★ ★ ★

POSITIVE END-EXPIRATORY PRESSURE AND CONTINUOUS POSITIVE AIRWAY PRESSURE

Krupesh N, Chandrashekar TR

Introduction of positive end-expiratory pressure (PEEP) into the practice for mechanical ventilation was among the most important milestones in ventilator therapy. Application of PEEP is expected to enhance both lung mechanics and gas exchange as it recruits lung units. It is not yet possible to determine clearly the balance between benefit and harmful effects of PEEP (mainly suppression of cardiovascular and other organ function). Setting PEEP at the bedside is still controversial at best.

Positive end-expiratory pressure (PEEP) is defined as pressure in the airway at the end of passive expiration that exceeds atmospheric pressure. The term PEEP is applicable to patients receiving mechanical ventilation. Many terms like expiratory positive airway pressure (EPAP in non invasive ventilation — NPPV) and continuous positive airway pressure (CPAP) are interchangeably used. CPAP is a term used in spontaneously breathing subjects where inspiratory and expiratory portions of the ventilatory cycle are pressurized above atmospheric pressure. Basically, "PEEP is mechanical CPAP and CPAP is spontaneous PEEP" (Fig 13.1). CPAP is not a mode of ventilation as there is no

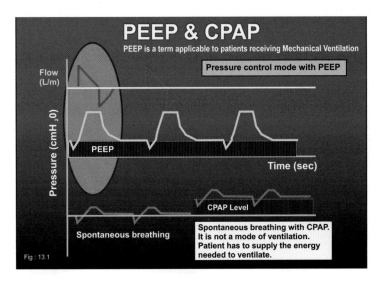
Fig: 13.1

inspiratory support. It is mainly used in NPPV applied for chronic conditions and the only application in acute patients is in cardiogenic pulmonary edema requiring NPPV support. Principles underlying PEEP and CPAP are identical. Hence, in all discussions that follow only PEEP application in mechanical ventilation is discussed.

Types of PEEP

External or Applied PEEP: PEEP that is provided by a mechanical ventilator (also called extrinsic PEEP).

Auto-PEEP or intrinsic PEEP: PEEP that develops secondary to incomplete expiration. Auto-PEEP can dramatically increase the work of breathing and provoke patient-ventilator dyssynchrony (Fig 13.2 and Fig 13.3).

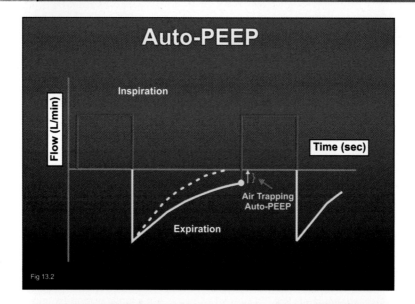

Fig 13.2

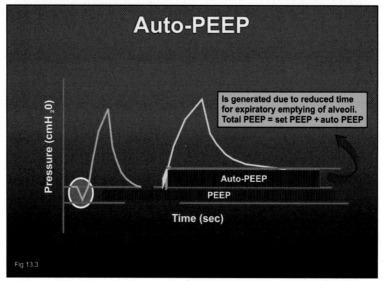

Fig 13.3

Commonly used strategies to minimize intrinsic positive end expiratory pressure include:

a. Aggressive bronchodilation
b. Secretion removal
c. Adequate pain and fever control to reduce CO_2 production
d. Minimization of inspiratory time and increase in expiratory time and inspiratory flow rate (decrease T_I)
e. Reduce tidal volume and respiratory rate (increase T_E)
f. Extrinsic PEEP can counter intrinsic PEEP and decrease the work of breathing. The effects of auto PEEP, how to quantify it at the bedside and how to manage it have been discussed in detail in 'Disease specific ventilation'.

Positive End-Expiratory Pressure

Physiological PEEP

A PEEP of 5 cm H_2O was routinely used in all patients as it was thought that the vocal cord closure at the end of expiration generates this amount of PEEP. This observation is not backed by any scientific data. Studies that followed this practice showed that prophylactic PEEP application did not prevent ARDS and hence it fell out of favor. Current knowledge of mechanisms that cause ventilator induced lung injury (VILI) and the alveolar stabilizing effect of PEEP makes it mandatory that a PEEP of 5 cm H_2O should be applied to all patients who are mechanically ventilated (except in acute severe asthma or unilateral / localized lung disease).

Prophylactic PEEP

Change from standing to supine posture leads to volume loss which is prevented by use of prophylactic PEEP (PEEP for 3 to 5 cm H_2O). Are the Physiological PEEP and the Prophylactic PEEP same or different, is an unanswered question.

Physiological rationale for using PEEP therapy

Airways become narrower during expiration. Airway closure is a normal physiologic phenomenon and is the effect of increasing pleural pressure during expiration. The volume above residual volume (RV) at which airways begin to close during expiration is called closing volume (CV), and the sum of RV and CV is called closing capacity (CC). Airway closure plays an even greater role in the supine position because FRC is reduced, whereas, CC is not affected by body position. The airways may be continuously closed if CC exceeds FRC. PEEP application results in increase in FRC. Therefore FRC will be more than CC and this prevents airway closure. If low lung compliance results in high CC, then higher PEEP (FRC) must be used to prevent alveolar collapse or partially reverse the collapse in parts of the lung. This is known as lung recruitment. This is illustrated in the figure below (Fig 13.4):

Increased FRC increases the number of alveoli recruited resulting in a larger surface area for gas

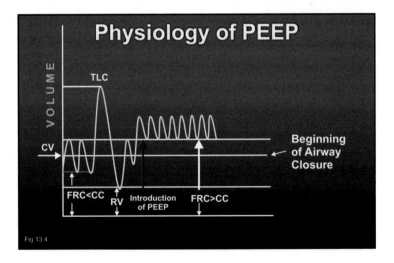

Fig 13.4

exchange. This leads to better oxygenation. Hence, PEEP reduces FiO_2 requirements and risk of oxygen toxicity (Fig 13.5). Perhaps more importantly, PEEP improves the distribution of alveolar liquid and translocates fluid from alveolar to interstitial spaces thereby lowering the diffusion distance for oxygen exchange. In the presence of alveolar edema, PEEP may prevent airway flooding by expanding the alveolar reservoir capacity. Abrupt withdrawal of PEEP in stiff lungs may precipitate translocation of alveolar liquid into the airways, impeding airflow and generating froth. Application of PEEP also prevents infected secretions from translocating into normal areas of the lungs. PEEP application leads to recruitment of alveolar units that were previously collapsed. This additional recruitment allows tidal volume to be distributed to more alveoli resulting in reduced peak airway pressure and increased compliance. Consequently the work of breathing is decreased.

PEEP levels that cause overdistention prove detrimental. The reasons for this are that the lung compliance may worsen as additional volume is forced into a fully recruited lung, increasing the elastic workload. High FRC results in flat diaphragm making the respiratory pump less efficient. The volume recruiting effect of PEEP is influenced by the chest wall compliance, tidal volume and the activity of the respiratory muscles. Any benefit from PEEP on oxygen exchange may be nullified by the expiratory muscle activity and can be restored by muscle relaxation.

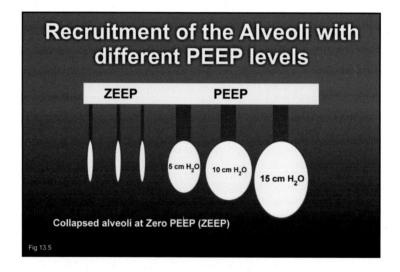

Fig 13.5

PEEP and VILI prevention

Recruitment of lung volume is a joint function of PEEP and the opening pressures generated in response to tidal volume (more so in low tidal volume ventilation). There is continuous collapse and re-expansion of the alveoli in the interface between collapsed and consolidated portion of the lung and normal lung. Sustained high pressure is required to open the adherent walls of collapsed airway which results in shear force on the thin tissue wall separating junctional alveoli (at the boundary between normal aerated and collapsed alveoli). This causes stress failure of alveolar membrane and disruption of the epithelium. The shear force depends on magnitude of recruitment and de-cruitment, cycling frequency and duration of exposure to high pressure. This injury is more in dependent regions of the lung because the diseased lung is oedematous and the superimposed weight of the oedematous alveoli (in non-dependent region) causes squeezing of the gas out of the alveoli and collapse of alveoli in the dependent region.

This is one of the reasons why V/Q matching improves on proning as there is more lung tissue in the dorsal region which now becomes non dependent and there is more homogeneous distribution of both ventilation and perfusion. Atelectrauma can be prevented by applying PEEP to avoid repeated opening and closing of the alveoli. PEEP reduces the number of lung units at risk for atelectrauma (Fig 13.6).

Positive End-Expiratory Pressure

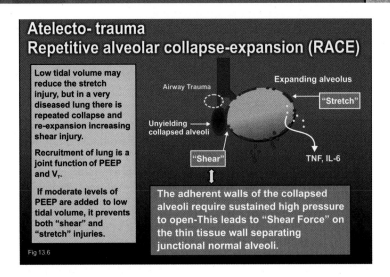

Fig 13.6

Cause for venous admixture: Effect of PEEP on PVR (pulmonary vascular resistance)

PVR and lung compliance are optimum at FRC. It increases at low lung volumes (collapsed alveoli causing hypoxic pulmonary vasoconstriction) and high lung volumes (over distension and compression of alveolar vessels) (Fig 13.7). Increasing PEEP increases PVR by causing over distension of alveoli and compression of the pulmonary vasculature. This is not offset by decreased resistance of extra alveolar vessels (high lung volumes cause dilatation of extra alveolar vessels due to tethering effect and reduced tortuosity). Positive end expiratory pressure may adversely alter the distribution of pulmonary blood flow, especially in patients with highly localized and

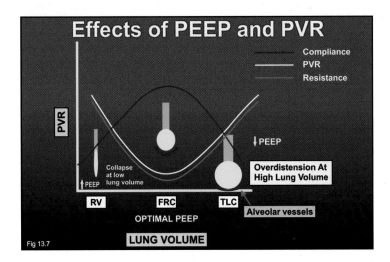

Fig 13.7

heterogeneous lung disease. Positive transpulmonary pressure has its greatest distending effect on compliant alveoli.

High PEEP levels result in disproportionate raise in resistance to blood flow through compliant lung units. This redirects blood flow towards stiffer, more diseased areas causing hypoxemia. At moderate levels of PEEP any such diversion usually does not outweigh the benefits of alveolar recruitment and hypoxic vasoconstriction. In a similar manner, PEEP can increase shunt flow in a patient with intrapulmonary or intracardiac right-to-left vascular communications. The end result of all this is increased venous admixture.

Effect of PEEP on different organ systems

Cardiovascular impairment due to PEEP

Approximately one half of the applied PEEP transmits to the pleural space (intrathoracic pressure-ITP). With abnormally stiff lungs, one fifth to one third is transmitted to the pleural space. In patients with normal lungs and stiff chest wall, more applied PEEP is transmitted to pleural space. PEEP reduces venous return due to increased right atrial pressure resulting in reduced gradient for venous flow (Fig 13.8). This effect is minimal if the patient is euvolemic. High levels of PEEP can

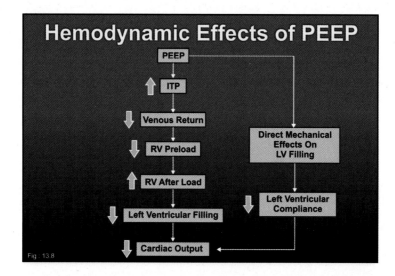

Fig: 13.8

compress the inferior vena cava at the thoracic inlet, thereby increasing the resistance to venous return. This seldom occurs in the prone position. Whether caval compression is important when the lungs are stiff and ITP changes are minimal, is an important unanswered question. In a diseased lung the cardiovascular effects due to increase in ITP is modest when compared to right ventricular dilation caused by alveolar overdistention, pulmonary hypertension, right ventricular afterload and left ventricular filling restrictions due to ventricular interdependence (ventricular septal-shifting effect).

After achieving euvolemic status, vasopressors may be added to achieve constriction of capacitance vessels and thereby improving the driving pressure for venous return. PEEP decreases left ventricular afterload by raising intrapleural pressure which aids ventricular contraction.

Effect on Cerebral Perfusion

PEEP increases jugular and intracranial pressures (ICP) by raising CVP. Predictably, these increments are less when the lungs are stiff. In normal cerebral circulation, a vascular waterfall has been postulated in which the intracranial pressure acts as the effective upstream pressure. PEEP must raise downstream venous pressure to increase intracranial pressure. If baseline intracranial pressure is greater than the increase in intrathoracic pressure caused by PEEP, the technique will not affect intracranial pressure. Abrupt withdrawal of PEEP can also be dangerous as it causes a surge

Positive End-Expiratory Pressure

in venous return and transient boosting of blood pressure and ICP. Despite its potential dangers, PEEP can be used safely if high levels are avoided and if it is applied and withdrawn in small increments.

Effects on Hepatobiliary system

PEEP causes decrease in hepatic perfusion by reducing the cardiac output. Liver has dual blood flow, hepatic artery and portal vein. Mechanical ventilation decrease both hepatic arterial and portal blood flow. The use of PEEP is also associated with decrease in hepatic arterial flow and increases resistance to bile flow through common bile duct. Decrease in the venous return by PEEP increase the hepatic venous pressure by elevating inferior venacaval pressure. All these effects could affect hepatic function which is often compromised in critically ill patients and increase plasma aminotransferase and LDH levels.

Effects on Gastrointestinal (GI) system

Main mechanism by which PEEP affects gastrointestinal system is by causing splanchnic hypoperfusion. Splanchnic hypoperfusion is caused by decreased mean arterial pressure (MAP)

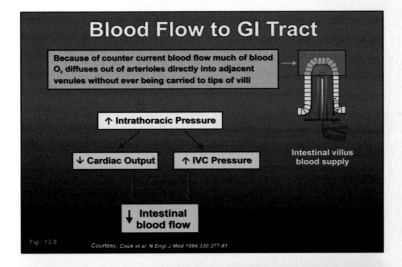

Fig: 13.9

Fig. 13.10

and increased resistance in GI vascular bed. Gut is more prone to ischemic injury because it has no autoregulation. Vascular architecture of gut mucosa is similar to renal medulla. Hypoxia is common at the tips of villi even during normal conditions because O_2 diffuses out of arterioles directly into adjacent venules without ever being carried in the blood to tips of the villi (counter current blood flow) and O_2 content in gut mucosal vessels is low because of dilution by absorbed fluids and nutrients (Fig 13.9). High level of PEEP decreases venous return resulting in decreased cardiac output. Also there is increased rennin angiotensin aldosterone activity and increased catecholamines (both endogenous and exogenous used for hemodynamic support). These can lead to vasoconstriction and redistribution of blood away from the splanchnic vascular bed. All these lead to relative O_2 deficit resulting in GI complications like mucosal damage and altered GI motility (Fig 13.10). In addition to this there is reperfusion injury and cytokines involved may affect many organs.

Acute respiratory failure requiring PEEP for more than 48 hr has been shown to be one of the two strongest independent risk factors for clinically significant GI bleeding in the ICU.

Effects on Renal system

The pulmonary and renal functions are closely interrelated and abnormality in either one or both of these organ systems is common in many critically ill patients. PEEP increases ITP and intra-abdominal pressures which result in various hemodynamic, neural, and hormonal responses that jointly act on the kidney. These mechanisms result in decreased renal perfusion, decreased glomerular filtration rate (GFR), and inhibit excretory function. This is manifested at bedside by deranged renal function tests, decreased urine output, positive fluid balance and edema formation. These effects are further aggravated depending on baseline cardiovascular status, intravascular volume status, preexisting chronic kidney disease, pulmonary disease like COPD.

PEEP induced decrease in cardiac output leads to decreased renal blood flow. These effects are enhanced in the presence of hypovolemia, preserved lung compliance. Studies show redistribution

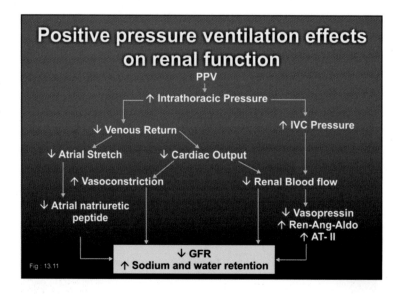

Fig: 13.11

of intrarenal blood flow from cortical region to medullary region. Increased intra-abdominal pressure and compression of inferior vena cava and renal veins results in obstruction to renal venous outflow and decreased renal perfusion pressure.

The main neurohormonal mechanisms thought to cause increased systemic and renal sympathetic nervous system activity are increased activity of renin-angiotensin-aldosterone system, increased secretion of vasopressin, and decreased release of atrial natriuretic peptide (ANP). Increased sympathetic nervous system activity can cause renal vasoconstriction and increased renal tubular reabsorption which can stimulate renin-angiotensin-aldosterone system directly. Also raised ITP can increase the activity of pulmonary endothelial angiotensin converting enzyme activity leading to increased levels of angiotensin II. ANP is released by the atria in response to an increase in atrial stretch and has potent diuretic and natriuretic properties. PEEP can decrease atrial distension, primarily by limiting venous return to the heart and decrease ANP level. This promotes sodium and water retention.

Antidiuretic hormone (ADH) is also responsible for some of the effects of PEEP on renal dysfunction. The increase in ADH levels associated with PEEP is a compensatory response towards decreased cardiac output. ADH increases the reabsorption of the glomerular filtrate from the collecting ducts of the nephron into the renal interstitium and then back into the systemic circulation. The net effect of salt and water retention is intravascular volume expansion which can alleviate the negative hemodynamic and neurohormonal consequences of PEEP on renal function. However, it may be detrimental in many patients especially those with poor underlying cardiac function or ARDS (Fig 13.11).

Setting PEEP

Choosing the optimum level of PEEP is an empirical process determined by response to multiple gas exchange parameters, mechanics and hemodynamic variables. Recruitment maneuvers are integral to this selection process.

Various methods of setting PEEP are listed below:

1. Best compliance (PEEP can be set incrementally or decrementally)
2. Best oxygenation (PEEP can be set incrementally or decrementally)
3. Stress index
4. Oesophageal pressure
5. CT scan

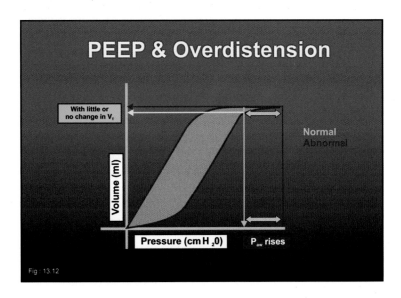

Fig: 13.12

Esophageal pressure reflects the pleural pressure which aids in estimating compliance of the lung. The chest wall component is removed out of the equation, if esophageal pressure is monitored. A recently published study which used esophageal pressure to estimate PEEP setting in ARDS patients showed reduced mortality. Esophageal pressure estimation is being incorporated into ventilators and should be available in near future. CT scan based PEEP setting is only experimental at this point of time.

Irrespective of the PEEP protocol used, oxygenation response, ventilatory efficiency, alterations of mechanics and hemodynamic response should all be considered together. Excess PEEP causes overdistension (Fig 13.12).

PEEP of best oxygenation or compliance are the two commonly used techniques. PEEP can be set incrementally starting from a level of 10 cm H_2O or decrementally stating at 20 cm of H_2O. The choice of incremental or decremental PEEP trial depends on the recruitability of the diseased lung.

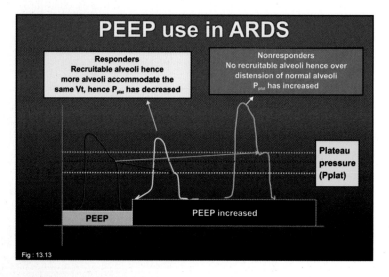

Fig: 13.13

Patient is considered a responder, if a recruitment test proves that PEEP manipulation leads to addition of new alveoli and not over distension of normal alveoli. Recruitment results in decreased plateau pressure and PCO_2. These patients are suitable for decremental PEEP trial. In non-responders, PEEP manipulation leads to over-distension of normal alveoli causing increased plateau pressure and PCO_2. These patients are candidates for incremental PEEP trial (Fig 13.13).

Additional selection criteria for incremental and decremental PEEP trials

Decremental PEEP trial: Decremental PEEP trials should be used in patients with lower inflection point (LIP) on PV curve, ground glass appearance on image studies (interstitial edema) and recruitment test producing decreased plateau pressure / PCO_2.

Incremental PEEP trial: Incremental PEEP trial should be used if the patient has no LIP on PV curve and has consolidation radiologically (alveolar edema) and if recruitment test produces increase in plateau pressure and PCO_2.

PEEP is manipulated in small installments whilst monitoring oxygenation and/or lung compliance. This is described below:

PEEP of Best oxygenation

Fundamental theory is 'when PEEP is decreased or increased (gradually 1 to 2 cm H_2O every 2–3 min)

Positive End-Expiratory Pressure

from a set value (20 or 10 cm of H_2O) arterial oxygenation (measured by arterial PaO_2 or SaO_2) will be reduced when decruitment or over stretching occurs'. At this juncture, a new recruitment maneuver is performed and PEEP is set about 1 cm H_2O above for decremental PEEP and 1cm below for incremental PEEP.

PEEP of Best compliance

In this method a recruitment manoeuvre is done and PEEP is set at 10 or 20 cm of H_2O. PEEP is then reduced or increased in steps of 1 or 2 cm of H_2O. Breath-by-breath compliance is estimated. It may first increase to a maximum and then decrease again. The PEEP at which compliance starts to

Decremental PEEP trail using oxygenation and compliance as indicators

PEEP	PaO_2 / SPO_2	Compliance
18	43 / 70%	26
16	67 / 92%	33
14	77 / 96%	37
12	83 / 98%	43
10	70 / 92%	38

Fig: 13.14

decrease is similar to the collapse pressure or over distending pressure. At this juncture, a new recruitment maneuver is performed and PEEP is set about 1 cm H_2O above for decremental PEEP and 1 cm below for incremental PEEP. Decremental PEEP trial is the method more in line with current understanding of pulmonary mechanics in ARDS patients (Fig 13.14).

Parameters like position, tidal volume, pressure control (with Pplat < 30 cm H_2O), appropriate sedation levels to tolerate high PEEP and/ or hypercarbia and FiO_2 (<60%) should be constant when PEEP trial is being carried out to assess PEEP induced recruitment.

PEEP and tissue oxygen delivery

Tissue oxygen delivery is a cardio-respiratory function. The improved oxygenation effect of PEEP can be offset by reduced oxygen delivery. Oxygen delivery may be reduced by PEEP due to following reasons:

- Decreased cardiac output
- Increased venous admixture
- Increased intracardiac or noncapillary shunt

Oxygen delivery declines, if the drop in cardiac output caused by PEEP outweighs the rise in arterial oxygen content. Whenever augmentation of PEEP is done, it is mandatory to follow the adequacy of tissue oxygen delivery by monitoring cardiac output as well as SaO_2. Whenever feasible, the determinants of tissue O_2 sufficiency, like central venous ($ScVO_2$) and serum lactate levels, should be tracked.

PEEP using pressure-volume curve (PV)

PV curves have been extensively studied to customize ventilator settings as per patient's individual respiratory mechanics and protect them from VILI (Fig 13.15). The PV curve helps in assessment of the mechanical properties of the respiratory system at different levels of lung inflation. The static PV curve of the respiratory system is done using super syringe technique. This method requires cessation of ventilation and is cumbersome. In modern ventilators, dynamic estimation of PV curves is possible. A number of studies and publications have shown that PV loops recorded during the course of ventilation correlate well with loops from standard procedures, so long as the inspiratory flow is constant. It has been hypothesized that proper PEEP can be determined by identifying PV curve inflection points.

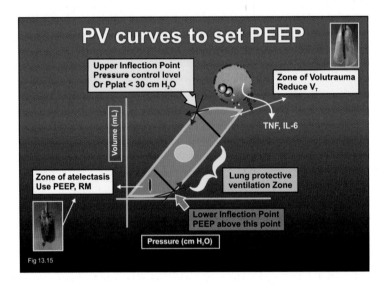

Fig 13.15

The lower inflection point of the inflation limb has been shown to be the point of massive alveolar recruitment and is therefore an option for setting PEEP. However, it is becoming widely accepted that the upper inflection point (UIP) of the deflation limb of the PV curve represents the point of optimal PEEP. The lower inflection point was believed to reflect the pressure level at which collapse of alveoli occurred during expiration and then re-opened during the next inspiration. This was considered to cause damage, referred to as atelectrauma. At the top of the PV curve, compliance decreased and this upper inflection point was considered to occur when the lung was overinflated. It was considered that tidal ventilation and PEEP should be set so that end expiratory pressure is above the lower inflection point to prevent cyclic collapse of alveoli and the end-inspiratory pressure be kept less than UIP to avoid over-distension.

PV curve limitations

The influence of volume history on recruitment, which considers PEEP, tidal volume and the respiratory rate, should be taken into consideration to better understand and interpret information reflected by the PV curve recorded from zero end-expiratory pressure.

PV curve represents the behavior of all alveoli within the heterogeneous lung. The contours of the static PV loop (comprised of two quite different inspiratory and expiratory limbs) obscure very important regional differences. Alveoli in dependent regions are most susceptible to collapse and those in nondependent regions are vulnerable to overdistention. This variability of opening pressures helps account for the zones (rather than points) of lower and upper inflection.

Positive End-Expiratory Pressure

Recruitment and overdistention coexist at virtually all lung volumes across the inspiratory capacity range. Although the expiratory curve contours have more appeal, there currently exists little evidence that it will prove to be the long-sought clinical tool for identifying the "optimum recruitment" point. Identifying "inflection points" on PV curve is difficult. LIP on the PV curve may be due to reflex broncho-constriction, pneumo-constriction, peri-bronchial edema or extreme expiratory flow limitation which diminishes the accuracy of the PV curves. The LIP is no longer considered a theoretically valid (or practically useful) guide to PEEP selection. LIP is used as starting point for PEEP application. PEEP settings are fine tuned empirically incorporating multiple indicators of response and recruitment maneuver (Fig 13.16).

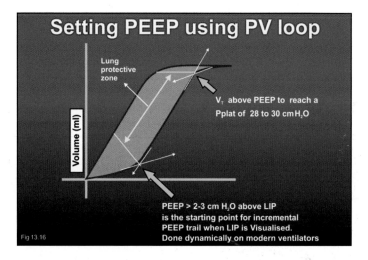

Fig 13.16

PEEP/ FiO$_2$ Table

Another way of setting PEEP is described by ARDS net which uses a protocolized alternating increase of PEEP and inspired oxygen fraction (FiO$_2$). This has been validated by studies. This approach is certainly user friendly, but there is some concern that it does not truly optimize the PEEP setting (Fig 13.17).

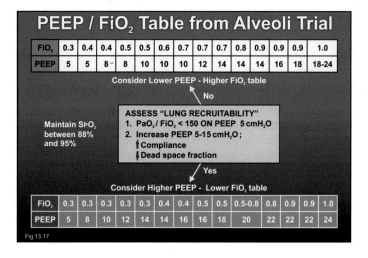

Fig 13.17

Limitations of PEEP/FiO₂ table

PEEP nonresponders recruit little (and arterial PaO$_2$ improves little) in response to higher levels of PEEP. Due to fixed pairings of PEEP and FiO$_2$ in these patients a FiO$_2$ rise which is optimal will result in higher PEEP and risk of overdistension. Whereas, in PEEP responders who recruit well in response to higher levels of PEEP, the PEEP rises which is required, comes along with higher FiO$_2$ and risk of oxygen toxicity.

"Stress index method"

Stress index is a method adopted in new generation ventilators (Maquet Servo-I) which helps in monitoring PEEP induced recruitment and avoids over distension. Stress index is done on a passive patient on volume controlled ventilation with constant flow and observing pressure over time graph. This method is based on the observation that during constant-flow insufflation, the rate of change of pressure at the airway corresponds to the rate of change in respiratory-system compliance. Accordingly, if the graph is linear it is considered as normal and stress index is equal to one. If the graph shows upward concavity it indicates decreased compliance due to lung over distension and stress index is more than one. If the graph shows downward concavity, it indicates increased compliance and potential for alveolar recruitment and the stress index is less than one (Fig 13.18).

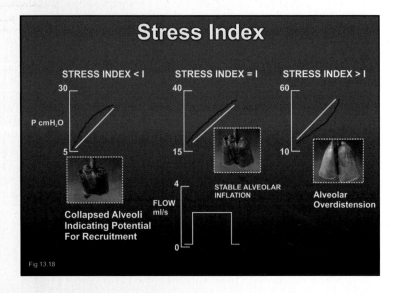

Fig 13.18

Stress index merely considers the inspiratory part of the breath. There may also be some doubts as to whether airway resistance is constant during inspiration.

Measurement of PEEP induced alveolar recruitment

The goal of PEEP therapy is to ensure that PEEP recruits "recruitable" alveoli but not over distends alveoli that are already open. This depends on the recruitability potential of the diseased alveoli. The question is, can it be measured at the bedside? Research is on and experts have proposed the following methods for doing this:

1. CT scan
2. P-V curve
3. Volumetric capnography

4. Dynamic estimation of FRC
5. Electrical impedance tomography
6. Positron emission tomography (PET) scan

'Gold standard' measurement of recruitment is End Expiratory CT scan, which is done by obtaining End Expiratory Spiral CT scan of whole lung at ZEEP and set PEEP. Then the respective volumes are compared. This method is cumbersome and carries a high risk of hypoxemia when PEEP is reduced to zero. There is additional risk involved in transporting the patient to radiology unit. The PV curve method needs construction of two static PV curves (at PEEP and ZEEP). These two curves must be plotted in the same volume-pressure coordinate system in order to relate both of them to the functional residual capacity (FRC) of the respiratory system at the time of testing. Therefore, the difference between the end-expiratory lung volume during mechanical ventilation at PEEP and the FRC must be assessed. This is achieved by disconnecting the patient from the ventilator and measuring the exhaled volume during a prolonged expiration at atmospheric pressure.

Electrical impedance tomography, Volumetric capnography, Dynamic FRC estimation and Positron emission tomography scan are being popularised for clinical practice. Is recruitment a therapeutic goal at all is controversial and warrants further clinical investigation.

Performing these measurements at bedside is difficult. ARDS network protocol for managing ALI/ARDS recommends monitoring of plateau pressures. Plateau pressures can be easily estimated at bedside and use of plateau pressure has been validated in many studies.

Weaning PEEP

PEEP should not be weaned in patients requiring a FiO_2 higher than 0.5 and those with worsening gas exchange. Attempts to wean PEEP should be initiated once there is partial reversibility of the disease process. PEEP should be withdrawn cautiously in steps of 2 cm H_2O with oximetry or arterial blood gas monitoring at each step change. A patient who has shown only marginal PEEP response is a possible exception to these guidelines. Abrupt or premature withdrawal of PEEP can cause deterioration of gas exchange which may respond slowly to reinstitution of PEEP. Sudden termination of PEEP also can cause cardiovascular overload and increase the work of breathing that will result in airway flooding with alveolar fluids. Once PEEP levels are below 10 cm H_2O, a spontaneous breathing trail (SBT) can be instituted after assessing other weaning parameters.

Conclusion

Since its introduction, PEEP has remained a topic of extensive study and intense debate. PEEP is used not only to enhance oxygenation but also to prevent VILI. It decreases the number units at risk for atelectrauma. PEEP should be applied to almost all patients requiring mechanical ventilation barring a few exceptions. The method of choosing optimal PEEP is still empirical. Optimum PEEP is one which does not decrease tissue oxygen delivery.

References

1. Principles and Practice of Mechanical Ventilation, 2nd edition. Martin J. Tobin.
2. Selecting the right level of positive end-expiratory pressure in patients with acute respiratory distress syndrome. JEAN
3. Jacques rouby, Qin lu, and Ivan Goldstein. Am J Respir Crit Care Med; Vol 165: pp 1182–1186, 2002
4. Measurement of pressure–volume curves in patients on mechanical ventilation: methods and significance. Qin Lu and Jean-Jacques Rouby. Crit Care 2000, 4:91–100

5. Measurement of PEEP-induced alveolar recruitment: just a research tool? Michele De Michele and Salvatore Grasso. Critical Care 2006, 10:148
6. Dynamic Functional Residual Capacity can be estimated using a Stress Strain Approach. Computer Methods and Programs in Biomedicine. Volume 101, Issue 2
7. Critical Care Medicine: The Essentials, John J. Marini, Arthur P. Wheeler

★ ★ ★

14. MECHANICAL VENTILATION

A : CHRONIC OBSTRUCTIVE PULMONARY DISEASE (COPD)

Krupesh N, *Senior consultant Department of critical care*
KR Hospital, Bangalore, India.
Chandrashekar TR

Global initiative for obstructive lung disease (GOLD) defines COPD as "a disease state characterized by airflow limitation that is not fully reversible". The airflow limitation is usually progressive and is associated with an abnormal inflammatory response of lungs to noxious particles or gases. COPD is a preventable and treatable disease. Still unfortunately, it is the only chronic disease that is showing a progressive upward trend in both mortality and morbidity.

COPD patients periodically suffer from mild to severe exacerbations. This leads to respiratory failure requiring ICU admission and subsequent mechanical ventilation. Exacerbations may be due to infections, fever or pollutants. These patients may require ventilator support if they undergo cardiac/thoracic surgeries, develop sepsis, suffer from drug over dosage or hyponatremia resulting in aspiration. These patients have some unique problems such as acid-base disturbances, a propensity for dynamic hyperinflation, auto-PEEP, barotrauma, difficult weaning and poor prognosis following mechanical ventilation. COPD is a lung disease with many systemic manifestations which have a bearing on mechanical ventilation and weaning. Figure 14A.1 below lists the systemic effects of COPD.

Extra-pulmonary manifestations of COPD

Loss of weight Cachexia	Cancer
Sleep disorders Depression Anxiety	Cardiac arrhythmias Ischemic heart disease Heart failure
Gastro-oesophageal reflux Chronic anemia or Polycythemia	Osteoporosis Peripheral muscle weakness

Fig : 14A.1

COPD patients already optimized with medical therapy and supplemental oxygen may still require mechanical ventilation under certain circumstances. They include unbearable breathlessness at rest, signs of respiratory distress like increased respiratory rate (> 30/min), accessory muscle usage, paradoxical breathing, increased heart rate and arterial blood gas findings of worsening hypercarbia and acidosis.

Goals of Mechanical Ventilation

- To support overloaded Ventilator pump
- To improve pH and arterial blood gases
- To relieve dyspnea and unload the respiratory muscles
- To "buy time" for the cause of acute exacerbation to resolve by using appropriate ventilator settings

Goals for Ventilator Settings

- Minimize air-trapping
- Avoid over-distention, (P_{plat} < 30 cm H_2O)
- Provide adequate oxygenation, (SpO_2 86% to 92%)
- Provide adequate ventilation (pH > 7.25)

Mechanical Ventilation is a challenge in COPD patients as they have a unique set of problems

- Disease may not have a reversible component
- Quantifying dynamic hyperinflation at bedside is difficult
- COPD patients are difficult to wean
- Steroid induced myopathy resulting in weaning difficulty
- Presence of co-morbidities

Pathophysiology of COPD and its significance

COPD patient have airway inflammation, damage and easy collapsibility. This causes expiratory flow limitation. These patients also have parenchymal destruction which leads to loss of alveolar attachments and decrease in elastic recoil (decreased ability to push out air). Consequent to these two problems there is an increase in functional residual capacity (FRC or EELV) and PEEPi. The relative importance of each component varies from patient to patient.

COPD patients with increased FRC have a higher alveolar pressure. The inspiratory muscles have to work against this pressure to push air into the alveoli. As long as they are capable of doing this, hypercapnia and respiratory failure do not ensue. As fatigue sets in, the patient goes into respiratory failure.

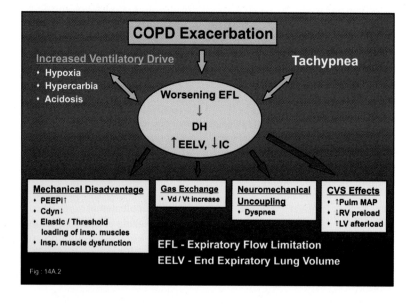

Fig : 14A.2

Mechanical factors like flattened diaphragm and horizontal ribs make the respiratory pump less effective compounding the problem (Refer Fig 14A.2). The mechanism of hypercapnia and hypoxia are illustrated in Fig 14A.3.

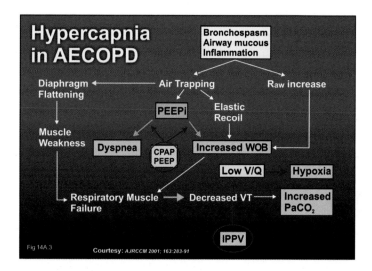

Fig 14A.3   Courtesy: AJRCCM 2001; 163:283-91

Increasing FRC encroaches on the total lung capacity (TLC) (Fig 14A.4). There is a decrease in space available for new tidal volume to enter the lung. Therefore a low tidal volume should be used. This leads to hypercapnia (permissible). According to current literature the risk of dynamic hyperinflation is much more than those of permissive hypercapnia. In fact providing sufficient ventilation to maintain pH more than 7.15 to 7.20 is the goal and not normalization of $PaCO_2$. Increasing the breath rate will shorten the time available for expiration (E-Time). Therefore, the breath rate should be maintained around 10-12/min.

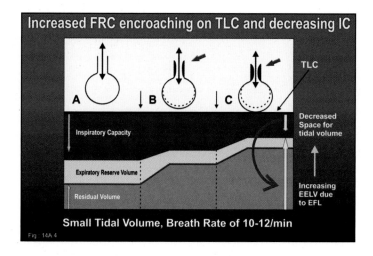

Fig 14A.4

Physiological rationale of mechanical ventilation in COPD

In COPD patients with increased FRC, breathing occurs on the flatter portion of PV curve leading to increased work of breathing (WOB) and dyspnea. This is corrected by application of external PEEP (EPAP). Inspiratory muscle loading and failure lead to respiratory failure. This is corrected by application of inspiratory positive pressure (IPAP). Simply put, "in COPD the load is expiratory but failure is inspiratory". We can ventilate COPD patients scientifically and appropriately, only if we understand the effects of gas trapping, quantify it and limit its effect.

Effects of intrinsic PEEP

- Hemodynamic compromise
- Increased WOB
- Failure to trigger results in missed breaths and wasted WOB

Hemodynamic changes due to gas trapping

Gas trapping leads to decreased venous return, reduced left ventricular preload and compression of heart resulting in decreased cardiac output. Compression of pulmonary vessels causes increased pulmonary vascular resistance causing right heart failure (corpulmonale) and V/Q mismatch. Also, interpretation of hemodynamic values is difficult.

Increased WOB and missed breaths

Mechanically compromised less effective respiratory pump and increased alveolar pressure increase the work of breathing (WOB). Increased FRC and PEEPi, in patients with pneumatic triggers lead to failure to trigger breaths, missed breaths and wasted WOB. This is illustrated in Fig 14A.5

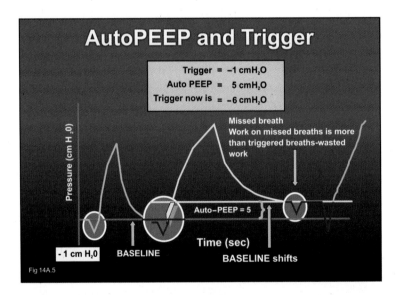

Fig 14A.5

Identifying PEEPi

Clinical circumstances in which PEEPi should be suspected:

- Unexplained tachycardia, hypotension or pulseless electrical activity, especially on initiation of mechanical ventilatory support
- Appearance of increased effort to trigger each breath
- Patient's inspiratory effort does not trigger airflow from the ventilator every time. Clinically, one

can observe active expiration or wheeze that continues up to the onset of inspiration
- If one is monitoring with a graphics display, expiratory flow would still be present at the time of initiation of next breath

In patients not actively attempting to breathe (passive patients):
- PEEPi (determination of end-expiratory occlusion pressure) should be measured by activating end-expiratory pause button on ventilator. 1 to 3 seconds occlusion time allows the trapped air to equilibrate across most obstructed airways (Fig 14A.6)
- Trapped volume is estimated by subtracting, tidal volume from volume estimated during apneic phase lasting for 30 to 50 seconds. This is illustrated in (Fig 14A.7)

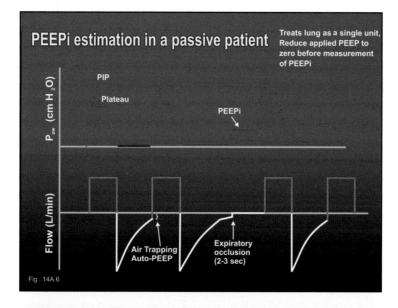

Fig : 14A.6

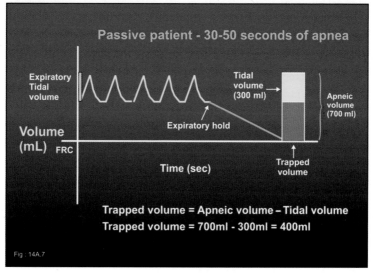

Fig : 14A.7

Due to wide spread airway closure, measured auto PEEP may not reflect the actual problem present in the patient (Fig 14A.8). This should be borne in mind as the measured auto PEEP and clinical scenarios may not correlate in many situations.

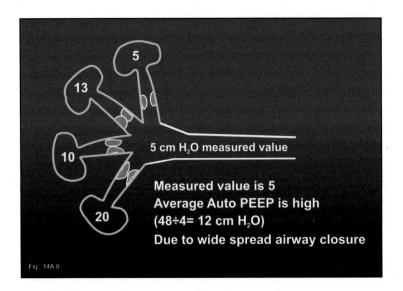

Fig: 14A.8

Modalities to limit PEEPi
- Low tidal volume
- Low breath rate
- Increase expiratory time
- Increase peak flow
- Addition of extrinsic PEEP
- Effective pain, anxiety and fever management to decrease CO_2 production
- Bronchodilators and optimal medical therapy

The 3 important factors which determine PEEPi are
1. Minute ventilation ($V_T \times RR$) - tidal volume is the most important determinant of PEEPi, respiratory rate is a minor culprit
2. I: E [Inspiratory: Expiratory] ratio
3. Expiratory time constants

In fact, rest of the parameters listed work by altering the above 3 parameters indirectly.

Minute ventilation

What is the most frequently changed ventilator settings if $PaCO_2$ increases in COPD patient?

Increase in minute ventilation (tidal volume or respiratory rate). Does this work?

Let us look at an example (Fig 14A.9).

A COPD patient on ventilator in volume control mode with the settings shown below had high $PaCO_2$ and pH. The minute ventilation was changed. Repeat ABG after 1 hr shows increased $PaCO_2$ and decreased PaO_2 and pH.

Why did this happen?

Mechanical Ventilation

Ventilator Settings	Initial Settings	New Settings
Tidal volume	400 ml	500ml
Breath rate	10/min	15/min
I:E ratio	1:2	1:2
PEEP	4 cm H$_2$O	4 cm H$_2$O
FiO$_2$	40%	40%
Minute ventilation (V$_T$ x RR)	400 x10=4L	500x15=7.5L
PaO$_2$/ PaCO$_2$/ pH	56 mmHg / 78 mmHg / 7.18	53 mmHg / 89mmHg / 7.09
Dead space	+	++

Fig 14A.9

We have learnt that CO$_2$ removal is proportional to Minute Ventilation. Is this statement always true? No. Let's analyze why (Fig 14A.10)?

Initial Settings	Changed Settings
Tidal volume - 400 ml, Breath rate - 10/min	Tidal volume - 500 ml, Breath rate - 15/min
E time= 4 seconds	E time= 2.6 seconds
One total cycle time (TCT) = 60 seconds / 10 breath rate = 6 seconds	TCT = 60 seconds / 15 breath rate = 4 seconds

Fig : 14A.10

The very reason for changing the settings of the ventilator was that patient had high PaCO$_2$. The reason for this was 400 ml could not come out in 4 seconds. What did we do? We increased the tidal volume (V$_T$) to 500 ml and reduced the E time to 2.6 seconds. This is the reason why both PaCO$_2$ and pH increased. (Can one expect 500 ml to come out in 2.6 seconds?). It is now apparent that increasing the breath rate will decrease the expiratory time (E time). So, a respiratory rate of 10-12/min is used with a low V$_T$ of 6 to 7ml per kg body weight.

Why does air trapping result in increased CO$_2$? There is less space for tidal volume (V$_T$) to be delivered as alveoli are distended. Distended alveoli in turn compress the alveolar vessels leading to increased pulmonary vascular resistance (PVR) and decreased compliance leading to V/Q mismatch (dead space). CO$_2$ removal is proportional to Effective Alveolar Ventilation.

(Effective Alveolar Ventilation = Minute Ventilation – Deadspace Ventilation).
Coming back to the example, what should have been changed? The answer is increasing I–E ratio to 1:3 or more, or even a decrease in tidal volume (V_T).

Expiratory time constant (ETC)

ETC calculations (Fig 14A.11) help determine the time required for the delivered V_T to empty from the alveoli. Serial tracking of ETC when expiratory time is increased or minute ventilation is decreased ($V_T \times RR$) helps the clinician to fine tune the settings. ETC estimation helps the bedside clinician to know the reversibility component of the disease and response to bronchodilators and other drugs.

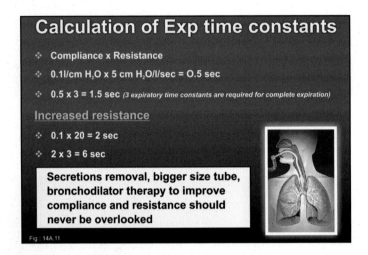
Fig : 14A.11

We have learnt that Flow × Time= Volume delivered. When volume is constant, if the flow is increased, time required to deliver that volume decreases (inspiratory time) giving more time for expiration. Consequently the peak pressure increases, but not the plateau pressure because most of the applied pressure is dissipated to overcome the airway resistance. Peak inspiratory pressures (PIP) up to 50 to 60 cm H_2O is acceptable in COPD patients. Same phenomenon is reflected as 'rise time' in pressure modes (Fig 14A.12).

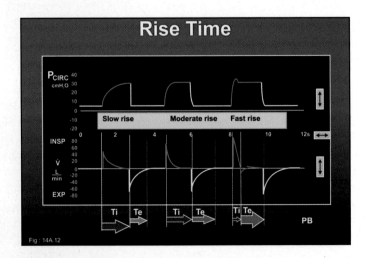
Fig : 14A.12

Mechanical Ventilation

In the example below (Fig 14A.13 and Fig 14A.14) the peak flow is increased from 30 L/min to 90 L/min. This decrease in number of missed breaths is because of decreased inspiratory time and long expiratory time.

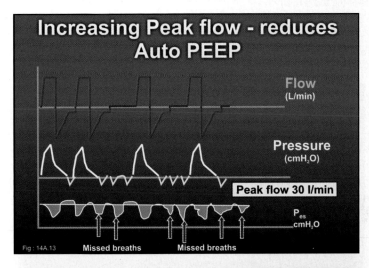

Fig: 14A.13

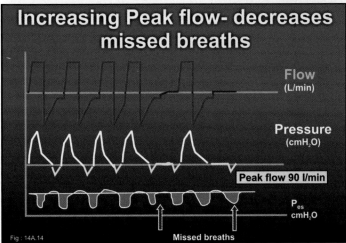

Fig: 14A.14

Applied or extrinsic PEEP in COPD

It is not well understood how extrinsic PEEP counteracts intrinsic PEEP. It is hypothesized that it works by splinting the airways, reducing the lung heterogeneity and opening up previously closed alveolar units. This is supposed to help in mucus clearance and efficaciously deliver bronchodilators to the diseased, constricted lung units.

To counteract the estimated PEEPi, 80% of it should be set as the extrinsic PEEP. Use of expiratory and accessory muscles by the patient during spontaneous breathing increase the force applied to airways. This causes collapse of airways and exaggerates the EFL. Hence, extrinsic PEEP is effective. There is no muscle activity during controlled ventilation. Therefore, applied PEEP should be used cautiously, if at all.

Setting PEEP to Counterbalance Auto-PEEP (Fig 14A.15)

PEEP is set by measuring peak inspiratory pressure (PIP) and plateau pressure (P_{plat}) while increasing PEEP in increments of 2 cm H_2O. If PIP and P_{plat} do not change, the set PEEP is below auto-PEEP. If PIP and/or P_{plat} go up with addition of external PEEP, auto-PEEP level has exceeded. PEEP has to be reduced by 2 cm of H_2O (only PIP can be measured if, patients are actively attempting to breathe). In spontaneously breathing patients, PEEP should be increased until there are no missed trigger efforts.

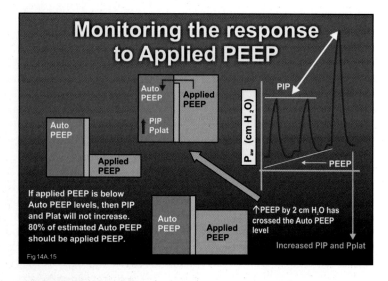

How to decide whether patient requires noninvasive ventilation (NPPV) or intubation and invasive ventilation (Fig 14A.16)?

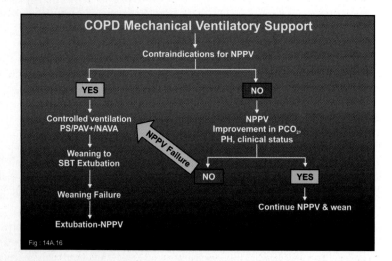

NPPV is the ventilation modality of first choice to treat properly selected patients with COPD exacerbations. Many studies have shown that NPPV decreases intubation rate and mortality.

NPPV prerequisites:
1. Establish the need for ventilatory assistance
2. Moderate-to-severe respiratory distress
   - Tachypnea (respiratory rate > 24 breaths/min)
   - Accessory muscle use or abdominal paradox
3. Blood gas derangement
   - pH < 7.35 and >7.25 show best benefit
   - $PaCO_2$ > 45 mm Hg or a 10 to 20 mm Hg increase from the baseline $PaCO_2$ values, or PaO_2/FiO_2 < 200 mm Hg
4. Exclude patients with contraindications to NPPV
   - Respiratory arrest
   - Medically unstable (septic or cardiogenic shock, uncontrolled upper GI bleed, acute myocardial infarction with planned intervention, uncontrolled arrhythmia)
   - Unable to protect airway
   - Excessive secretions
   - Uncooperative or agitated
   - Unable to fit mask
   - Recent upper-airway or upper-gastrointestinal surgery

Mode and Settings

Controlled and assisted modes can be used for NPPV in COPD patients. Pressure support is the commonest mode used for NPPV. PAV+ has been studied for NPPV use and the results are encouraging. NAVA is a very promising mode with its unique electrical triggering (EAdi). It scores over all other modes in circumventing triggering issues due to leaks and PEEPi. COPD patients are mouth breathers, so full-face mask should be used initially, changing to a nasal mask after 24 hours as the patient improves. If the patient is likely to deteriorate within minutes after removal of the mask, a closely monitored setting such as an intensive care unit should be used for instituting NPPV. A selection of different sizes and types of interfaces should be available for success of NPPV. A helmet interface is preferable as studies have proved good result with this interface in COPD patients. Refer Fig 14A.17 for example of NPPV setting.

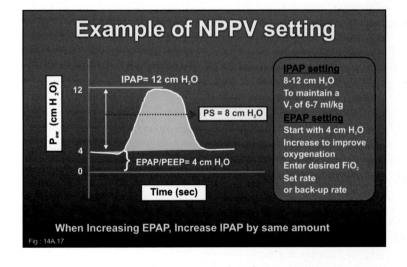

Fig: 14A.17

Indications for Invasive Mechanical Ventilation

1. NPPV failure
2. NPPV contraindicated
   - Inability to protect airway
   - Hemodynamic instability
   - Impaired consciousness
   - Confusion/agitation/vomiting
   - Copious respiratory secretions
3. Life-threatening hypoxemia
4. Severe acidosis (pH < 7.1)
5. Respiratory arrest
6. Somnolence, impaired mental status
7. Cardiovascular complications (hypotension, shock, heart failure).

A prompt and decisive decision has to be made to intubate patients with NPPV failure or if the patient is not a candidate for NPPV to prevent increased morbidity and mortality. Caution should be exercised when using manual bag ventilation. Tidal insufflations must be small (1/3rd the volume of the ventilation bag = a tidal volume of around 450 ml). Insufflation rate should be low. Rates can be as low as 6–8 per minute. The sound of the exhaled air through the ventilation bag is a good indicator when deciding to initiate the next insufflation. NPPV is not a replacement for intubation or invasive MV. Indications for both forms of support are different.

Ventilatory settings in passive patient

Mode - pressure or volume modes can be used, as we have already learnt, the settings required and their physiological rationale putting them into numbers is easy.

- Tidal volume = 6-7 ml/kg (Reduced space for fresh gas flow- V_T)
- Breath rate =10-12 breaths/min
- I–E ratio =1:3 or more (I time of 0.8-1.2 sec)
- Flow = 80-90/min or high rise time in pressure modes (To shorten I time)
- A PIP = Up to 50-60 cm H_2O acceptable (High flow)
- P_{pl} pressure < 30 cm H_2O
- Minimal sensitivity-Pressure or Flow trigger (NAVA preferable)
- PEEP setting- Start at 3 cm H_2O, and for any further increase always look at PIP and plateau pressure
- Any increase in these pressures, decrease PEEP (Keep a close watch on hemodynamics)
- Adequate fluid resuscitation before induction is mandatory, and a small dose of an inotrope can be administered if patient has cor pulmonale. If patient is administered neuromuscular blockers the same may be continued for a day more.

Ventilatory settings in spontaneously breathing patients

- Pressure support is the commonest mode used, if available NAVA and PAV+ preferable
- Pressure support to generate a tidal volume of 7 ml/kg
- Minimal trigger setting-flow or pressure

- High rise time
- PEEP can be added starting at 3 cm H$_2$O in an increment of 2 cm H$_2$O, rarely more than 8 cm H$_2$O is required
- In pressure support mode Expiratory sensitivity can be set much above the default setting of 25% (>40%) to shorten inspiratory time and add more time for expiration.

Weaning begins when the precipitating factor of the respiratory failure is partially or totally reversed. Factors which increase resistance like size of the tube, deposition of secretions in the tube, kinking or curvature of the tube, presence of elbow-shaped parts and HME filters in the circuit should be avoided.

- Heated humidifiers and metered dose inhalers (MDI) delivered through spacer is essential
- Role of tracheostomy in COPD weaning is uncertain. In presence of marginal respiratory mechanics in COPD, tracheostomy may aid in weaning
- Weaning can be done with PS mode to spontaneous breathing trail (SBT)
- When weaning becomes difficult extubation and use of NPPV is an option
- Weaning corpulmonale patients can be accomplished with a small dose of inotrope, diuretic and low fluid strategy.

Summary of ventilatory settings in COPD (Fig 14A.18)

Summary of setting in COPD patients

COPD patient on controlled or assist mode	Spontaneous breathing COPD patient on ventilator (PS)
Tidal volume- 6-7 ml / kg	Adjust PS level to achieve a Tidal volume of 6-7 ml / kg
Breath rate =10-12/min I: E ratio =1:3 or more (I time of 0.8-1.2 sec)	Increase expiratory sensitivity to more than 40%
Flow = 80 - 90l/min, PIP = 50 - 60 cm H$_2$O	High rise time
Ppl pressure < 30 cm H$_2$O Minimal trigger sensitivity	Ppl pressure < 30 cm H$_2$O Minimal trigger sensitivity
PEEP setting - Start at 2 cm H$_2$O, increments of 2 cm H$_2$O, watch PIP and plateau pressure, any increase in these pressures, decrease PEEP	PEEP can be added starting at 3 cm H$_2$O in an increment of 2 cm H$_2$O, Increase PEEP until there are no missed trigger breaths. More than 8 cm H$_2$O is rarely required.

Fig 14A.18

Conclusion

Mechanical ventilatory support allows patients who have COPD to gain time for pharmacologic treatment to act and to avoid (or recover from) respiratory muscle fatigue. The cornerstone to avoid associated morbidity with mechanical ventilation is to prevent dynamic hyperinflation of the lung. This can be achieved by limiting minute ventilation, maximizing time for expiration and by inducing synchronization between the patient and mechanical ventilator. Two major changes have been advocated in COPD ventilation. The first is use of extrinsic PEEP to counter balance PEEPi. The second is use of NPPV as a standard of care whenever indicated.

References

1. Clinical concise review: Mechanical ventilation of patients with chronic obstructive pulmonary disease.

Nicholas S. Ward, Kevin M. Dushay. Crit Care Med 2008 vol. 36: No. 5.

2. Noninvasive Ventilation for Chronic Obstructive Pulmonary Disease. Nicholas S Hill. Respiratory care. January 2004 vol 49: No 1

3. Exacerbations in COPD: Role of invasive mechanical ventilation. L. Appendeni, A. Pattessio, and C.F. Donner: 2005 Annual update

B : MECHANICAL VENTILATION IN ASTHMA

Asthma and COPD both are diseases characterized by expiratory flow limitation (EFL) but pathophysiologically they are different. In Asthma there is no airway destruction, fibrosis and collapsibility. Airway inflammation causes edema, smooth muscle contraction, increased mucus production, resulting in rigid airway obstruction. Asthma patients exhibit hyper-irritability of airways, exacerbated by injury from viruses, inhaled toxins which denudes airway epithelium and exposes nerve endings causing, increased sensitivity to irritants, viruses, etc (Fig 14B.1 and Fig 14B.2). Asthma is more common in females and younger patients, and the disease is reversible. Due to rigid airway obstruction, ventilator settings have to be set in accordance to this.

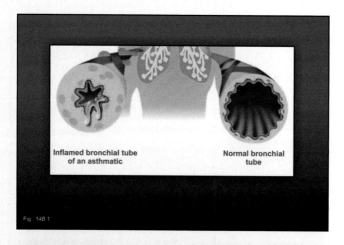

Fig : 14B.1

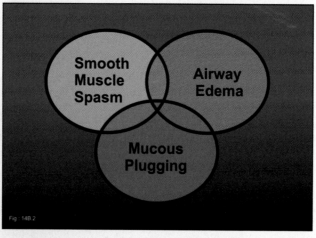

Fig : 14B.2

Mechanical Ventilation

Two major differences in ventilator settings are

A breath rate of 7-12/min is appropriate. When baseline respiratory rate is already low, further reductions will probably have less impact on the improvement of air trapping, because expiratory flow is slower at end-expiration and the prolongation of expiratory time will not significantly improve alveolar emptying. With rigid airway obstruction, no chance for airway collapsibility and absent forced expiratory efforts, zero PEEP (ZEEP) or very low PEEP is advisable in passively ventilated patients. Indeed addition of low levels of PEEP to paralyzed asthmatic patients did not show benefit, higher levels of PEEP that raised FRC being detrimental.

In spontaneously breathing, extrinsic PEEP can be of help by reducing the superimposed WOB caused by PEEPi, and by keeping the airway open against the dynamic collapse caused by forced expiratory efforts. Only when some degree of COPD coexists, as in older asthmatics and cigarette smokers, does the use of PEEP contribute to compensate for the loss of elastic recoil, keeping small airways open against adjacent hyperinflated lung units? The reaction of airway pressure and expiratory flow to a PEEP trial will help to decide if it has a role in reducing hyperinflation or if its use will be detrimental. If airway pressure rises proportionally to the amount of PEEP added and expiratory flow does not approach zero at end-expiration, PEEP should be removed. Conversely, if total pressure does not increase and expiratory flow improves, the level of PEEP that reverses auto PEEP should be maintained. Rest of the settings and principles of ventilation are same as in COPD patients.

Use of NPPV in asthma

There is no strong evidence supporting the use of non-invasive pressure support ventilation for severe asthmatic exacerbations. Non-randomized, observational studies have shown improvement in clinical parameters (heart and respiratory rate), and gas exchange (PCO_2) using non-invasive pressure support ventilation with low levels of PEEP (3 to 5 cm H_2O) and moderate levels of pressure support (8 to 12 cm H_2O). Therefore, before intubation is finally required, it seems reasonable to perform a trial of non-invasive pressure support ventilation in selected patients.

As when using non-invasive pressure support ventilation for other indications, the time of initiation and the comfort of the patient with the mask are key elements for the success of the technique.

Weaning should occur as soon as the patient's condition allows. Barring contraindications, patients should be extubated once they successfully complete spontaneous breathing trial.

Conclusion

Accurate management of mechanical ventilation in acute asthma is extremely important, since mechanical ventilation is fraught with the occurrence of life-threatening complications frequently, and has a great influence on outcome. Extreme caution is required during endotracheal intubation and manual bag ventilation, particularly avoiding high insufflation volumes and allowing sufficient time for expiration. Identification and accurate measurement of air trapping allows correct setting of the ventilator, the analysis of the expiratory flow trace and the identification of alveolar and end expiratory pressures being essential. Minute ventilation must be low, as well as respiratory rate, in order to reduce hyperinflation.

References

1. Mechanical Ventilation for Acute Asthma Exacerbations. D. De Mendoza, M. Lujan, and J. Rello. Yearbook of Intensive Care and Emergency Medicine.

2. Management of Life-Threatening Asthma in Adults. Praveen Mannam and Mark D. Siegel. Journal of Intensive Care Medicine, 25(1): 3-15: 2010.
3. Clinical review: Mechanical ventilation in severe asthma. David R Stather and Thomas E Stewart. Critical Care; December 2005; Vol 9; No 6.

C : MECHANICAL VENTILATION IN SEVERE BRAIN INJURY

Severe head injury patients having a Glasgow coma scale (GCS) of less than or equal to 8, need intubation and mechanical ventilation because they are unable to protect the airways and are at high risk of developing aspiration of oropharyngeal contents leading to aspiration pneumonias, atelectasis, and patients who develop acute lung injury due to neurogenic pulmonary edema require mechanical ventilation.

Goals of mechanical ventilation of (acute) severely brain injured patients:

1. Maintaining adequate oxygenation (Normal PaO_2 levels)
2. Maintaining eucapnia (Normal $PaCO_2$ levels)
3. Minimizing intrathoracic pressure.
4. Protect cerebral perfusion (CPP = MAP−ICP)

(Cerebral perfusion pressure = Mean arterial pressure−Intracranial pressure)

Traditional ventilation strategy for severe brain injury and lung protective ventilation strategy have conflicting paradigms as mentioned in Fig 14C.1

Historical "Brain-directed" strategy	Lung Protective Ventilation

❖ Optimize oxygen delivery
❖ Control of PCO_2
   (higher V_T and V_E)
❖ Minimize potential effects of PEEP
	❖ Avoid overdistention
	   (Volutrauma)
	❖ Open the lung
	❖ Avoid cyclical collapse
	   (Atelectrauma)

Fig 14C.1

Two Parameters, most concern in severe head injury

1. $PaCO_2$
2. PEEP

$PaCO_2$ is of a concern because, hypercarbia may worsen cerebral hyperemia and which in turn raises intracranial pressures leading to herniation, in order to prevent this prophylactic hyperventilation was considered in earlier days but recent studies have shown that prolonged pulmonary hyperventilation must be avoided in the absence of high ICP as sustained vasoconstriction reduces

CBF to deleterious levels and could generate brain ischemia. The consensus is that optimized hyperventilation for a short time is considered for patients with high ICP and the causal factor for increase of ICP must be sought and efforts be made to treat it. The ideal value for $PaCO_2$ is the one that keeps ICP < 20 mm Hg and $PaCO_2$ must be kept at 35 mm Hg to 40 mm Hg while hyperventilation is reserved for cases with high ICP and herniation risk. Prophylactic hyperventilation ($PaCO_2$ of 25 mm Hg or less) is not recommended

Role of PEEP in severe brain injury

Brain injured patients may have associated lung, chest complications as a part of primary injury or as secondary complication and may need significant levels of PEEP to maintain oxygenation. In normal cerebral circulation, a vascular waterfall has been postulated in which the intracranial pressure acts as the effective upstream pressure. To increase intracranial pressure, PEEP must raise downstream venous pressure. Consequently, if baseline intracranial pressure is greater than the intrathoracic pressure caused by PEEP, the technique will not affect intracranial pressure. Similarly, if the head is elevated 30° above the heart it promotes intracranial venous drainage via anterior neck veins, as well as the vertebral venous system which is not majorly affected by ITP. Jugular veins collapse and act as resistors to some of the ITP transmitted and increase in PEEP will not increase intracranial pressure (Fig 14C.2).

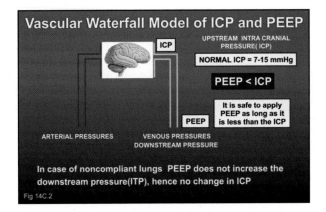

Fig 14C.2

Hemodynamic Effects of PEEP on intracranial pressure (ICP) (Fig 14C.3)

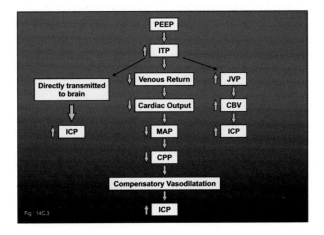

Fig: 14C.3

Bed side management flow chart (Fig 14C.4)

	NORMAL ICP	RAISED ICP
Begin with	Normocapnia Low V_T (6 ml/kg) Limit Pplat <30 cm H_2O	Normocapnia Low V_T (6 ml/kg) Limit Pplat<30 cm H_2O
Raising $PaCO_2$	Moderate Hypercarbia Follow ICP Remove excess dead space Sedation / Ensure synchrony Drain large effusions / ascites	Consider increasing V_T Normocarbia Follow ICP Remove excess dead space Sedation / Ensure synchrony Drain large effusions / ascites
Next	Alternative modes, prioritizing lung protection (but following ICP)	Alternative modes, prioritizing CO_2 elimination

Fig : 14C.4

Conclusions

1. Prolonged hyperventilation must be avoided if ICP is not high and hyperventilation for short period can be used if ICP is very high with high risk of herniation. Brain oxygenation should be monitored if hyperventilation is used.
2. PEEP can be used safely up to 15 cm H_2O to improve oxygenation but a high level of PEEP needs ICP monitoring.
3. Protective lung ventilation when indicated must be considered without hesitation. Studies have proved that high levels of PEEP increase ICP but do not cause reduction in CPP.
4. Increasing the oxygen supply to supraphysiological levels is not recommended.

References

1. Management of mechanical ventilation in brain injury: hyperventilation and positive end expiratory pressure. Rev Bras Ter Intensiva.
2. Mechanical ventilation and the injured brain. South Afr J Anaesth Analg 2011;17(1) 009; 21 (1): 72-79.
3. Transmission of intrathoracic pressure to intracranial pressure. Koehler RC, Michael JR. Clin Crit Care 1985; 1:212-214
4. The lung and the brain: a dangerous cross-talk. Pelosi and Rocco. Critical Care 2011 15:168

D : MECHANICAL VENTILATION IN CHEST TRAUMA

Chest trauma is a significant cause of morbidity and mortality across the globe. The lethality of isolated chest traumas is about 5% to 8%. Up to 25% of all deaths caused by trauma are related to chest injuries, direct forces, abrupt deceleration and other mechanisms can cause injury to thoracic structures like major intrathoracic vessels, lungs or the heart. Chest injuries often occur in combination with other severe injuries, such as extremity, head, brain and abdominal. The most common causes among these are Flail chest, pulmonary contusion and bronchoplural fistula (Fig 14D.1).

Non - Penetrating Chest Injuries	Penetrating Chest Injuries
Rib facture (flail chest)	Pneumothorax
Pneumothorax	Aortic tears
Pulmonary and cardiac contusion	Vena caval tears

Fig 14D.1

Flail chest

A flail chest, by definition, involves 3 or more consecutive rib fractures, in 2 or more places, which produces a free-floating, unstable segment of chest wall. Separation of the bony ribs from their cartilaginous attachments, termed costochondral separation, can also cause flail chest. Patient complains of pain at the fracture sites, pain upon inspiration and dyspnea. Examination reveals paradoxical motion of the flail segment. The chest wall moves inward with inspiration and outward with expiration. A significant amount of force is required to produce a flail segment and most of the times will be associated with underlying lung contusion. Goals of management in chest wall injury are directed towards protecting the underlying lung and maintaining adequate oxygenation, ventilation and pulmonary toilet. All patients with flial chest should initially be placed on 100% oxygen via a non-rebreathing face mask and analgesia is the main stay of treatment, however, some of the patients will have increased work of breathing even after adequate pain control. In such patients, according to the recent Canadian guidelines use of NPPV is not recommended, because of a lack of RCTs. Many experts advocate a trial of NPPV in properly selected patients. Intubation and IPPV is rarely indicated for chest wall injury alone. Whenever ventilation is necessary it is usually for hypoxia due to underlying pulmonary contusions.

Pathophysiology of respiratory failure in chest trauma (Fig 14D.2)

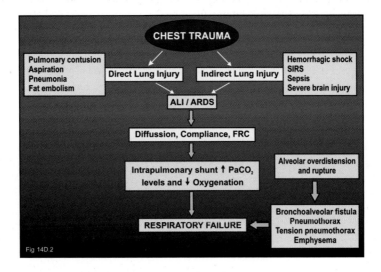

Fig 14D.2

Pulmonary contusion

Pulmonary contusion is an injury to lung parenchyma, leading to edema and blood collecting in alveolar spaces and loss of normal lung structure and function. This blunt lung injury develops over the course of 24 hours, leading to poor gas exchange, increased pulmonary vascular resistance and decreased lung compliance. There is also a significant inflammatory reaction to blood components in the lung and 50-60% of patients with significant pulmonary contusions will develop bilateral ARDS. In younger patients, severe pulmonary contusion can occur without fractures of the bony thorax due to the compliant nature of the thoracic cage. Conversely in elderly patients severe rib fractures and flail segments can be present with minimal underlying pulmonary contusion due to the brittleness of the bones. It is important therefore to recognize pulmonary contusion as a serious but potentially isolated complication following blunt thoracic trauma.

Practical approach to mechanical ventilation in chest trauma (Fig 14D.3)

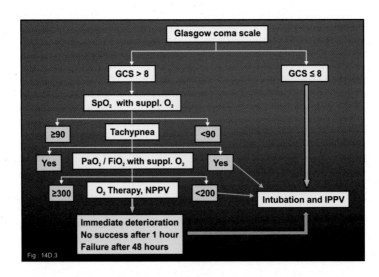

Fig : 14D.3

All patients with pulmonary contusion should be treated with supplemental oxygenation, in patients who do not respond to oxygen therapy, NPPV is an option, which delivers continuous PEEP or CPAP, and prevents atelectasis, maintains functional residual capacity and increases cardiac output. Indications for intubation in case of pulmonary contusion may be worsening oxygenation in spite of CPAP therapy, very high levels of PEEP needed on NPPV. If intubated these patients may need long term management as it takes 2-3 weeks for the lung to recovery. Ventilating strategies in pulmonary contusion is done with lung protective ventilation. Low tidal volumes (tidal volumes of 6 mL/kg of predicted body weight), plateau pressure of less than 30 cm of H_2O, optimal PEEP, and permissive hypercapnia should be followed.

Bronchopleural fistula (BPF)

Bronchopleural fistula may be seen in trauma patients as a part of direct penetrating injury or blunt injury to lungs. BPF occurs after thoracocentesis for hemo/pneumothorax if air bubbling continues even after 24 hr. BPF offers a pathway of least resistance which leads to incomplete lung expansion, loss of tidal volume, loss of PEEP, leading to hypoxemia, respiratory acidosis, V/Q mismatch, and inappropriate cycling of ventilator. Goals of mechanical ventilation in these patients is to reduce mean airway pressure by ventilating with lowest effective tidal volume, shorten inspiratory time, least number of mechanical breaths, limited PEEP. If patients do not respond to conventional ventilation then unconventional ventilation like independent lung ventilation with double lumen tube and conventional ventilation for normal lungs (CPAP) and high frequency jet ventilation for the affected lung can be tried (Fig 14D.4).

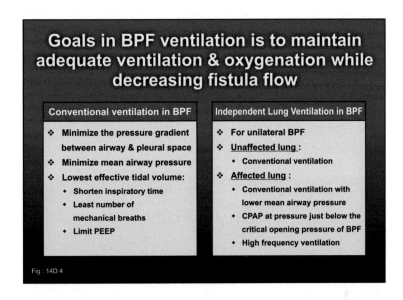

Fig: 14D.4

References

1. British Thoracic Society Standards of Care Committee: Non-invasive ventilation in acute respiratory failure. Thorax 2002;57:192–211.
2. Management of flail chest. Aaron M Ranasinghe, Jonathan AJ Hyde and Timothy R Graham. Trauma ventilation. 2001; 3: 235-247
3. Management of bronchopleural fistula in patients on mechanical ventilation. David J Pierson. 1998
4. Principles and Practice Of Mechanical Ventilation. 2nd edition. Martin. J. Tobin.

E : MECHANICAL VENTILATION IN NEUROMUSCULAR DISEASE (NMD)

Neuromuscular diseases that affect the respiratory system are a major cause of morbidity and mortality in both acute and long-term settings. Long standing congenital and acquired neurological disease can cause respiratory failure requiring ventilator support.

Causes of neuromuscular diseases frequently referred to the ICU (Fig 14E.1)

Neuromuscular Diseases in ICU

ICU - Acquired Weakness (ICU-AW)
- Critical illness polyneuropathy (CIP)
- Critical illness myopathy (CIM)

Pre - Existing
- Guillian-Barré syndrome
- Myasthenia Gravis
- Stroke / drugs
- Tumour
- Multiple sclerosis
- Muscular dystrophies
- Trauma/Spinal cord injuries

Fig 14E.1

Patients with NMD usually have normal respiratory drive and normal lungs. The main problem with these type of patients is respiratory muscle weakness (Fig 14E.2).

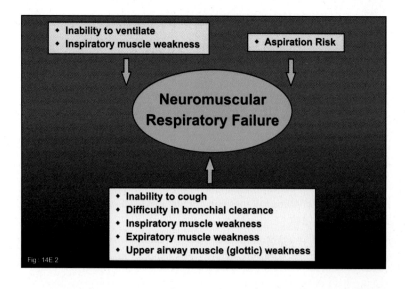

Fig : 14E.2

ICU-acquired weakness (ICU-AW)

ICU-acquired weakness (ICU-AW) is recognized as a major complication of critical illness. Both functional and structural abnormalities in muscle and nerve causing critical illness polyneuropathy and myopathy (CIP and CIM), have been implicated in the development and maintenance of the generalized progressive muscle weakness and atrophy seen in ICU-AW. Neuromuscular weakness typically becomes apparent when an attempt is made to wean the patient from the ventilator, although there are earlier clues, which include grimacing without movement with noxious stimuli before recovery of consciousness, relative lack of movement after regaining consciousness and (not inevitably) loss of deep tendon reflexes that had been present earlier. The presence of severe muscle abnormalities that cannot be fully explained by disuse atrophy or compressive neuropathies suggests that ICUAW may be a primary myogenic problem. It is associated with longer time on ventilator, increased length of stay and increased morbidity and mortality.

Diagnosis

Experts advocate physical examination as the primary determinant of ICU-AW. Symmetric weakness and facial sparing are classical findings, along with difficult to wean and profound weakness despite return of sensorium that causes quadriplegia gives a clue that the patient has developed ICU-acquired weakness (ICU-AW). Patients demonstrating the characteristic examination combined with any evidence of recovery on serial examination usually require no further investigation. Patients with a protracted altered sensorium or fixed motor deficit should undergo further testing for CNS pathology. When a reliable motor examination is not possible muscle biopsy and electrophysiological studies may be warranted.

Risk factors associated with increased incidence for ICU-acquired weakness, are severe systemic inflammation, medications (specifically, corticosteroids and neuromuscular blocking agents), glycemic control and immobility.

Management protocol for ICU-acquired weakness (ICU-AW) (Fig 14E.3)

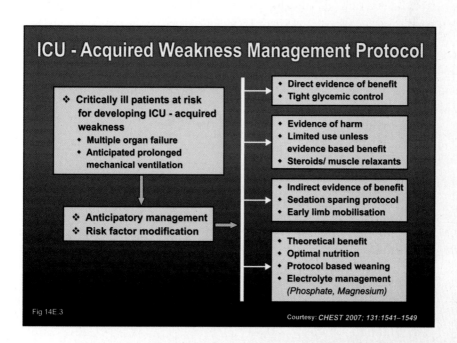

Fig 14E.3

Courtesy: *CHEST 2007; 131:1541–1549*

The most common pre-existing NMD referred to ICU are Guillain-Barré syndrome (GBS) and myasthenia gravis (MG).

Guillain-Barré syndrome (GB syndrome)

Neuromuscular respiratory failure requiring mechanical ventilation occurs in 20% to 30% of GBS patients. The clinician must monitor for clinical signs of impending respiratory failure, including tachypnea, use of accessory muscles of respiration, asynchronous movements of the chest and abdomen and tachycardia. A vital capacity below 20 ml/kg, maximal inspiratory pressure (PI_{max}) less than 30 cm H_2O, or maximal expiratory pressure (PE_{max}) less than 40 cm H_2O predicts imminent respiratory arrest. Time from onset to admission of less than 1 week, facial weakness, inability to cough, inability to lift head off the pillow and atelectasis on chest radiograph are other factors associated with respiratory failure and need for mechanical ventilation. BTS guidelines have advocated the use of NPPV in GBS patients if there are no contraindications. Invasive mechanical ventilation with lung protective strategies is warranted when used. The mean duration of mechanical ventilation for GBS is 2 to 6 weeks. Weaning from the ventilator should follow improvement in serial pulmonary function tests and strength. Plan for tracheostomy should be based on the status of the individual in the context keeping in mind the advantages of the procedure.

Myasthenia gravis (MG)

Complaints of shortness of breath and bulbar dysfunction, especially dysphagia, in patients with MG, especially if they are of recent onset, along with other clinical signs of respiratory failure must be taken very seriously. When accurate measures are possible, patients with a peak negative inspiratory force (NIF) of less than 20 cm (absolute value) H_2O or positive expiratory force (PEF) of < 40 cm H_2O often require tracheal intubation. In general, a low forced vital capacity (especially < 25–30 ml/kg) is worrisome and carefully following FVC in a closely monitored setting is important. Patients with marked bulbar dysfunction that compromises airway protection should be admitted to the intensive care unit even in the absence of overt respiratory failure. It is important to note that endotracheal intubation may be necessary to maintain airway patency in such patients who are having difficulty handling oral secretions even in the absence of overt respiratory failure. Earlier elective intubation may avert the likelihood of requiring emergency intubation and its inherent risks. Use of NPPV, ventilator setting, weaning and tracheostomy principles are same as discussed in GB syndrome section.

Goals of mechanical ventilation in chronic neuromuscular disease:

1. Maintain pulmonary compliance
2. Support muscles of respiration to maintain normal alveolar ventilation

These goals can be achieved with respiratory muscle training with frequent spontaneous breathing trails, cough assist techniques, when respiratory failure ensues, patients may require NPPV and intubation with mechanical ventilation if contraindications to NPPV are present. Ventilator support in chronic NMD patients can be provided with NPPV.

The indications for NPPV are symptoms of fatigue, dyspnea, orthopnea, and early morning headache with either $PaCO_2$ of more than 45 mm Hg or nocturnal desaturation with SpO_2 of less than 88% for 5 consecutive times. The advantage of NPPV includes respiratory muscle rest, improves alveolar ventilation, lung compliance, ventilation/perfusion matching and also avoidance of complications associated with intubation and complications of long term IPPV.

Selection of settings for NPPV in patients with neuromuscular disease is often done based on symptoms of the patient. Initially the NPPV settings are selected based on short-term symptoms such as chest expansion, accessory muscle use, and patients comfort and adjusted later for long term goals. Initially started with low settings and gradually titrated to the patients requirements.

Lung protective ventilator protocols should be implemented when they have acute deterioration in lung status. The ultimate goal in these patients on NPPV is to improve symptoms of morning headache, fatigue and daytime sleepiness (Fig 14E.4).

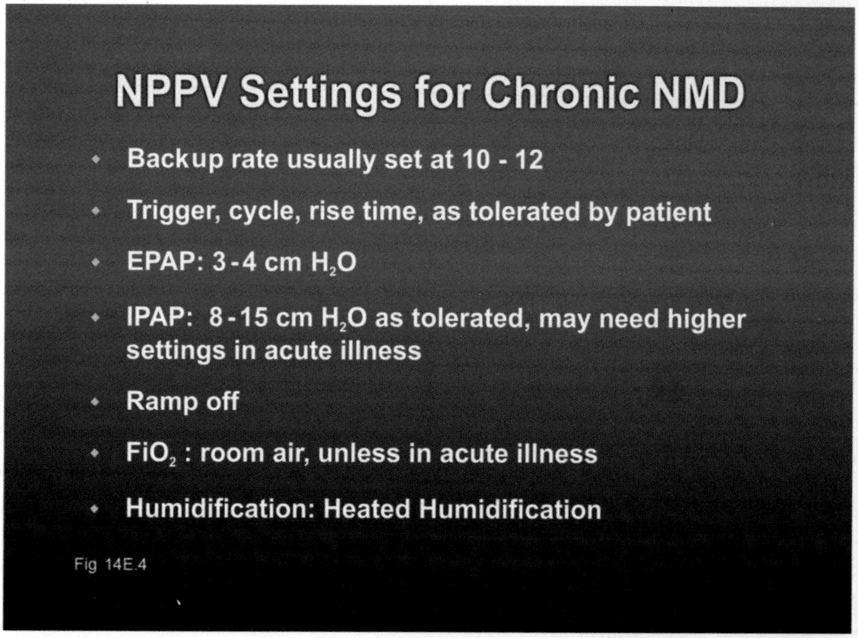

NPPV Settings for Chronic NMD

- Backup rate usually set at 10 - 12
- Trigger, cycle, rise time, as tolerated by patient
- EPAP: 3-4 cm H_2O
- IPAP: 8-15 cm H_2O as tolerated, may need higher settings in acute illness
- Ramp off
- FiO_2: room air, unless in acute illness
- Humidification: Heated Humidification

Fig 14E.4

Conclusion

Many patients with NMD require mechanical ventilation for a short duration till the acute cause is resolved. In some chronic conditions mechanical ventilation may be instituted in the ICU if there is an acute deterioration in the respiratory status with lung protective settings. NPPV and airway clearance in properly selected patients can be life prolonging. Cough and secretions are important determinates of extubation success.

References

1. Noninvasive Ventilation in Neuromuscular Disease. Dean R Hess. Respiratory care: August 2006 vol 51 no 8.
2. Neuromuscular Disease in Respiratory and Critical Care. Nicholas S Hill: Respir Care 2006; 51 (9): 1065–1071.
3. Principles and Practice of Mechanical Ventilation. 2nd edition. Martin.J.Tobin.
4. ICU-Acquired Weakness. William D. Schweickert and Jesse Hall. Chest 2007; 131:1541–1549.

★ ★ ★

NON INVASIVE POSITIVE PRESSURE VENTILATION (NPPV)

Negative pressure ventilators (Iron lung) were used widely in 1950s' during the poliovirus epidemic. These were the fledgling steps of ventilatory management. With improvement in medical knowledge and ventilator technology, positive invasive ventilation became the main stay of ventilator support. In the last decade, non-invasive positive-pressure ventilation (NPPV) has reemerged as the first-line intervention, especially in properly selected patients with certain forms of acute respiratory failure (ARF).

Definition

Non invasive ventilation refers to the delivery of mechanical ventilation to the lungs using techniques that do not require a tracheal airway. Support is provided through patient's upper airway using mask or similar devices.

Advantages of NPPV (Fig 15.1)

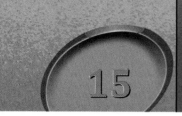

Fig 15.1

Above figure lists the obvious advantages of NPPV over tracheal intubation. NPPV avoids complications of tracheal intubation like airway trauma, sedation, anesthetic usage and stress response. Similarly, complications of endotracheal tube like VAP, gastric aspiration, tracheal stenosis, hoarseness of voice etc. are avoided.

NPPV delivery considerations

Interface

Interfaces are devices that connect ventilator tubing to the patient, facilitating the entry of pressurized gas into the upper airway during NPPV. Interface intolerance and NPPV failure is common because of anatomical variations in patients. Proper sizing of the interface is essential to achieve the best clinical results. Hence, different types of interfaces of various sizes are available in ICUs, administering NPPV as shown in the Fig 15.2.

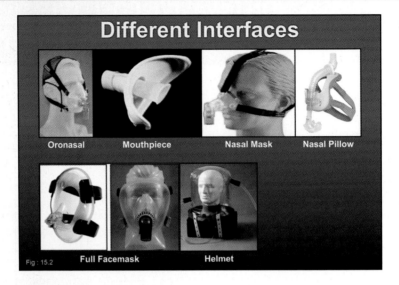

Fig : 15.2

Securing interface devices is essential to maintain comfort as well as safety for the patient. Repeated disconnection or twisting of the interface may decrease patient tolerance of NPPV. Figure 15.3 explains the securing system in face mask type interface.

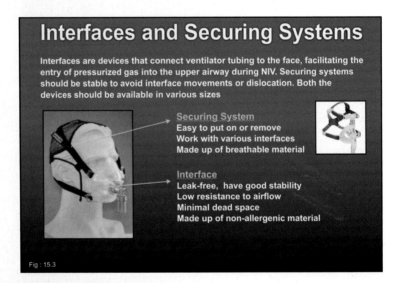

Fig : 15.3

Which Interface system is best for patients?

Guidelines recommend the use of an oronasal mask rather than a nasal mask in patients who have acute respiratory failure, as very dyspneic patients are mouth breathers. A full-face mask should be used initially, changing to a nasal mask after 24 hours as the patient improves.

Whichever mask is chosen, a comfortable fit is of paramount importance. Care must be taken to use the minimum strap tension that achieves an adequate air seal so that pressure sores are avoided. The need for excessive tightening is an indication that the mask is not of the appropriate size or shape to the face. Mask cushions help in increasing comfort and preventing leaks from mouth.

Non Invasive Positive Pressure Ventilation

The choice of NPPV interface requires careful evaluation of the patient, the ventilation mode and of the clinical setting. Individualization is the key in making the right choice of NPPV interface. Care givers must be prepared to try different types and sizes of masks in an effort to enhance patient comfort and NPPV success.

Advantages and disadvantages of different interfaces used for NPPV application (Fig 15.4)

Oronasal Mask

Advantages
- No Mouth leaks
- Less patient cooperation required
- High ventilatory targets tolerated

Disadvantages
- Skin breakdown
- Vomiting & Aspiration
- Increased deadspace
- Claustrophobia

Nasal Mask

Advantages
- Less interference with speech and eating
- Allows cough
- Less danger with vomiting
- Claustrophobia uncommon
- No risk of asphyxia if ventilator malfunctions
- Less likely to cause gastric distension

Disadvantages
- Mouth leaks & dry mouth
- Ineffective ventilation
- Nasal congestion

Fig : 15.4

Similarly, Helmet interface has certain advantages over oronasal mask (Fig 15.5)

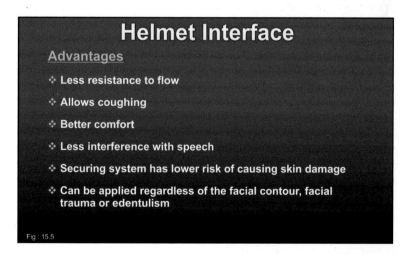

Helmet Interface

Advantages
- Less resistance to flow
- Allows coughing
- Better comfort
- Less interference with speech
- Securing system has lower risk of causing skin damage
- Can be applied regardless of the facial contour, facial trauma or edentulism

Fig : 15.5

Use of helmet has disadvantages like claustrophobia, risk of rebreathing and increased deadspace. Both the external and middle ear are directly exposed to inspiratory positive pressure. This could theoretically expose the middle and inner ear to the risk of mechanical damage. There are also potential ventilator triggering and cycling issues caused by the large compressible volume within the circuit. Helmet is less effective compared to standard interfaces in situations of resistive load and has worse CO_2 clearance. HME filters and earplugs reduce the high noise levels present during helmet usage.

Interface dead space and CO_2 elimination

The issue of dead space is an inherent problem in larger, non-invasive interfaces when directly compared with an endotracheal tube. The dead space volume of the helmet is 10,000 ml and volume of total-face mask is 1500 ml which are relatively large when compared to volume of nasal mask (100 ml), oronasal mask (205 ml) and full-face mask (250 ml). Carbon dioxide rebreathing leads to hypercapnia resulting in higher respiratory drive and increased WOB. For nasal masks or nasal pillow, CO_2 rebreathing is relevant to a lesser extent. The greatest effect is seen in full-face masks, total-face masks and helmet. Effective dead space is not related to the internal gas volume included in the interface suggesting that this internal volume should not be considered as a limiting factor for its efficacy during non-invasive ventilation. CO_2 rebreathing can be reduced by taking a few key factors into consideration. It has been shown that continuous flow throughout the expiration phase reduces total dynamic dead space to almost physiological levels in most face masks. The exhalation port located within the full-face mask was found to be more effective in eliminating CO_2 than the exhalation port located within the circuit.

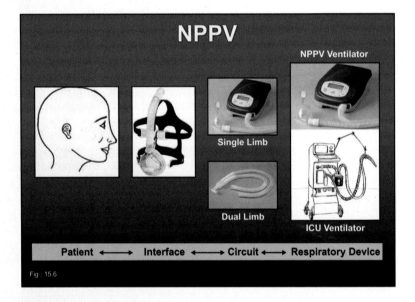

Fig : 15.6

Ventilator circuits

Circuits connect interface to the ventilator. These can be single limb in dedicated NPPV ventilators and dual limb in ICU ventilators (Fig15.6). Carbon dioxide rebreathing is seen in ventilators with a single gas delivery circuit and no true exhalation valve. Dual limb circuits use non-vented mask and do not require exhalation devices. Exhalation devices vent the expired air to the exterior and also introduce an intentional leak in the system to flush the mask and circuit thereby preventing rebreathing. These could either be simple exhalation ports built into the mask or could take the form of a separate attachment in the circuit (whisper Swivel, plateau exhalation valve or non-rebreathing valve). It is important to remember that CO_2 rebreathing can occur with NPPV using standard exhalation valves. Moreover, masks add significant dead space. This should be considered in patient on NPPV who develop unexplained rise of CO_2 (or decrease of CO_2). It can be tackled by either using a non-rebreathing valve or by increasing the level of EPAP, which flushes the mask and circuit. It is important to remember that at commonly used levels of EPAP, especially when the respiratory rate is high, a substantial rebreathing volume may still be present. NPPV breathing is not a closed system. Air leak occurs between the mask and face (unintentional) and through exhalation devices (intentional leak). Air leaks may reduce the efficiency of NPPV by causing reduced tolerance, increased patient-ventilator asynchrony (through loss of triggering sensitivity) and sleep fragmentation. During pressure-support ventilation (PSV, flow cycled) leaks can hinder achievement of the inspiration-termination point. These air leaks can be minimized by various measures (Fig 15.7)

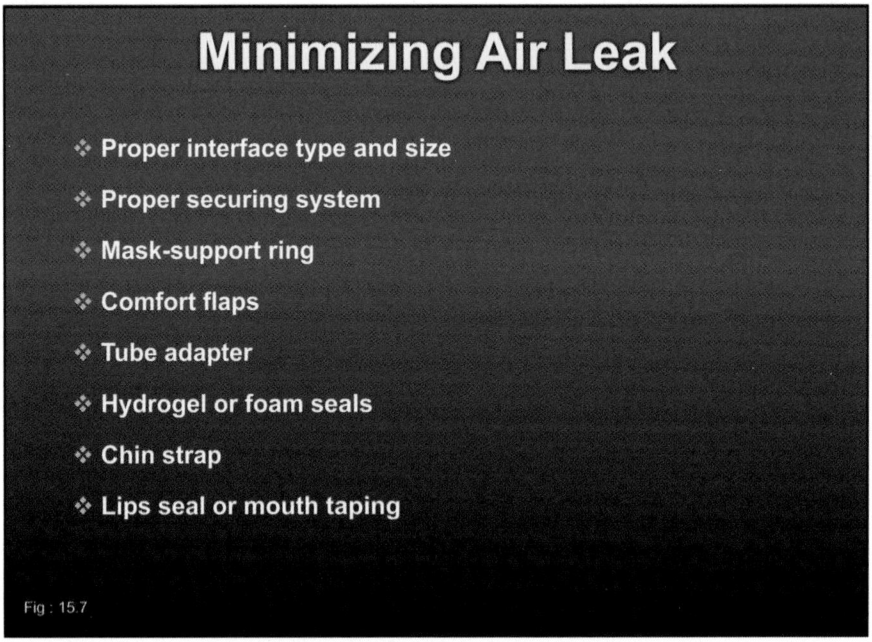

Minimizing Air Leak

- Proper interface type and size
- Proper securing system
- Mask-support ring
- Comfort flaps
- Tube adapter
- Hydrogel or foam seals
- Chin strap
- Lips seal or mouth taping

Fig : 15.7

The leak related issues have been solved by innovations in ventilator technology and these are discussed below.

Leak compensation

One of the technical challenges of any NPPV ventilator is to evolve strategies for dealing with leaks. Leak compensation is available in dedicated NPPV and hybrid ICU ventilators. Leaks up to 65 l/min can be compensated in these ventilators. NPPV ventilators utilize a smart algorithm which eliminates leak and triggering related problems. As described previously, triggering and cycling issues may occur if an interface from one manufacturer is matched with a ventilator from a different manufacturer. Other bi-level ventilators allow the user to test the leak port as a part of the pre-use procedure. Leak-detection algorithms must adjust for changes in leak with inspiratory and expiratory pressure changes, as well as changes that may occur from breath-to-breath due to 'fit' of the interface. An example is illustrated below (Fig 15.8).

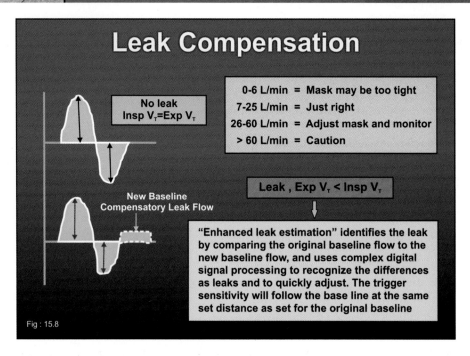

Fig: 15.8

Dyssynchrony due to leak (triggering, flow and cycle dyssynchrony)

Trigger asynchrony with NPPV may be the result of leaks, which can produce either auto-triggering or ineffective triggers. Ineffective triggers can also be due to the underlying disease process such as those that occur with auto-PEEP in patients with COPD, and weak inspiratory efforts in neuromuscular disease. Dyssynchrony can be minimized by treating underlying disease process (bronchodilators to decrease airways resistance and auto PEEP), reducing unintentional leak and correcting ventilatory settings to promote synchrony.

Trigger Synchrony is attained by following measures:

- Adjust trigger sensitivity for the best balance between trigger effort and auto-triggering. Appropriately set trigger sensitivity, either pressure or flow is acceptable
- Increase PEEP (EPAP) to counterbalance auto-PEEP

Flow Synchrony

- Adjust inspiratory pressure with pressure-targeted ventilation or adjust flow and tidal volume with volume-targeted ventilation
- Adjust rise time (pressurization rate) as per patient comfort. A faster rise time has been reported to better unload the respiratory muscles of patients with COPD during NPPV, but this may be accompanied by substantial air leaks and poor tolerance. Thus, the physiologic benefit that might occur with rise-time adjustment should be balanced against patient comfort.
- Reduce respiratory drive (increase ventilation to treat acidosis, sedation)

Cycle Synchrony
- Reduce pressure support setting
- An inspiratory termination trigger, adjustable from 5-70% of the maximal inspiratory flow, must be set.

Mode Synchrony
- Use backup rate if apnea or periodic breathing occurs

Sleep and sedation

Inability to sleep well can be due to many causes such as anxiety, frequent disruptions of the patient at night during normal sleeping hours, discomfort caused by the mask or ventilating pressures (leaks). All this lead to sleep fragmentation, oxygen desaturation and decreased REM sleep. Appropriate interface and less ventilating pressures (reduced leak) should be considered. If all this fail then using an appropriate medication to reduce anxiety, and promote sleep may be appropriate. Sedation may also be required due to mask intolerance, claustrophobia, delirium and agitation. Before sedation is administered be sure that the patient is able to the protect airway and is not likely to aspirate. In COPD patients increased CO_2 and sedation may have additive effects hence, should be used with caution.

Leak-compensation capabilities of most of the intermediate and newer ICU ventilators with "NPPV modes" are good at improving patient-ventilator synchrony with a large mask leak. Unlike the situation in the past, when using modern ventilators, trigger asynchrony is probably more often due to issues with pathophysiology of the disease process rather than ventilator performance.

The goals of NPPV are listed in Fig 15.9

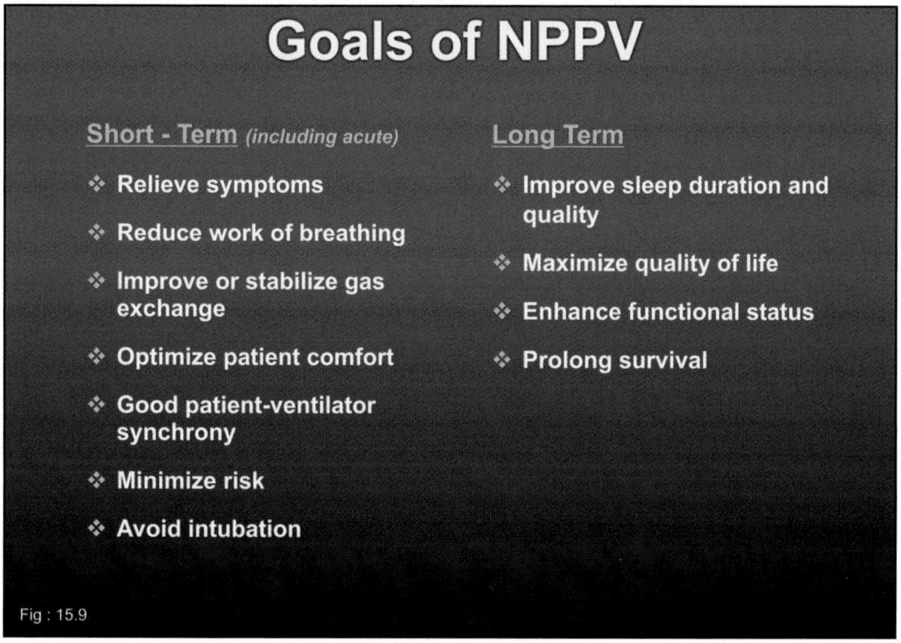

Goals of NPPV

Short - Term *(including acute)*
- Relieve symptoms
- Reduce work of breathing
- Improve or stabilize gas exchange
- Optimize patient comfort
- Good patient-ventilator synchrony
- Minimize risk
- Avoid intubation

Long Term
- Improve sleep duration and quality
- Maximize quality of life
- Enhance functional status
- Prolong survival

Fig : 15.9

Ventilators used for NPPV can be of three types (Fig 15.10)

1. ICU ventilators
2. Hybrid ICU ventilators
3. NPPV dedicated ventilators

The choice of a ventilator may be crucial for the success of NPPV in the acute setting, because intolerance and excessive air leaks are significantly correlated with NPPV failure.

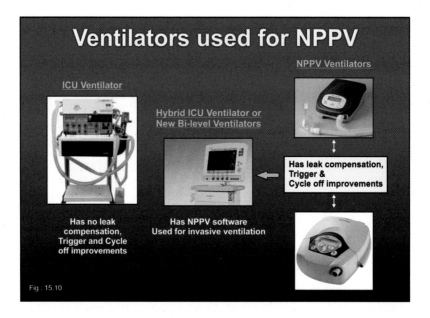

Fig : 15.10

Patient-ventilator asynchrony and discomfort can occur if the clinician fails to adequately set NPPV to respond to the patient's ventilatory demand. So clinicians need to be fully familiar with the ventilator's technical peculiarities (e.g., efficiency of trigger and cycle systems, speed of pressurization, air-leak compensation, CO_2 rebreathing, reliability of fraction of inspired oxygen) and disease pathology.

The advantages and disadvantages of all three types of ventilators are mentioned in Fig 15.11

Modes used in NPPV

All modes used for invasive ventilation can theoretically also be used for NPPV. However, NPPV is usually delivered in the form of assisted ventilation where every breath is supported. Pressure support ventilation is the commonest mode used. Rarely controlled mechanical ventilation is used, when patient is sedated or has no effort. On NPPV machines this is referred to as 'timed' mode (T). CPAP is mainly used in cardiogenic pulmonary edema (CPE) where pressure is applied to the airway throughout the respiratory cycle. It is not a ventilatory mode. In proportional assist ventilation (PAV) the ventilator assists the patient by generating volume assist or flow assist in proportion to patient's effort creating a ventilatory pattern that matches metabolic demands on a breath-by-breath basis. The guidelines make no recommendation about the use of proportional assist ventilation versus pressure support ventilation in patients who are receiving NPPV for acute respiratory failure, because of insufficient evidence.

The advantages and disadvantages of all three types of ventilators

Settings	ICU ventilators	Hybrid or new Bi-level ventilators	NPPV ventilators
FiO$_2$	FiO$_2$ accurate Blender present	FiO$_2$ accurate Blender present	FiO$_2$ Inaccurate Depends on many factors
Alarms and monitoring	Sophisticated Graphics monitoring present Alarms sound inappropriately	Sophisticated Graphics monitoring present Use only essential alarms	Alarms less sophisticated Graphics are being added Use only essential alarms
Circuit	Dual limb Less CO$_2$ rebreathing	Dual limb Less CO$_2$ rebreathing Better leak estimation	Single limb Increased CO$_2$ rebreathing
Leak compensation	Absent	Present	Present
Rise time	May be present	Present Interface need not be tight Better patient comfort	Present Interface need not be tight Better patient comfort
Battery	Absent	Present	Present / lasts longer
High inspiratory pressures	Possible	Possible	Less than 25 cm H$_2$O
Compactness	Less compact	Less compact	Compact
Cost	Expensive	Expensive	Less expensive
Location	ICU	ICU	ICU/Ward/Home

Fig 15.11

Aerosol bronchodilator delivery during NPPV

Although it seems that, during NPPV, inhaled drugs (e.g. bronchodilators) could be efficiently delivered via either nebulizer or MDI spacer, there is not enough consistent evidence about the ventilator features (settings, circuit, and interface) specifically designed and approved for application in everyday practice. But studies have shown optimum drug delivery is achieved if nebulizer position is between the leak port and patient connection, administering high inspiratory pressure, low expiratory pressure, and a breath rate of 20/min.

FiO$_2$

Accurate FiO$_2$ delivery is possible in ventilators with oxygen blenders (21% to 100%). Such ventilators should be used in hypoxemic failure. In NPPV devices FiO$_2$ cannot be estimated accurately due to leaks and bias flows. Titrate oxygen flow to maintain SpO$_2$ of more than 90%. Oxygen flows of 10 to 15 L/min are used for this purpose. Many factors affect delivery of FiO$_2$ during NPPV. FiO$_2$ is decreased as IPAP and EPAP pressures are increased.

Humidification during NPPV

From a pathophysiologic view point, spontaneously breathing patients without a tracheal tube or tracheostomy necessarily do not require additional strategies for conditioning respiratory gases. In NPPV there are large leaks around the mask, high inspiratory flow of dry medical gases which overwhelm mucosal humidification capacity and worsen secretion problems and fluid depletion. So, it is advisable to use active humidifier because of their large capacity to produce heated and humidified air. Well humidified air at a temperature between 25°-30°C is an attributing factor for success in NPPV therapy.

This improves both secretion clearance and the tolerance of the NPPV therapy. Passive humidification is not recommended for NPPV.

Alarm adjustment

Set alarms for pressure, minute volume, tidal volume and frequency according to the ventilation settings and patient range. For modern ventilators equipped with NPPV option, it is possible to turn off the alarms for low minute volume, high V_T in order to avoid nuisance alarms. Additionally, a delay time can be set for low airway pressure, allowing short disconnections for skin care, alimentation or speaking without triggering a disconnect alarm.

Backup or apnea ventilation

Set the apnea time, minimum minute volume setting, V_T and frequency as a backup in case the patient stops breathing spontaneously.

Position of the patient

The patient should be in a semi-recumbent position of about 45°. This position promotes spontaneous breathing as abdominal pressure is reduced and FRC is therefore increased. There is less risk of upper airway obstruction and coughing is facilitated, improving airway clearance.

Nasogastric tube and NPPV

NPPV can cause gastric distension which can lead to discomfort and vomiting. Pressure required to overcome the gastro-esphageal sphincter is more than 20-25 cm of H_2O. Commonly used IPAP is less than 20 cm of H_2O, hence gastric distension is rare. Moreover NG tube increases leaking around the mask, the tube itself blocks the nasal passage. Compression of tube against the skin by the mask may increase risk of skin breakdown. If the risk of vomiting and aspiration are high then NG tubes can be used. If an NG tube is required a fine bore NG tube with a NG sealing pad which interfaces between the tube and skin and mask should be used.

Steps in application of NPPV are described below (Figs 15.12 and 15.13) and is discussed in detail in the text that follows it.

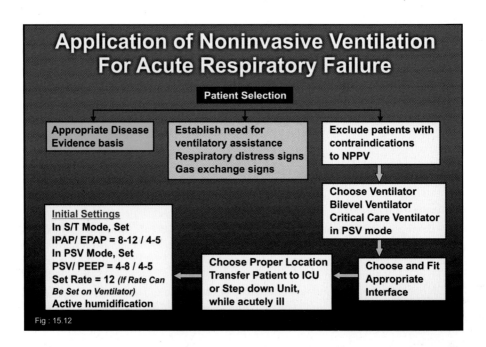

Fig : 15.12

Non Invasive Positive Pressure Ventilation

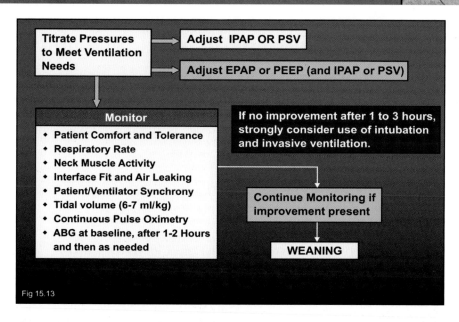

Fig 15.13

Selection criteria for NPPV in the acute setting (Fig 15.14):

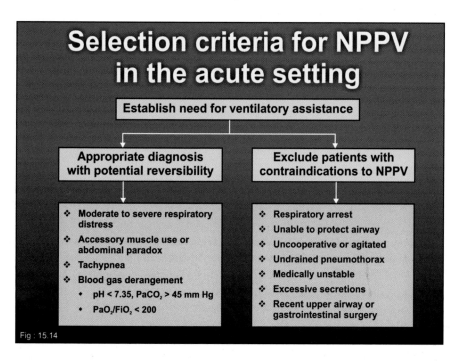

Fig : 15.14

The contraindications for NPPV listed above are the exclusion criteria used in most studies. These are not considered as absolute contraindications. NPPV can be applied in some of these patients depending upon the clinician's expertise and facility for swift intubation and invasive ventilation. An example is listed below (Fig 15.15).

COPD Patient with Respiratory Failure

- COPD patient was shifted for tertiary care is drowsy, looks dehydrated, BP 80/60 mmHg, RR 38/min, Accessory muscle use+, pH 7.09, PaCO$_2$ 95 mm Hg, bilateral crepitations+, HR 140/min, Bicarb 35 mmol.

- Do we intubate?

Trial of NPPV given- PSV 12 cm H$_2$O and PEEP of 5 cm H$_2$O, Fluid resuscitation done - BP 120/70 mmHg, RR 25/min, HR 110/min, Mentation better, synchronising well, ABG after 1 hr -pH 7.18, PCO$_2$ 65 mmHg - continue NPPV	Trial of NPPV given- PSV 12 cm H$_2$O and PEEP of 5 cm H$_2$O Fluid resuscitation done- BP 100/60 mmHg, RR 38/min, HR 120/min Drowsy, not synchronising well, ABG after 1 hr - pH 7.05, PCO$_2$ 105 mmHg - Intubate

Fig 15.15

NPPV for patients with exacerbation of COPD

COPD patients are prone for acute exacerbations and respiratory failure with increased mortality and morbidity. Intubation and ventilation was a standard method in managing these patients. It was associated with significant complications and mortality. In last decade many studies were published comparing patients with NPPV on standard medical therapy with acute hypercapnic respiratory failure versus invasive ventilation. The results were analyzed in a meta-analysis which showed reduction in the rate of endotracheal intubation, in-hospital mortality and complications like nosocomial pneumonia with NPPV. The recently published guidelines recommend the use of noninvasive positive-pressure ventilation in addition to usual care in patients who have a severe exacerbation of COPD (pH less than 7.35 and relative hypercarbia). Patients with relatively mild exacerbation of COPD (pH more than 7.35) may not benefit from NPPV. However, it does not seem to cause harm in these patients. At the time of presentation, all patients with acute exacerbation of COPD should have arterial blood gas analysis besides clinical evaluation. Patients on NPPV should be closely monitored during the first 1-2 hours and ABG should be repeated, preferably, at the end of 1-4 hours. For the first 24 hours NPPV should be given for as much time as possible except during feeding and physiotherapy. Later on, the duration can be decreased depending upon the clinical condition and physiological parameters (SpO$_2$ and ABG).

Cardiogenic pulmonary edema (CPE)

Guidelines recommend the use of either noninvasive positive-pressure ventilation or continuous positive airway pressure (CPAP/NPPV are equally effective in CPE) by mask in patients who have cardiogenic pulmonary edema and respiratory failure in the absence of shock or acute coronary syndrome requiring urgent coronary re-vascularization.

Immunosuppression

Immunosuppressed patients are at greater risk of developing serious nosocomial infections when ventilated through an invasive route. Guidelines suggest that noninvasive positive pressure ventilation be used for immunosuppressed patients who have acute respiratory failure, particularly in those with hematological malignancies.

Asthma

One may assume that NPPV should be as effective in asthma as in COPD, both being disorders of airway resistance. However, this has not been confirmed by any randomized controlled trials. This may be due to the fact that the natural history and pathophysiology of asthma is entirely different. It has also been suggested that aerosolized medicines may be delivered more effectively by NPPV. Further studies must be done before recommending NPPV for the routine therapy of severe asthma exacerbations. Hence, NPPV is not recommended for routine use of asthma exacerbation. Though experts advocate a trial of NPPV in properly selected patients in closely monitored ICU setting in patients of acute severe asthma and have no contraindication.

Adjunct to early liberation

Guidelines recommend use of NPPV to facilitate early liberation from mechanical ventilation in patients who have COPD. The use of noninvasive positive-pressure ventilation for this indication requires both considerable expertise and the ability to closely monitor the patients, because urgent reintubation may be required. Guidelines do not recommend the use of NPPV to facilitate early liberation from mechanical ventilation in patients who do not have COPD, because of insufficient evidence.

Recommendations of NPPV in disease states are summarized below (Fig 15.16):

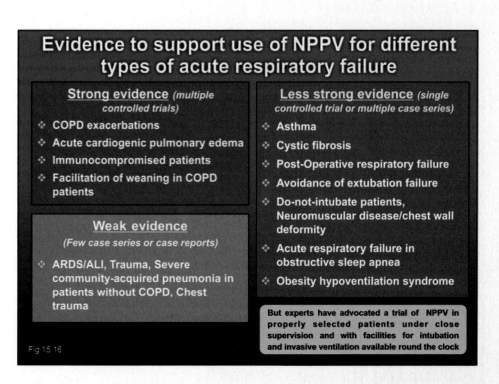

Fig 15.16

Protocol for initiation and maintaining NPPV

NPPV should be administered in appropriately monitored location with pulse oximetry. Vital signs should be recorded. Select and fit the interface. Ventilator settings are based on bedside assessment and ABG findings. Explain the procedure to the patient, encourage and reassure frequently. Apply headgear avoiding excessive strap tension (should be able to pass one or two fingers under strap) or encourage patient to hold mask. Start with low pressures/volumes in spontaneously triggered mode with backup rate. Standard ventilator settings can be as described below (Fig 15.17):

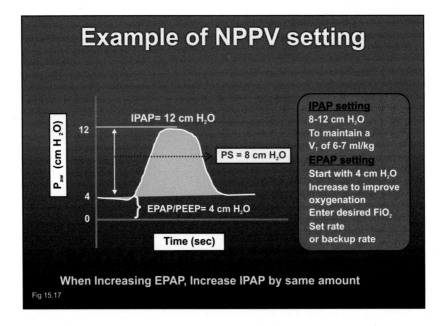

Fig 15.17

Begin with a low pressure support level of about 4-6 cm H_2O and increase in steps of 2-3 cm of H_2O until the desired support level is reached. This allows the patient to become accustomed to the ventilatory support. Start with a low PEEP of 2-3 cm H_2O and increase with steps of 1-2 cm H_2O at an interval time of about 10 minutes to get the patient accustomed to NPPV (increasing EPAP without increasing IPAP leads to decrease in the driving pressures). Alleviation of dyspnea, decreased respiratory rate, increased tidal volume (if being monitored) and good patient-ventilator synchrony are the goals. Provide O_2 supplementation as needed to keep O_2 saturations of 90%. Increase PEEP till either each breath is triggered or appropriate level is achieved. Check the mask for leaks and reduce them if necessary by repositioning the mask, using supporting cushions or molding it to better fit the patient's facial contours. Motivate the patient to breathe quietly through the mask and provide feedback. Inform the patient that he or she is doing well and provide encouragement and praise. Due to the learning curve involved with assisted breathing, it is very important to communicate with the patient on his/her performance particularly during the first hour. Add a heated humidifier as indicated. Consider mild sedation (i.e. intravenously administered Lorazepam 0.5 mg) in agitated patients. After NPPV initiation, monitor blood gases within 1 to 2 hours and then as needed. The predictors and determinants of success of NPPV are mentioned in Fig 15.18.

Non Invasive Positive Pressure Ventilation

Predictors of success of NPPV in acute setting	Determinants of success for NPPV in the acute setting
Younger age	Synchronous breathing
Lower acuity of illness (APACHE score)	No pneumonia
Able to cooperate; better neurologic score	Dentate
Able to coordinate breathing with ventilator	pH > 7.10
Less air leaking, intact dentition	Lower APACHE score $PaCO_2$ < 92 mm Hg
Hypercarbia, but not too severe ($PaCO_2$ >45 mm Hg but < 92 mm Hg)	Less air leaking
	Better neurologic score
Acidemia, but not too severe (pH < 7.35 but > 7.10)	Less secretions
Improvements in gas exchange, heart and respiratory rates within first 2 hr	Better "compliance" or "tolerance" refers to the clinician's assessment of the patient's acceptance of the technique

Fig 15.18

In the initial phase, check the profile of breaths delivered by varying the T_i, ramp/rise time, termination criteria and trigger sensitivity. Ask the patient what is more comfortable following each change. Setting up NPPV is somewhat more labor intensive, but maintaining NPPV therapy requires the same amount of nursing time as invasive ventilation. If there are major tolerance problems which cannot be solved in the first 1 to 2 hours with no improvements, discontinue NPPV and switch over to invasive ventilation. Unfortunately, many patients do not have a standalone oxygenation or a ventilation problem. Usually, a combination of both can be observed. This is why it is important to have a good understanding of the cause of each of them, how they are related to each other and how to treat the condition most effectively (Fig 15.19)

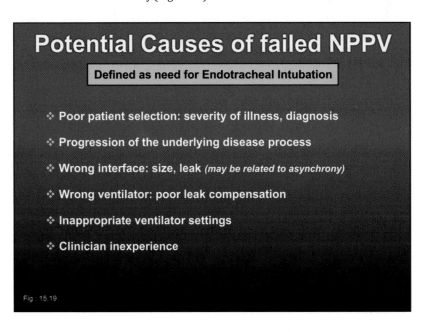

Fig : 15.19

Monitoring

Subjective responses

Patient comfort is a very important sign of NPPV success. Clinicians should ask patients repeatedly about discomfort related to the mask or airflow, and observe for nonverbal signs of distress or discomfort (Fig 15.20).

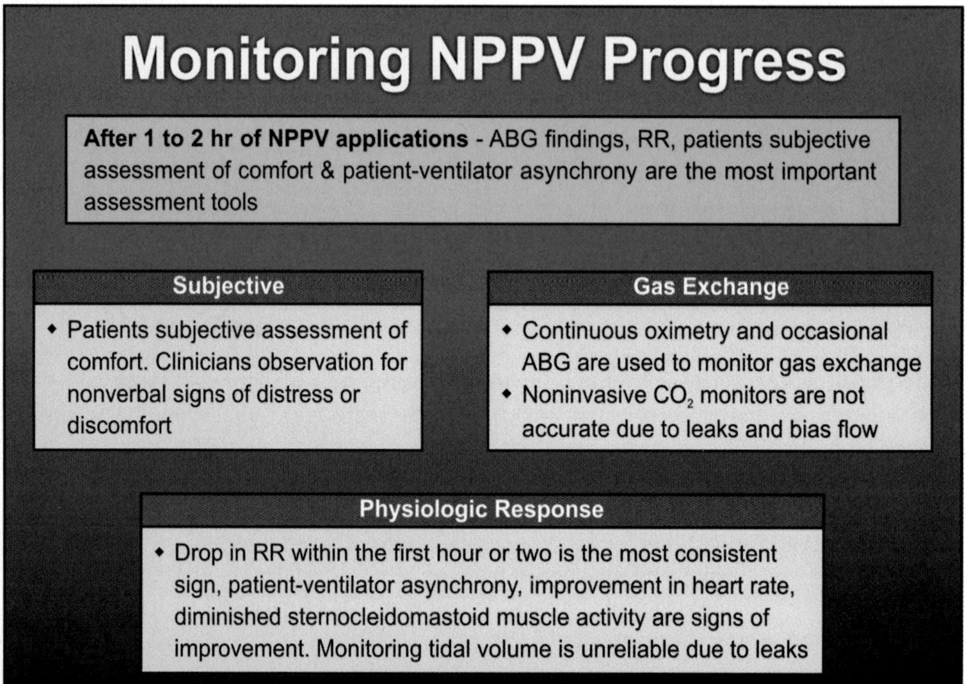

Monitoring NPPV Progress

After 1 to 2 hr of NPPV applications - ABG findings, RR, patients subjective assessment of comfort & patient-ventilator asynchrony are the most important assessment tools

Subjective
- Patients subjective assessment of comfort. Clinicians observation for nonverbal signs of distress or discomfort

Gas Exchange
- Continuous oximetry and occasional ABG are used to monitor gas exchange
- Noninvasive CO_2 monitors are not accurate due to leaks and bias flow

Physiologic Response
- Drop in RR within the first hour or two is the most consistent sign, patient-ventilator asynchrony, improvement in heart rate, diminished sternocleidomastoid muscle activity are signs of improvement. Monitoring tidal volume is unreliable due to leaks

Fig 15.20

Weaning from NPPV

In acute setting the inspiratory pressures are raised quickly as tolerated. The aim is to assist ventilation promptly. With underlying condition improving the patient has increasing periods of time off the ventilator.

Sequential use where in periods of use alternate with lengthy ventilator-free periods and total daily use averages only 6 hours. Ventilator assistance is discontinued when no respiratory distress recurs during ventilator-free intervals.

The total duration of ventilator assistance depends on the speed of resolution of the respiratory failure. Patients with COPD have an average ventilator time of 2 days or more, and acute pulmonary edema requires an average of 6 to 7 hours. Some patients may continue nocturnal ventilation after discharge from the hospital, although there are no guidelines for selection of such patients (Fig15.21).

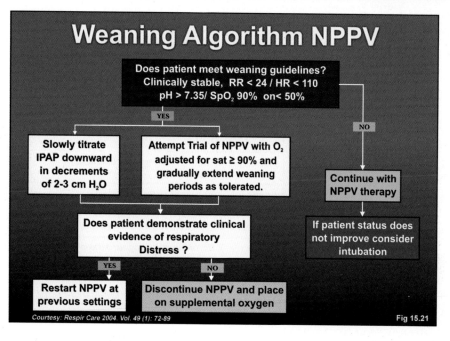

Fig 15.21

The most frequently encountered adverse effects and complications are minor. They are related to the mask (leaks) and ventilator airflow (nasal congestion, nasal/oral dryness, gastric insufflation, eye irritation and sinus/ear pain) or pressure (discomfort, nasal bridge ulceration, etc.). Rarely life threatening complications (less than 5%) like aspiration, pneumothorax and respiratory arrest can happen, hence, constant vigil has to be maintained (Figs 15.22 and 15.23).

Complications of NPPV Interface Related

Adverse Effect	Remedy
Discomfort	Check fit, adjust straps, change interface
Excessive air leaks	Realign interface, check strap tension, change to full face mask
Nasal bridge redness or ulceration	Use artificial skin, minimize strap tension, use spacer, alternate interface
Skin irritation or rashes	Use skin barrier lotion and/or topical corticosteroids, change to mask made from a different material, properly clean mask
Claustrophobic reactions	Try nasal interface or total face mask, sedate judiciously

Fig : 15.22

Complications of NPPV: Airflow / Pressure Related

Adverse Effect	Remedy
Nasal congestion	Try nasal steriods, decongestant, antihistamine or humidification
Nasal or oral dryness	Add humidification, nasal saline, oral/nasal hygiene or decrease leak
Sinus or ear pain	Lower inspiratory pressure
Gastric inflation	Avoid excessive inspiratory pressures (over 20 cm H_2O), administer Simethicone
Eye irritation	Check mask fit, readjust headgear straps
Failure to ventilate	Use sufficient pressures, optimize patient-ventilator synchrony

Fig 15.23

Conclusion

NPPV constitutes a significant therapeutic advance for certain forms of acute respiratory failure and critical care applications are expanding. It is considered as a safe and effective way to successfully ventilate or oxygenate many patients without intubation. Innovations in ventilator technology have enhanced patient comfort, safety and have extended ventilatory care to patients home. Centers not using NPPV should be encouraged to gain training and experience with the modality because evidence indicates that this improves patient outcomes.

References

1. Noninvasive Ventilation. Sangeeta mehta and Nicholas s. hill. Am J Respir Crit Care Med vol 163: pp 540–577, 2001
2. Clinical practice guidelines for the use of noninvasive positive-pressure ventilation and noninvasive continuous positive airway pressure in the acute care setting. CMAJ 2011. DOI: 10.1503/cmaj.100071
3. Guidelines for noninvasive ventilation in acute respiratory failure. Rajesh Chawla, G. C. Khilnani, J. C. Suri, N. Ramakrishnan, R. K. Mani, Shirish Prayag, Shruti Nagarkar, Sudha Kansal, U. S. Sidhu, Vijay Kumar. Indian J Crit Care Med April-June 2006 Vol 10 Issue 2
4. 42nd Respiratory care Journal Conference, "Noninvasive Ventilation in Acute Care: Controversies and Emerging Concepts," held–March 7-9, 2008, in Cancun, Mexico.

★★★

16. ARDS AND VENTILATORY CHALLENGES

ARDS and ALI are a spectrum of lung diseases diagnosis of which is mainly clinical. They are one of the most common causes of respiratory failure seen in the intensive care unit (ICU). Even with advanced medical care, morbidity and mortality still remain high (30-50%). Early recognition and appropriate treatment are vital to reduce adverse outcome. Etiology of ARDS and ALI is manifold and patients can present to any medical or surgical specialty with acute respiratory deterioration. sepsis, pneumonia, aspiration, and multiple traumas account for most cases.

Mechanical ventilation (MV) is critical for survival of patients with ALI and ARDS. Ventilatory support provides more time to the clinician for administration of specific therapies and the therapies to take effect. However, MV can also cause additional iatrogenic lung injury (ventilator-induced lung injury - VILI). This may delay or prevent recovery from acute respiratory failure. Clinicians are challenged to use MV in a manner that maintains acceptable gas exchange but also avoids VILI.

Definition of ARDS/ALI

In 1967, Ashbaugh and colleagues first described a syndrome of acute respiratory distress in adults that closely resembled respiratory distress in infants. The patients had an acute onset of tachypnea, hypoxemia, pan-lobular infiltration on chest X-ray and loss of lung compliance. Since, its initial description in 1967, ARDS definition has been the focus of intense scrutiny and attempts are still on to improve it.

The American–European Consensus Conference on ARDS (1994) formally defined ARDS as

1. of acute onset which may follow a catastrophic event
2. bilateral infiltrates on chest radiograph
3. no cardiac causes for pulmonary edema (pulmonary artery wedge pressure of less than 18 mm Hg)
4. hypoxia- PaO_2/FiO_2 ratio < 200 (PaO_2/FiO_2 ratio < 300 is ALI)

ALI is considered as a milder form of ARDS. The limitation of this definition is, it is a broad definition and may include many non ARDS patients who will be enrolled into clinical trials thereby degrading the inference drawn from data obtained. Other limitations of the definition include

1. A lack of explicit criteria for defining the term 'acute'
2. Sensitivity of PaO_2/FiO_2 to different ventilator settings
3. Poor reliability of the chest radiograph criterion
4. Difficulties distinguishing hydrostatic edema

Despite the limitations, ease of use has kept this definition popular with bedside clinician. Even if non ARDS patients are provided lung protective ventilation (LPV) it does not cause any harm. Inclusion of non ARDS patients may be the reason for differences in data and conclusions of different studies.

Hence, an attempt has been made to improve the definition. Delphi definition and lung injury scores are a few examples of these attempts. Valid and reliable definitions are essential to conduct epidemiological studies successfully and to facilitate enrollment of a consistent patient phenotype into clinical trials. Clinicians also need such definitions to implement the results of clinical trials, discuss prognosis with families and plan resource allocation.

In March 2012, a consensus conference on ARDS proposed a new definition called Berlin ARDS definition which has addressed most of the limitations present earlier. See below:

The Berlin Definition of Acute Respiratory Distress Syndrome

Timing - Within 1 week of a known clinical insult or new or worsening respiratory symptoms

Chest imaging (chest radiograph or CT scan) - Bilateral opacities which are not fully explained by effusions, lobar/lung collapse, or nodules

Origin of edema - Respiratory failure which cannot be fully explained by cardiac failure or fluid overload. Need objective assessment (e.g. echocardiography) to exclude hydrostatic edema if no risk factor present.

Oxygenation

1. **Mild** - PaO_2/FiO_2 of less than 200 mm Hg or less than or equal to 300 mm Hg with PEEP or CPA more than or equal to 5 cm H_2O

2. **Moderate** - PaO_2/FiO_2 of less than 100 mm Hg or less than or equal to 200 mm Hg with PEEP or CPAP more than or equal to 5 cm of H_2O

3. **Severe** - PaO_2/FiO_2 of less than or equal to 100 mm Hg with PEEP or CPAP more than or equal to 5 cm of H_2O

(CPAP- continuous positive airway pressure, FiO_2- fraction of inspired oxygen, PaO_2- partial pressure of arterial oxygen, PEEP- positive end-expiratory pressure. CPAP may be delivered noninvasively in the mild acute respiratory distress syndrome group).

Definitions are important as even a few hours delay in identifying and implementing LPV can produce ventilator induced lung injury (VILI). Berlin definition is easy to use and aids in quantifying the oxygenation defect. This narrows down discrepancies between different clinical trials and also helps in prognostication. Any definition of ARDS becomes more accurate when restricted to acute non-cardiogenic pulmonary edema in the background of certain characteristic features (listed below):

1. Delay between the precipitating event (24 to 48 hr) and rapidly developing dyspnea
2. Decreased respiratory system compliance and reduced aerated lung volume (20% to 30%)
3. Refractory hypoxemia even with modest levels of FiO_2 and PEEP
4. Delayed resolution

ALI patients also require LPV as it is a milder form of ARDS. Pathophysiology, physiological rationale of ventilation and causes are same for both ALI and ARDS. Therefore, only ARDS will be discussed henceforth.

ARDS and Ventilatory Challenges

Causes of ARDS (Fig 16.1)

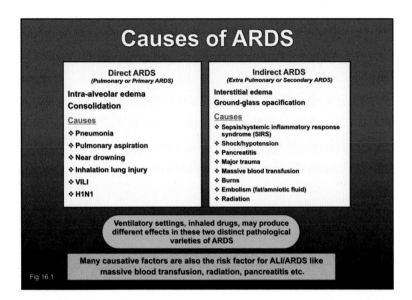

Fig 16.1

Weather direct and indirect ARDS are different or one and the same is debatable with no definite answer available as yet. Some authorities believe the two have to be differentiated and studied separately to answer many unresolved questions in ARDS.

ARDS prevention

Patients with preexisting risk factors are more prone to ARDS, if exposed to additional insult as a part of treatment for the primary pathology. Lung Protective Ventilation should also be used to prevent ARDS in high risk patients. An example is illustrated in Fig 16.2.

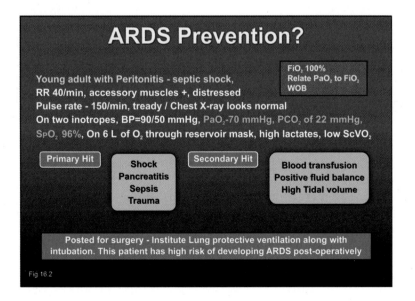

Fig 16.2

Pathophysiology of ARDS (Fig 16.3)

Lung injury can occur either from alveolar side (air) or vascular (blood) side resulting in ARDS. Neutrophil activation and proliferation is central to initiating an inflammatory cascade and release of mediators. If it is from the vascular side, then the alveolar capillary endothelial damage results in disruption and interstitial edema. The capillary alveolar distance increases and the injury propagates into alveolar side. The type II cells which produce surfactant are damaged leading on to alveolar collapse and hypoxemia.

If the injury is from alveolar side, type II cell damage occurs and alveolar epithelial injury results in alveolar edema. Widespread alveolar flooding impairs alveolar ventilation and inactivates surfactant. This in turn causes decreased lung compliance, increased ventilation and perfusion mismatch and produces intrapulmonary shunt. Intrapulmonary shunt becomes apparent when hypoxemia does not improve despite oxygen administration. The lung's response to injury can be divided into exudative phase, proliferative phase and fibrotic phase. Hypoxemia refractory to treatment is the hallmark of ARDS. Only 20 to 30% of the alveoli are normal in ARDS and can participate in gas exchange ("baby lung").

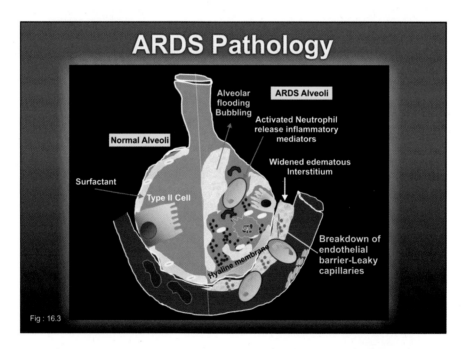

Fig : 16.3

Contrary to commonly accepted notion, decreased respiratory compliance is due to reduced number of normal alveoli (baby lung) indicating the smaller portions of lung capable of accepting tidal volume and is not related to the amount of "diseased" lung tissue. Whereas hypoxemia in ARDS is related to the amount of "diseased" lung tissue (collapsed alveoli). The reason for severe hypoxemia is not due to perfusion of collapsed alveoli but due to mechanical compression of the blood vessels by collapsed alveoli and worsening hypoxic pulmonary vasoconstriction (HPV).

A basic understanding of stress and strain is essential to understand the injury potential of ventilatory setting used in ARDS patients. Stress is defined as, "force per unit area acting on a plane within a body". Strain is any forced change in length in relation to the initial length (Fig 16.4).

ARDS and Ventilatory Challenges

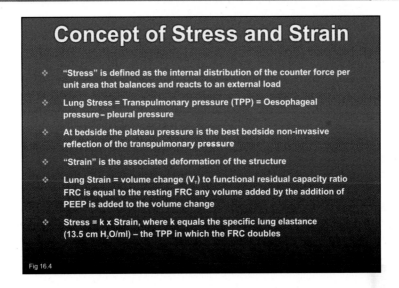

Fig 16.4

Lung stress is proportional to transpulmonary pressure (TPP) which is the difference between esophageal pressure and pleural pressure. At bedside plateau pressure is the best non-invasive reflection of the transpulmonary pressure (Fig 16.5).

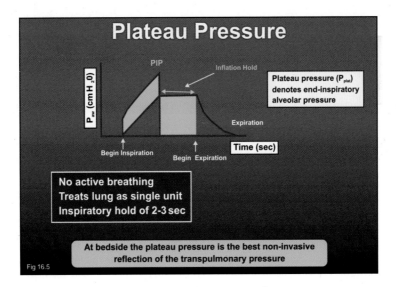

Fig 16.5

ARDS lung has following features

1) Reduction in number of alveoli that can accept tidal volume (baby lung)
2) Areas of normal and collapsed alveoli lie side by side
3) The pressure required to open the diseased and collapsed alveoli is more than that required to open normal alveoli
4) Dependent alveoli are difficult to open in previously diseased lungs due to both preexisting pathology and to superimposed pressure applied by the non-dependant alveoli

These features have to be taken into consideration when applying mechanical ventilation in ARDS. Strategies have been developed in LPV to prevent VILI.

Lung Protective Ventilation (LPV) or Open Lung Ventilation (OLV).

Reduced lung volume, rationale for using low tidal volume and implications in mechanical ventilation

Air always chooses the path of least resistance. Normal tidal volume is used when lung volume is reduced, the air will go to more compliant normal alveoli causing their overdistension. Gas exchange and patient survival hinge on keeping the baby lung intact as this leads to increased tidal stretch (volutrauma) resulting in alveolar damage, increased epithelial permeability, capillary permeability, alveolar flooding and interstitial edema (Fig 16.6).

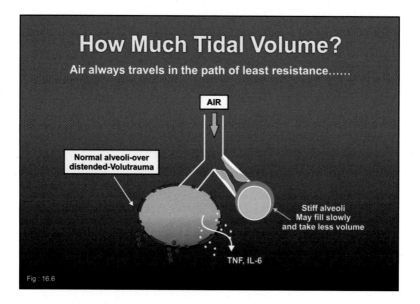

Fig: 16.6

It is obvious that low tidal volume has to be used. How low, will be discussed in detail with supporting studies later in this chapter.

Rationale for PEEP use and prone positioning

Areas of normal and collapsed alveoli lie side by side. The pressure required to open the diseased and collapsed alveoli is more than the normal alveoli. The implications of this in mechanical ventilation is that if unsupported by PEEP, certain collapsible alveoli may wink open and close with every tidal cycle generating shearing stresses on the thin tissue wall separating junctional alveoli and tending to deplete surfactant. This causes stress failure of alveolar membrane and disruption of the epithelium (Fig 16.7). The shear injury increases with cycling frequency and duration of exposure to adverse ventilatory patterns. The magnitude of blood flow in these stressed areas also may play an important role. Injury is more in dependent regions of the lung because the diseased lung is edematous and the superimposed weight of the edematous alveoli (in non-dependent region) causes squeezing of the gas and collapse of alveoli in the dependent region. This is one of the reasons why V/Q matching improves on proning since, there is more lung tissue in the dorsal region which now becomes non-dependant. PEEP reduces the number of lungs units "at risk" for atelectrauma. Recruitment of lung volume is a joint function of PEEP and the opening pressures generated in response to tidal volume (more so in low tidal volume ventilation).

ARDS and Ventilatory Challenges

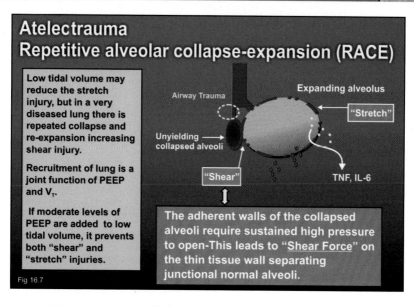

Fig 16.7

Rationale for recruitment maneuvers (RM)

As discussed previously, diseased and dependent alveoli are difficult to open and very high pressure may be required to recruit these alveoli. These high pressures will most definitely impact normal and compliant alveoli first leading to VILI. Two things become obvious now. Firstly RM should be used only in life threatening refractory hypoxemia. Secondly it should be applied for a very short time (1 to 2 minutes). Amount of pressure required in keeping the alveoli open after RM is much less compared to pressure required to force it open, as once the alveoli are forced open the surfactant monolayer may spread resulting in increased compliance.

The LPV is summarized in Fig 16.8

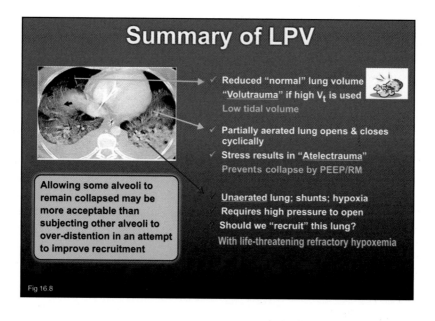

Fig 16.8

The ventilatory strategies used in ARDS listed below will be discussed.

1. Mode of ventilation
2. FiO_2
3. Tidal volume and plateau pressure
4. PEEP
5. Prone positioning
6. Recruitment maneuvers
7. High frequency oscillation
8. ECMO
9. Non-ventilatory strategies like nitric oxide, steroids, surfactant, etc

Mode of ventilation

Either volume or pressure control mode can be used. Guidelines for lung protection should be employed in any mode employed and the clinician should remain alert to the potential shortcomings and complications of the mode in use. The ARDS net recommends use of volume control mode. When using volume modes, pressures have to be monitored and vice versa.

Volume control mode (VC) was used in the three RCTs, of ARDS in which significantly reduced mortality was noted. The ease of teaching this to bed side clinicians (4 to 8 ml/ kg of IBW) have been the reason for the popularity of this mode. The availability of decelerating flow for volume ventilation in modern ventilators has made this mode more attractive.

Pressure control mode (PC) is advocated as a better mode by many experts. The reason for this is that with a fixed pressure limit the incidence of VILI is reduced. The decelerating flow used leads to better distribution of tidal volume, reduced overdistension and decreased incidence of VILI.

Many believe reducing tidal volumes with worsening compliance acts as a safety feature in preventing VILI. When using pressure-control modes, clinicians must remember that the ventilator reports only the pressure at the airway opening. If a patient has spontaneous inspiratory efforts, transpulmonary pressure can be considerably augmented and may cause substantial overdistension even with normal airway opening pressure reading (refer to chapter on VILI).

Inverse ratio ventilation (APRV and BI-Level) (Fig 16.9)

These modes work by using long T_I to recruit lung units having increased inspiratory time constants. Short T_I is used to prevent easily de-recruitable lung units with short expiratory time constants.

The resultant intrinsic PEEP can have the same effect as applied PEEP but the distribution of intrinsic PEEP (most pronounced in lung units with long time constants) may be different from that of applied PEEP and the resultant V/Q effects may also be different. Spontaneous breathing is possible during both phases of ventilation and these result in better hemodynamics.

Both these modes use two pressure levels, pressure high (P_{high}) with a goal of improving oxygenation and pressure low (P_{low}) which facilitates ventilation or CO_2 clearance. Also they use two time periods $T_{inspiratory}$ and $T_{expiratory}$, with synchronized patient triggering and cycling to change phases.

ARDS and Ventilatory Challenges

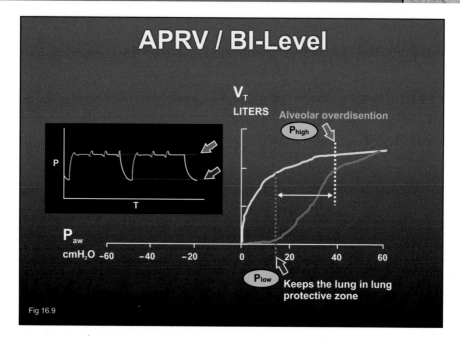

Fig 16.9

Spontaneous breathing is allowed at both levels. APRV uses very short expiratory time (I–E ratio-4:1 or more) than BI-Level which has an I–E ratio of 1:1 or more. Very short expiratory time in APRV leads to patient ventilator dyssynchrony. BI-Level has less synchrony problems. In BI-Level ventilation, spontaneous effort at upper pressure are provided with pressure support if pressure support is set higher than P_{High}, otherwise only at lower level. Whichever mode is chosen it is important to use them with the principles of LPV.

FiO_2 and oxygen toxicity

Increasing FiO_2 is an option if patients with already high plateau pressure develop refractory hypoxemia (plateau pressure > 30 cm of H_2O). An FiO_2 of less than 60% is considered safe in ARDS patients. Reducing the FiO_2 to the lowest tolerable limit is a good principle for all patients. In practical terms, oxygen should be administered to achieve a PaO_2 of 60 to 65 mm Hg (SaO_2 of approximately 90 %). FiO_2 should be reduced to below 60% as soon as the patient's condition allows and then to 40%, as at this level, oxygen can be tolerated for prolonged period without any deleterious consequences. In very sick ARDS patients, clinician may be faced with the difficult choice of choosing very low level of arterial oxygenation or increasing the airway pressures (PIP, P_{plat} pressures) and risk VILI. The immediate risks of systemic hypoxia or VILI are clearly more established and devastating than potential future risk of hyperoxia induced lung injury.

Ironically in several ways the disease process of ARDS may itself provide some degree of protection against O_2 toxicity. Areas of greatest injury (atelectatic units) may not be exposed to hyperoxia. By definition, ARDS has low PaO_2 and hence, systemic toxicity is unlikely. Exudates in ARDS are known to have antioxidant properties. Oxygen toxicity is both concentration and time dependent. As a rule, very high inspired fractions of oxygen can be used safely for brief periods while efforts are being made to reverse the underlying process.

Tidal volume and plateau pressure

Low tidal volume ventilation has been discussed previously. The incidence of VILI due to overdistension is reduced when a tidal volume of 4 to 8 ml/kg of predicted body weight is used while limiting the stretch pressure (plateau pressure) below 25 to 30 cm of H_2O. In most ARDS patients a starting tidal volume of 6 ml/kg of PBW is advised. Higher tidal volumes are reserved for patients who experience severe respiratory acidosis, especially when there is elevated intracranial pressure. The severity of "stretch injury" seems greatest when these maximum transalveolar pressures exceed 25 to 30 cm H_2O and insufficient PEEP fails to keep lung units fully recruited. Unsupported by PEEP, certain collapsible alveoli may wink open and close with every tidal cycle, generating shearing stresses within junctional tissues and tending to deplete surfactant. Recruitment of lung volume is a joint function of PEEP and the opening pressures generated in response to tidal volume (more so in low tidal volume ventilation).

It is unscientific and dangerous to guess the weight of the patient. Using formulas to estimate either predicted body weight (PBW) or ideal body weight for setting tidal volume should be included in LPV protocol.

PBW formula

Males = 50+ 2.3 (Height in inches-60)

Females = 45.5+ 2.3 (Height inches-60)

Plateau Pressure (P_{Plat}) is a better determinant than tidal volume for preventing VILI. Patients with lower plateau pressures have better outcome (Fig 16.10). A clinical guide for setting tidal volume in proportion to estimated plateau pressure is given below:

1. P_{Plat} of more than 28 cm H_2O, use tidal volume of 4 to 5 ml/kg PBW
2. P_{Plat} of 25 to 28 use tidal volume of 6 ml/kg PBW
3. P_{Plat} less than 25 cm H_2O maintain a tidal volume of 6 to 8 ml/kg PBW

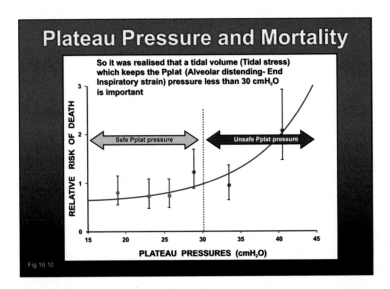

Fig 16.10

Permissive hypercapnia

Deliberate induction of alveolar hypoventilation (low tidal volume ventilation) and acceptance of hypercapnia to prevent VILI is referred as permissive hypercapnia. Studies have shown that

ARDS and Ventilatory Challenges

permissive hypercapnia is well tolerated. Some authorities have used the term therapeutic hypercarbia as it has shown a decreased mortality. This was noticed only when high tidal volumes with potential for VILI were used. Threshold of safe or hazardous levels of PCO_2 is unknown. A pH range of 7.10 or more should be the target irrespective of PCO_2 levels. There is evidence that the protective effect of hypercapnic acidosis in ARDS is a function of the acidosis rather than elevated CO_2 per se.

Buffering of hypercapnia induced acidosis in ARDS patients is common, albeit controversial. Controversy stems from the fact that both hypercapnia and acidosis per se may exert distinct biologic effects. Buffering with sodium bicarbonate was permitted in the ARDS net study. Buffering with bicarbonate raises systemic CO_2 levels and may worsen intracellular acidosis. Another option is the use of tromethamine acetate which does not increase CO_2 production. There are no long-term clinical outcome data (e.g. survival, duration of hospital stay etc.) to support the practice of buffering in hypercapnic acidosis. If the clinician chooses to buffer hypercapnic acidosis, the indication should be clear, such as to ameliorate potentially deleterious hemodynamic consequences of acidosis.

The implementation of permissive hypercapnia may initially require deep sedation and/or paralysis. Permissive hypercapnia is not advisable (or may be impossible to implement safely) in coexisting metabolic acidosis, renal failure, raised intracranial pressure or cardiac disease.

Respiratory Rate (RR)

Shear injury is dependent on cycling frequency and hence, the target in severe ARDS should be to set the lowest RR that can maintain a pH above 7.10. Tidal volume is set with a plateau pressure less than 25 to 30 cm of H_2O and adjustments are made to RR to maintain pH of 7.30-7.45. Do not exceed RR of 35 per minute (can cause auto-PEEP).

PEEP

Firm numerical guidelines for PEEP and tidal volume selection are invalid in the background of contribution of chest wall component for plateau pressure and difficulty in quantifying the amount of recruitable lung tissue at bedside. Use of PV curves (LIP or P_{flex}, UIP) may fare little better (refer to PEEP chapter) (Fig 16.11).

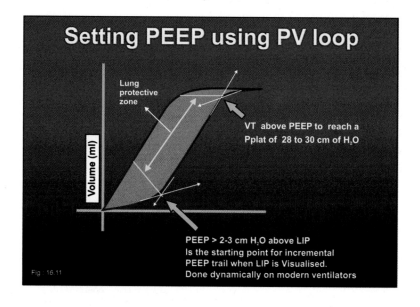

Fig. 16.11

At present, an empirical approach that incorporates multiple indicators of response and the recruitment maneuver in PEEP selection appears most rational. Common practice is to use PEEP/FiO$_2$ tables (Fig 16.12) targeting a conservative range of PaO$_2$ or SpO$_2$ values. This approach is certainly user friendly, but there is some concern that it does not truly optimize the PEEP setting.

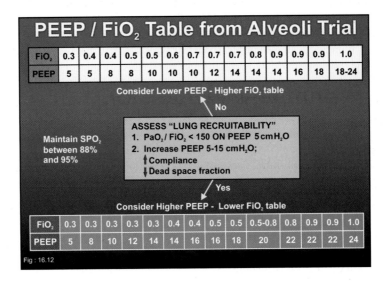
Fig : 16.12

PEEP non-responders recruit little (and arterial PaO$_2$ improves little) in response to higher levels of PEEP. Due to fixed pairings of PEEP and FiO$_2$ in these patients, a FiO$_2$ rise which is optimal will result in higher PEEP and risk of overdistension. Whereas, in PEEP responders who recruit well in response to higher levels of PEEP, the PEEP rise which is required comes along with higher FiO$_2$ and risk of oxygen toxicity. Hence, we recommend an approach that attempts to distinguish PEEP responders from non-responders, and to apply higher levels of PEEP in the responders with lower levels in non-responders (Fig 16.13).

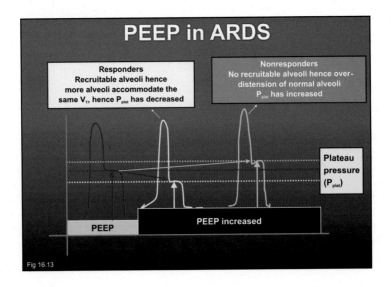
Fig 16.13

PEEP of best oxygenation or compliance are the two commonly used techniques. PEEP can be set incrementally starting from a level of 10 cm H_2O or decrementally starting at 20 cm of H_2O. The choice of incremental or decremental PEEP trial depends on the recruitability of the diseased lung. Patient is considered a responder if a recruitment test proves that PEEP manipulation leads to addition of new alveoli and not over distention of normal alveoli. Recruitment results in decreased plateau pressure and PCO_2. These patients are suitable for decremental PEEP trial. In non-responders, PEEP manipulation leads to over-distension of normal alveoli causing increased plateau pressure and PCO_2. These patients are candidates for incremental PEEP trial.

Additional selection criteria for incremental and decremental PEEP trial

Decremental PEEP trial: Decremental PEEP trails should be used in patients with lower inflection point (LIP) on PV curve, ground glass appearance on image studies (interstitial edema) and recruitment test producing decreased plateau pressure / PCO_2.

Incremental PEEP trial: Incremental PEEP trial should be used if the patient has no LIP on PV curve and has consolidation radiologically (alveolar edema) and if recruitment test produces increase in plateau pressure and PCO_2. PEEP is manipulated in small installments whilst monitoring oxygenation and / or lung compliance. This is described below:

PEEP of Best oxygenation

Fundamental theory is 'when PEEP is decreased or increased (gradually 1 to 2 cm H_2O every 2–3 min) from a set value (20 or 10 cm of H_2O) arterial oxygenation (measured by arterial PaO_2 or SaO_2) will be reduced when decruitment or over stretching occurs'. At this juncture, a new recruitment maneuver is performed and PEEP is set about 1 cm H_2O above for decremental PEEP and 1 cm H_2O below for incremental PEEP.

PEEP of Best compliance

In this method a recruitment manoeuvre is done and PEEP is set at 10 or 20 cm of H_2O. PEEP is then reduced or increased in steps of 1 or 2 cm of H_2O. Breath-by-breath compliance is estimated. It may first increase to a maximum and then decrease again. The PEEP at which compliance starts to decrease is similar to the collapse pressure or overdistending pressure. At this juncture, a new recruitment maneuver is performed and PEEP is set about 1 cm H_2O above for decremental PEEP and 1 cm below for incremental PEEP. Decremental PEEP trial is the method more in line with current understanding of pulmonary mechanics in ARDS patients.

Whichever PEEP protocol is used, oxygenation response, ventilatory efficiency, alterations of mechanics and hemodynamic response should be considered together. Three studies comparing low PEEP versus high PEEP (ALVEOLI, LOVS, EXPRESS studies) have shown no mortality difference between high and low PEEP groups but have shown less rescue therapies and duration of ventilation in high PEEP group. In very low PaO_2/FiO_2 patients there was a mortality benefit.

Prone positioning

The prone position (Fig 16.14) may dramatically improve the efficiency of arterial oxygenation for an unchanging ventilatory pattern and level of applied PEEP. Proning can be instituted on a regular ICU bed and does not require any specialized equipment.

In the prone position, the pleural pressure gradient is more uniform between dependent and non-dependent regions. This is because heart, mediastinum, and abdominal contents now "hang" from the vertebral structures rather than lying upon them which result in less atelectrauma (less VILI). The regional ventilation/perfusion ratio is more uniform and better matched resulting in shunt reduction. Proning allows the diaphragm to assume a more normal curvature, which may improve the muscle function. The prone position should be considered in patients with severe ARDS from the outset of management. Prone positioning generally offers its greatest oxygenation benefit when used early in the course of illness.

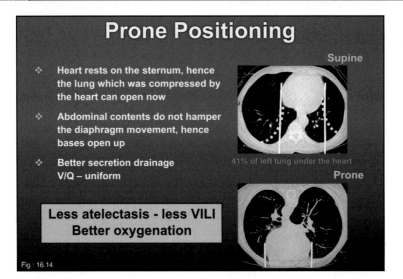

Fig: 16.14

In the prone position, pressure of the bed surface against weight-bearing ventral bony prominences can result in skin breakdown. Heightened vigilance and use of soft foam supports to pressure areas are generally sufficient to prevent serious ulceration when standard beds are employed. Hemodynamic instability and inotrope dependency are relative contraindications and should be considered on an individual risk-benefit basis. Spinal fractures, spinal instability and pregnancy are contraindications for the use of the prone position in ventilated patients. More recent studies document the benefit of extended prone position therapy (for more than 20 hours per day) in ARDS. Meta-analyses of all published studies on the efficacy of prone position in ARDS concluded that prone ventilation was associated with reduced mortality in patients with severe hypoxemia, defined as PaO_2/FiO_2 ratio less than 100 mm Hg.

Recruitment Maneuvers (RM)

Recruitment maneuvers (RM) is a ventilatory strategy to increase the transpulmonary pressure transiently (30 seconds–2 minutes) with the goal to open up atelectatic alveoli. It is pressure increment procedure leading to a volume increment in the lungs. The recommendations for RM are summarized in Fig 16.15.

Recommendations

- Repeat recruiting maneuver after position change, circuit break, or deterioration of Mechanics or PaO_2
- Depends on ARDS type/duration of disease, RM time
- Employ RM in Prone Position and/or PEEP to consolidate RM benefit
- Use closed suction, MDI and Heated humidifiers
- Do not always work

Fig 16.15

ARDS and Ventilatory Challenges

RMs should be reserved only for life threatening hypoxemia. There are no studies that clearly define a role for RMs in ventilatory management of ALI/ARDS. There are various approaches to recruitment of the lung. These are listed in Fig 16.16.

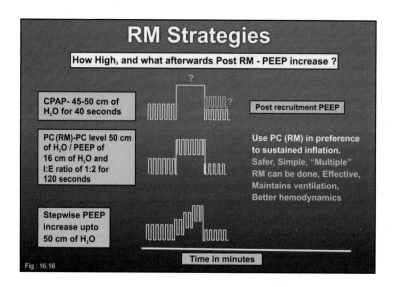
Fig: 16.16

Increased PC level with raised PEEP is preferred to sustained inflation. PC (RM) is safer, simpler, effective, maintains ventilation and multiple RM can be done. In a study PC (RM) had better preserved hemodynamics. An example of PC (RM) is illustrated in Fig 16.17.

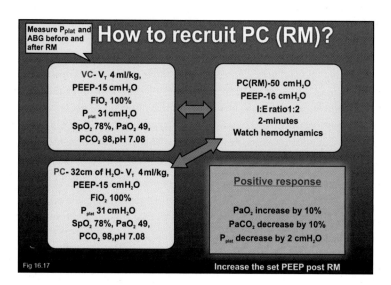
Fig 16.17

Some key considerations in ARDS ventilation

1. Profound bradycardia develops during ventilator disconnections in some patients with refractory hypoxemia during airway suctioning. Hence, suctioning is done under supervision and strict protocol only when indicated. Although hypoxemia occasionally contributes, this bradycardia

usually is reflex in nature and responds to prophylactic atropine or prompt reapplication of positive airway pressure. Closed suctioning systems are a standard of care as they do not interrupt tidal breath delivery or PEEP during suctioning.

2. Paralysis reduces oxygen consumption and improves PaO_2 in patients who remain agitated or fight the ventilator despite more conservative measures. In patients with severe ARDS short term neuromuscular blockade with cisatricurium (e.g. $PaO_2/FiO_2 \leq 120$) is probably safe and likely beneficial (first 48 hr).
3. Conservative fluid management strategy leads to reduced mortality.
4. Liberation from mechanical ventilation is carried out after disease resolution and when weaning protocol deems the patient fit for weaning with daily interruption of sedation, daily screen for spontaneous breathing trial (SBT)
5. Steroids may be used in ARDS treatment. A loading dose of 1 mg/kg, followed by an infusion of 1 mg/kg/day from day 1 to day 14, 0.5 mg/kg/day from day 15 to day 21, 0.25 mg/kg/day from day 22 to day 25, and 0.125 mg/kg/day from day 26 to day 28 can be used.

Corticosteroid use in late stage of ARDS probably will have negative effect on final outcome.
6. Many physiologically attractive pharmacological therapies like nitric oxide, surfactant etc have all been studied for use in ARDS. But no morality benefit has been proved. Many ongoing studies using these drugs are in different stages of completion. Once they are complete more drugs may be available for ARDS treatment.

High-frequency oscillatory ventilation (HFOV)

HFOV utilizes higher frequencies of 120 to 600 breaths per minute. This allows the use of smaller tidal volumes. The principle goals for ventilating a patient with ARDS using HFOV are to prevent VILI and to achieve adequate ventilation and gas exchange with as low FiO_2 as possible. The key features of HFOV that are thought to be responsible for decreasing the incidence and severity of VILI are smaller tidal volumes, higher mean airway pressure, smaller differences between inspiratory and expiratory pressures which helps prevent atelectrauma and lower peak pressures. The risks of HFOV relate to barotrauma and hemodynamic compromise is due to sustained elevation in mean airway pressure. Current data suggest HFOV is best considered a rescue regimen for patients with intractable hypoxemia. Recently, studies have shown HFOV is safe and equivalent to conventional ventilation in adult patients with ARDS, but no mortality benefit has been demonstrated. Ongoing clinical trials hope to address more specifically the role of this therapy in patients with ARDS.

Extracorporeal membrane oxygenation (ECMO)

Extracorporeal life support is a strategy to achieve lung rest. The potential benefit of (ECMO) is offset by an incremental bleeding risk related to the need for anticoagulation, and an additional infection risk due to intravascular catheters. The CESAR trial showed reduced mortality in ARDS patients with ECMO. Although the CESAR trial provides some guidance for the use of ECMO, it is not clear which patients with ARDS are the best candidates for ECMO. The most favorable timing for the initiation of ECMO has not been established, and it is not clear whether patients who have required more than 7 days of high-pressure or high FiO_2 ventilation should be excluded from receiving ECMO. Because of the extreme cost of the intervention, additional studies will be needed to define the role of extracorporeal support in the management of severe ARDS patients.

Lung protective ventilation strategies are summarized in Figs 16.18 and 16.19.

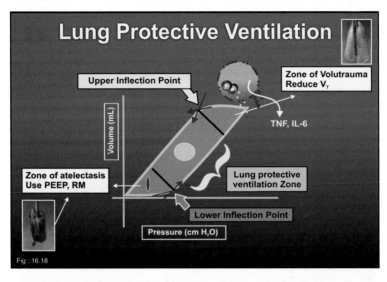

Fig : 16.18

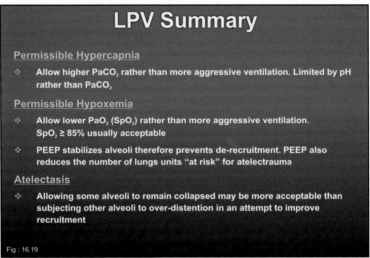

Fig : 16.19

Conclusion

ARDS is a common cause of respiratory failure in critically ill patients. With such a varied etiology patients can present to surgical, medical and other specialized units handling trauma and burns. Even with improved care mortality remains around 30%. LPV is the only intervention which has showed reduction in mortality and should be implemented in patients with ALI/ARDS and also in patients with risk factors for developing ARDS.

References

1. Acute Respiratory Distress Syndrome, The Berlin Definition, The ARDS Definition Task Force. JAMA. June 20, 2012; vol 307: No. 23
2. Lung Recruitment in Patients with the Acute Respiratory Distress Syndrome. Luciano Gattinoni, Pietro Caironi, Massimo Cressoni, Davide Chiumello, V. Marco Ranieri et al. N Engl J Med 2006; 354:1775-86.

3. Lung injury—Settle for a sketch or design a blueprint? John J. Marini, MD, Crit Care Med 2008; vol. 36, No. 10

4. Permissive hypercapnia–role in protective lung ventilatory strategies. Intensive Care Med 2004; 30:347–356

5. Prone ventilation - more questions than answers by John Marini. Focus Journal Sep/Oct 2008

6. Non-ventilatory Interventions in the Acute Respiratory Distress Syndrome. Kevin M. Schuster, Reginald Alouidor and Erik S. Barquist. J Intensive Care Med 2008; 23; 19,

7. Stress and strain within the lung. Luciano Gattinonia, b, Eleonora Carlessoa, and Pietro Caironi. Curr Opin Crit Care 2012, 18:42–47,

8. Lung opening and closing during ventilation of acute respiratory distress syndrome. Caironi P, Cressoni M, Chiumello D, et al. Am J Respir Crit Care Med 2010; 181:578–586.

9. Lung stress and strain during mechanical ventilation: any safe threshold? Protti A, Cressoni M, Santini A, et al. Am J Respir Crit Care Med 2011; 183:1354.

★★★

17. HAZARDS OF MECHANICAL VENTILATION

A : VENTILATOR INDUCED LUNG INJURY

Chandramohan M, *Senior consultant Department of critical care*
KR Hospital, Bangalore, India
Chandrashekar TR

Mechanical ventilation is required by many critically ill patients during the course of treatment. It may be required either for primary pathology in the lungs or for lung involvement secondary to other disease states. Mechanical ventilation provides time for the disease process to improve. It is not without complications. Positive pressure applied may worsen preexisting lung damage leading to ventilator associated lung injury (VALI).

Ventilator induced lung injury (VILI) is defined as acute lung injury proven to be caused by mechanical ventilation only. If a causative relationship cannot be proven, then it is called ventilator associated lung injury (VALI).

VILI can be caused when high tidal volumes are used in normal lungs or by ventilation with medium or even smaller tidal volumes in diseased lungs. It is difficult to differentiate VALI from

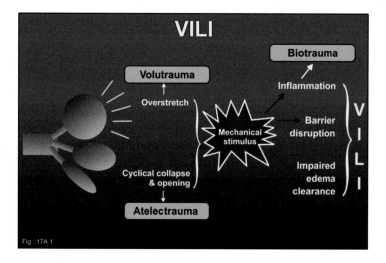

Fig: 17A.1

ARDS not only radiologically, but also functionally and histologically. It is comprised of following components: barotrauma, volutrauma, atelectrauma, biotrauma and oxygen toxicity (Figs 17A.1 and A.2).

VILI results due to complex interaction between the following components:
1. Lung volume (determined by tidal volume)
2. Alveolar pressure
3. Capillary pressure
4. Surface tension
5. Flow through pulmonary vessels
6. Lung expansion rate (determined by rate)

Components of ventilator-associated lung injury

Volutrauma	It is the damage caused by over - distension. It is sometimes called high volume or high end - inspiratory volume injury
Atelectrauma	It is caused by repeated recruitment and collapse. It is also called low volume or low end - expiratory volume injury
Biotrauma	It is the pulmonary and systemic inflammation caused by the release of mediators from lungs subjected to injurious mechanical ventilation
Barotrauma	It is high pressure induced lung damage
Oxygen toxicity	It is damage caused by high FiO_2

Fig 17A.2

Pathogenesis

Baby lung concept and heterogenous lung involvement in ARDS/ALI patients (Fig 17A.3)

VALI is more common in the lungs of patients with ALI or ARDS because the lungs are not uniformly diseased. Some areas, especially in the dependent regions, may be atelectatic, consolidated and less compliant making them difficult to ventilate. Non-dependent alveoli may be normal. Air follows the path of least resistance and functionally normal alveoli (baby lung) may get overdistended leading to barotrauma or volutrauma even when volume and pressure judged to be normal for the whole lung are used. Shear forces generated by repeated opening and closing at the junction of normal and diseased alveoli cause atelectrauma. Both these injuries can lead to production of cytokines which cause systemic side effects and finally result in multisystem organ failure (biotrauma).

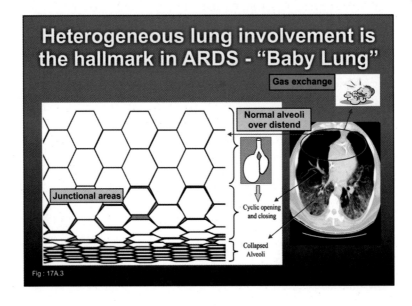

Fig : 17A.3

Respiratory mechanics: pertinent concepts

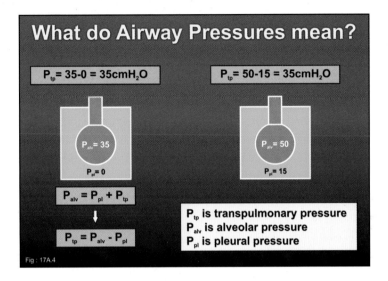

Fig: 17A.4

It is not the airway pressure that is directly responsible for causing VILI. Transpulmonary pressure (P_{tp}), which is the distending pressure of the lungs, causes VILI. Plateau pressure is the non-invasive bed side estimate of P_{tp} (Fig 17A.4). Alveolar pressure or the plateau pressure should be limited to less than 30 cm H_2O to minimize VILI. Depending on the chest wall elastance the transpulmonary pressure can vary. Therefore, Ptp may not be always equal to plateau pressure (Fig 17A.5). Chest wall elastance increases in extrapulmonary ARDS, but the transpulmonary pressure is less. Simply put, increased stiffness of the chest wall tries to oppose the alveolar distension caused by alveolar pressure. But if a patient makes spontaneous respiratory effort when on assist/control mode of ventilator support, the transpulmonary pressure is comparatively more. Here, the negative pleural pressure because of spontaneous effort adds to the distending force of the alveolar pressure. Therefore, the risk of VILI also increases accordingly even though the plateau pressure is same in both situations.

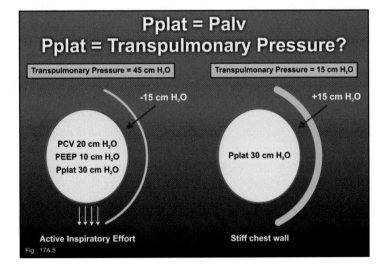

Fig: 17A.5

Studies have shown that increased transpulmonary pressure may not cause VILI as much as predicted. The reasons may include:
- recruitment of dependent atelectatic lung regions, reducing shear stress forces
- more homogeneous distribution of regional transpulmonary pressures
- variability of breathing pattern
- redistribution of perfusion towards non-atelectatic injured areas
- improved lymphatic drainage

In clinical practice the pleural pressure is measured as esophageal pressure by using an esophageal balloon. However, the pressure measured in the esophageal balloon does not reflect the absolute value of the pleural pressure because it varies in different regions of the lungs.

Risk factors

VALI is more common in patients receiving ventilatory support for:
- Acute lung injury or acute respiratory distress syndrome (ALI/ARDS) because of previous injury and heterogeneous distribution of disease
- Restrictive lung disease
- Blood product transfusions
- Patients receiving high tidal volumes

Diagnosis of VALI/VILI

Definitive diagnosis of VILI/VALI is difficult because of lack of pathognomonic features. But it is not necessary to differentiate it from ARDS/ALI as management strategies are same for both the conditions.

Types of ventilator-induced lung injury

Volutrauma

As explained above, whatever be the amount of tidal volume delivered, it preferentially enters the alveoli in the aerated region which is small compared to diseased and collapsed alveoli resulting in overdistension of normal alveoli. This causes increased stretch leading to alveolar damage, increased epithelial and capillary permeability, and pulmonary oedema. This can be minimized by using low tidal volume strategy (6 ml/kg predicted body weight) and limiting end-inspiratory plateau pressure to less than 30 cm H_2O. The resulting hypercarbia is acceptable as long as the pH is more than or equal to 7.15 and patient is haemodynamically stable (permissive hypercarbia).

Atelectrauma

Shear forces on the thin tissue wall separating junctional alveoli causes stress failure of alveolar membrane and disruption of the epithelium (Fig 17A.6). The shear force depends on recruitment and de-recruitment, cycling frequency and duration of exposure to high pressure. This injury is more in dependent regions of the lung because the diseased lung is edematous and the weight of the edematous alveoli (in non-dependent region) causes squeezing of the gas out of the dependant alveoli leading to collapse. This is one of the reasons why V/Q matching improves on proning since, there is more lung tissue in the dorsal region which now becomes non-dependent and there is more homogeneous distribution of both ventilation and perfusion. Atelectrauma can be prevented by applying PEEP to avoid repeated opening and closing of the alveoli (Fig 17A.7).

Hazards of Mechanical Ventilation

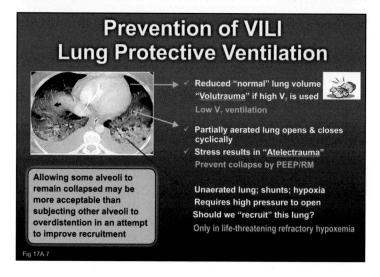

Fig 17A.6

Fig 17A.7

Biotrauma

Direct physical consequences of mechanical ventilation were given more importance in the past. Of late, it has become clear that there are other potentially dangerous mechanisms in addition to direct mechanical effects. Ventilation leads to mechanical stress resulting in release of inflammatory mediators from lung tissue. These mediators in addition to causing direct injury to lung tissue also cause injury to other organs. This response is called biotruama (Fig 17A.8).

Normally, there is a balance between proinflammatory cytokines [tumour necrosis factor (TNF)-α, interleukin (IL) -1 etc] and anti-inflammatory cytokines (IL-10). When there is a mechanical stress during ventilation the proinflammatory cytokines induce NF- κB activation which in turn results in transcription of genes necessary to sustain immune response and finally lead to activation and extravasation of granulocytes. There is delayed apoptosis of these cells mediated by proinflammatory cytokines. These inflammatory cytokines cause surfactant dysfunction or deficiency. Proinflammatory cytokines also cause coagulopathy by stimulating the coagulation cascade through tissue factor and inhibiting fibrinolytic system.

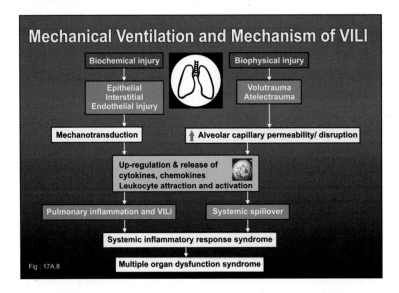

Fig : 17A.8

The mediators are released during mechanical ventilation by many mechanisms:
- Mechanotransduction
- Stress failure of alveolar membrane and plasma membrane
- Effects on vasculature

Mechanotransduction is the conversion of physical deformation to chemical response. The important structures involved in this process are transmembrane receptors such as integrins, stretch-activated ion channels and the cytoskeleton. These structures sense the mechanical stress and initiate various intracellular processes including gene transcription which lead to increased cytokine synthesis. Because of damage to alveolar and epithelial cells there is release of cytokines into both alveolar space and systemic circulation. Also, there is propagation of bacteria and endotoxins from alveolar space to systemic circulation and cause MODS. This passage of endotoxins and bacteria to systemic circulation will cause death in many ARDS patients and not hypoxemia.

Most studies give importance to injurious ventilatory practices that cause mechanical stress to minimize the incidence of VILI. But biotruama is actually thought to play a major role in development of MODS and finally cause mortality in many ARDS patients. This gives an opportunity to develop new treatment strategies based on curtailing the inflammatory response and apoptosis to decrease the deleterious consequences of mechanical ventilation and improve the survival rates in ARDS patients.

Vascular contribution to VALI

The alveolar capillary membrane offers a delicate interface between blood and gas. Alveolar pressure applied to alveolar epithelium can also impact capillary endothelium. Similarly, the intraluminal pressure and flow within the blood vessels can play a role in the development of VILI.

The pulmonary circulation from pulmonary artery to left atrium comprises of two types of vessels:
- Alveolar vessels (capillaries in alveolar wall primarily exposed to alveolar pressure) and
- Extra-alveolar vessels (vessels in corner of alveolar junction, larger vessels feeding capillaries, pulmonary arteries and veins mainly exposed to pleural pressure).

Under normal circumstances extra-alveolar vessels contribute most to overall pulmonary vascular resistance. The effect of alveolar pressure on alveolar vessels is responsible for change in the pulmonary

Hazards of Mechanical Ventilation

vascular resistance (PVR) during ventilation. During expansion of a normal lung, the capillaries in the alveolar wall are compressed by the expansion of adjoining alveoli, while extra-alveolar vessels dilate and elongate (Fig17A.9). Pulmonary vascular resistance rises in proportion to the lung volume at all lung volumes above FRC because the effects of compression of alveolar vessels and elongation of extra-alveolar vessels (increase PVR) outweigh the effects of dilatation of the extra-alveolar vessels (decrease PVR). These effects are exaggerated by heterogeneous lung involvement in injured lungs and are more in the dependent regions of the lungs.

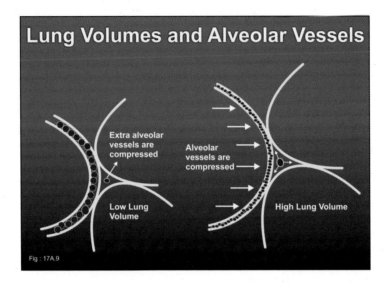

Fig: 17A.9

Even trivial increase in pulmonary microvascular pressure will increase edema formation considerably during the early stage of ALI/ARDS because of increased capillary permeability due to inflammatory changes. The resulting alveolar edema adversely affects gas exchange and edematous airways obstruct airflow and secretion clearance. However, alveolar edema may produce opposing effects from the perspective of VILI. The shear forces acting on collapsed alveoli are proportional to

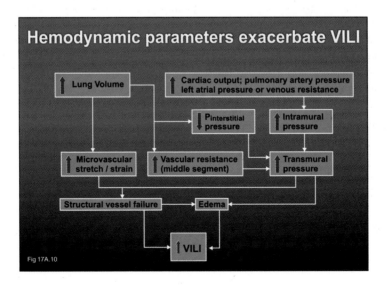

Fig 17A.10

the difference in the size between the collapsed alveolus and adjoining distended alveoli. Completely fluid-filled (edematous) alveoli are subjected to lower shearing stresses than collapsed alveoli as the gas-liquid interface is eliminated and alveolar size increases. At the same time, oedema fluid causes elimination of surface tension which causes capillaries in the alveolar walls to bulge further into the interior causing rupture. The increased weight of the edematous lung may cause small airway compression and increase the tendency for tidal opening and closure to occur.

It is difficult to tell which of these opposing effects predominates in a given scenario. Some animal studies have shown that increasing the cardiac output could lead to increased pre-alveolar microvascular pressure and a higher vascular pressure gradient across the lung. This magnifies tensile forces external to the microvessels or gives rise to shearing stresses within the vascular endothelium predisposing for VILI (Fig17A.10).

Lower respiratory rate and/or lower pulmonary vascular pressure would both be expected to reduce the risk of VILI as reducing the respiratory rate decreases the number of stress cycles and allows sufficient time between adjacent cycles for repair to take place. Targeting just adequate cardiac output to maintain end organ perfusion rather than supra physiologic levels and by reducing the physiologic requirements for ventilation will reduce the vascular stress and reduce the risk of VILI. But further studies are required to substantiate this.

Pulmonary barotrauma

Positive pressure ventilation results in increased transalveolar pressure (alveolar pressure - pressure in the adjacent interstitial space). When this overcomes the structural integrity of the alveolar membrane it results in alveolar rupture and extra alveolar air. This is barotrauma. The incidence of barotrauma is decreasing due to lung protective ventilation (LPV). The common consequences of barotrauma include pneumothorax, pulmonary interstitial emphysema, pneumomediastinum, pneumoperitoneum and subcutaneous emphysema.

Patients with pulmonary barotrauma may not show any signs and symptoms. Depending on the complication, patients manifest a variety of symptoms and signs. Commonly they present with dyspnoea, tachypnea, chest pain, tachycardia, hypotension and desaturation. In addition, local distension and tenderness may be present. It is important to suspect and identify the patients with pneumothorax early because it can develop into tension pneumothorax and lead to cardiac arrest in a very short time. A sudden increase in the peak inspiratory pressure and deterioration in static compliance may indicate development of pneumothorax although it is also possible in other situations like pulmonary oedema. There are two types of airway pressure: peak airway pressure (PIP) and plateau pressure. It is the plateau pressure that is most indicative of alveolar pressure and not peak inspiratory pressure. It is recommended to maintain plateau pressure below 30cmH2O because lower plateau pressure result in lesser incidence of barotrauma.

Assessment of oxygenation, ventilation and acid base status by ABG evaluation gives a clue to consequences of barotrauma but may not always indicate the diagnosis of barotrauma.Next Section: Epidemiology Even in the absence of signs and symptoms, portable chest x-ray may show evidence of barotrauma. Presence of previous opacities in the chest x-ray may make it difficult to identify barotrauma. Sometimes small pockets of extra alveolar air may be missed on regular chest x-ray, in which case, lateral chest x-ray and CT thorax may help.

Whenever barotrauma is suspected, immediate measures to decrease plateau pressure like decreasing the tidal volume or PEEP, increasing the level of sedation, paralyzing the patient and further intensifying the treatment of underlying medical condition should be undertaken.

Hazards of Mechanical Ventilation

In addition to this, specific management of various consequences of barotrauma should be instituted. For example, pneumothorax due to barotrauma may require insertion of chest tube especially if it is progressing to tension pneumothorax or compromising gas exchange or is persistent. Otherwise, the patient should be closely monitored because any pneumothorax can progress to tension pneumothorax. Other complications are usually self limiting and require only supportive care. Surgical intervention may become necessary only if tension physiology develops.

Lung-protective mechanical ventilation with small tidal volumes is becoming the standard of care for patients with ALI/ARDS (Fig17A.11)

In order to minimize VALI, it is important not to target achieving the physiological goals of gas exchange. A fine balance should be struck between maintaining life sustaining adequate gas exchange and minimizing injurious effects to lungs. This goal is achieved by balancing the opening and maintaining patency of as many alveoli as possible to maintain oxygenation and at the same time ventilating (distending) the alveoli as gently and as minimally as possible, thereby maintaining carbon dioxide level within acceptable pH level (≥ 7.15, if haemodynamically stable).

Two main management strategies during mechanical ventilation to minimize VALI are:

1. Restricting the inflation volume and pressure to prevent overdistension of alveoli
2. Applying adequate PEEP to prevent repetitive opening and collapse of alveoli

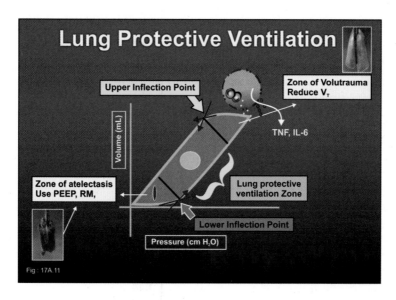

Fig: 17A.11

By using above strategies it is possible to bring the lung into zone of safety. Management strategies for refractory hypoxemia like recruitment maneuvers, alternate modes of ventilation like high frequency ventilation and adjunctive therapies to lung protective ventilation have been discussed in the chapter on ARDS.

Oxygen toxicity

The term "oxygen toxicity" is usually reserved for tracheobronchial and pulmonary parenchymal damage. Patients exposed to inspiratory oxygen fraction (FiO_2)>50% may experience oxygen toxicity, particularly if the exposure is prolonged. Oxygen toxicity is related to free radicals. The major end product of normal oxygen metabolism is water. Some oxygen molecules, however, are converted into highly reactive species called free radicals, which include superoxide anions, perhydroxy radicals and hydroxyl radicals. These are toxic to alveolar and tracheobronchial cells. When the production of these reactive species increases and/or the cell's antioxidant defenses are depleted, oxygen radicals can react with and impair the function of essential intracellular macromolecules, resulting in cell death.

There is no well-defined threshold FiO_2 or duration of supplemental oxygen therapy below which oxygen toxicity cannot occur. Lung tissue is exposed to the highest concentrations of oxygen in the body, placing cells that line the tracheobronchial tree and alveoli at the greatest risk for hyperoxic cytotoxicity. Hyperoxia may also increase susceptibility to mucous plugging, atelectasis and secondary infection by impairing both mucociliary clearance and the bactericidal capacity of immune cells.

High fractions of inspired oxygen (FiO_2) have been associated with several pulmonary consequences such as increased intrapulmonary right-to-left shunt fraction, diminished lung volumes due to absorptive atelectasis, accentuation of hypercapnia and damage to airways and pulmonary parenchyma.

Hyperoxic hypercarbia

It is described as increase in $PaCO_2$ level in COPD patients with compensated respiratory acidosis when FiO_2 is increased. There has been an overemphasis that administration of oxygen may lead to respiratory drive depression which in turn causes hypercapnia with resulting respiratory acidosis. The main mechanism is now thought to be due to V/Q mismatch leading to increased dead space ventilation because of abolition of hypoxic pulmonary vasoconstriction reflex. This has caused some clinicians to be overly timid about prescribing oxygen. Oxygen-induced hypercapnia does rarely occur, but it is even rarer that respiratory acidosis occurs. Hence, supplemental oxygen should not be withheld in COPD patients presenting with hypoxia.

Prevention

There is no single threshold of FiO_2 defining a safe upper limit for prevention of oxygen toxicity. The relative importance of the duration and magnitude of hyperoxic exposure also has not been clearly defined. Some factors which cannot be easily quantified, such as the adequacy of a given patient's antioxidant defenses probably also play a role in determining individual susceptibility. Reducing the FiO_2 to the lowest tolerable limit is a good principle for all patients, in particular those likely to be at risk of hyperoxia-induced lung injury because of a prolonged duration of oxygen therapy or prior therapy with bleomycin (patients who receive bleomycin appear to be more susceptible to diffuse alveolar damage following oxygen exposure, based upon *in vitro* data and uncontrolled clinical experience). In practical terms, oxygen should be administered to achieve a PaO_2 of 60 to 65 mm Hg (SaO_2 approximately 90 percent). FiO_2 should be reduced to below 60% as soon as the patient's condition permits and then to 40% because at this level, oxygen can be tolerated for prolonged period without any deleterious consequences.

Additional strategies to maximize oxygenation and reduce FiO_2 (e.g. diuresis, bronchopulmonary hygiene, prone positioning, inhaled nitric oxide, recruitment maneuvers and/or optimal PEEP) should be considered when FiO_2 exceeds 60 percent for more than six hours. Antioxidant and immunomodulator use have remained experimental. According to available data, known immediate risks of systemic hypoxia or VILI are clearly more established and devastating than potential future risk of hyperoxia induced lung injury.

Hence, one should not hesitate to use higher FiO_2 levels if need be when hypoxemia becomes life threatening despite the use of moderate PEEP, recruitment maneuvers, proning and other adjuvant therapies.

Conclusion

Lung protective ventilation strategy is the only intervention that has shown significant and sustained short term mortality benefit probably by reducing VALI. So, it is advisable to implement this strategy in all mechanically ventilated patients. In spite of lung protective ventilation, VALI can still occur and progress indicating in addition to mechanical stretch, cytotoxic and proinflammatory mediators play a major role. More and more studies are supporting this and in future controlling and targeting these proinflammatory mediators may provide new modality of treatment to further improve the outcome.

References

1. Cytokines and biotrauma in ventilator-induced lung injury: a critical review of the literature. F.J.J. Halbertsma, M. Vaneker et al. The journal of medicine, The Netherlands. November 2005; vol. 63, no.10,
2. Methods to prevent ventilator-associated lung injury: a summary, Sarah J. Cooper, Intensive and Critical Care Nursing 2004; 20, 358—365
3. Mechanical Ventilation with Lung Protective Strategies: What Works? Carl F. Haas. Crit Care Clin 27, 2011; 469-486
4. Bench-to-bedside review: Microvascular and airspace linkage in ventilator-induced lung injury: John J. Marini, John R; Hotchkiss, et al. Critical Care. December 2003; vol 7 No 6
5. Bench-to-bedside review: Chest wall elastance in acute lung injury/acute respiratory distress syndrome patients; Luciano Gattinoni, Davide Chiumello et al. Critical Care October 2004; vol 8 No 5
6. ARDS net
7. Ventilator-associated lung injury: Liao Pinhu, Thomas Whitehead, Timothy Evans et al. Lancet 2003; 361: 332-40
8. Pathophysiology of ventilator-associated lung injury: Patricia R.M. Roccoa, Claudia Dos Santosb et al. Curr Opin Anesthesiol 2012; 25:123-130
9. Physical and biological triggers of ventilator-induced lung injury and its prevention: L. Gattinoni, E. Carlesso et al. Eur Respir J 2003; 22: Suppl. 47, 15s-25s

B : VENTILATOR ASSOCIATED PNEUMONIA

Ventilator associated pneumonia (VAP) forms a part of hospital acquired pneumonia (HAP). Among HAP patients, ventilator associated pneumonia (VAP) has the highest morbidity and mortality. VAP is one of the most common ICU-acquired infections in patients requiring mechanical ventilation over 48 hr and its estimated incidence is 10–20%. Even though it is called ventilator associated pneumonia it is not associated with ventilator but with artificial airways (endotracheal tube and tracheostomy tube). The crude ICU mortality rates for VAP range from 24% to 76%. Besides being an independent determinant of mortality, VAP is associated with longer ICU and hospital stays, prolonged mechanical ventilation, and attributable costs.

Definition of VAP

Ventilator-associated pneumonia is defined as pneumonia occurring more than 48 hr after patients have been intubated and received mechanical ventilation.

Classification of VAP (Fig 17B.1)

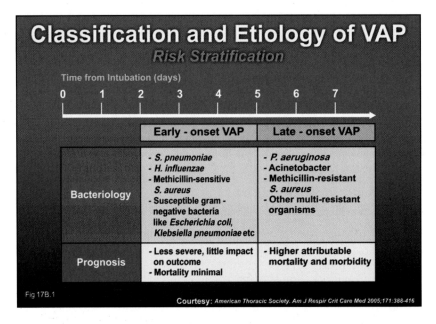

Fig 17B.1

The time of onset of pneumonia is important because it determines risk of infection with MDR pathogens and outcomes in patients with VAP. Early onset VAP is usually caused by antibiotic sensitive pathogens and carries better prognosis. Late onset VAP is usually caused by MDR pathogens and carries poor prognosis.

Pathogenesis and etiology of VAP (Fig 17B.2)

VAP is commonly caused by bacterial pathogens and rarely by fungal and viral pathogens in immunocompetent hosts. The common organisms include gram negative aerobic bacilli like *P. aeruginosa, E. coli, Klebsiella* and acinetobacter species. Infections due to gram positive cocci like *Staphylococcus aureus* especially methicllin resistant is also on the rise.

The common sources for these organisms are health care devices, air, water, equipment, fomites and also transfer of organisms from other patients and health care staff.

Hazards of Mechanical Ventilation

The organisms gain entry into lower respiratory tract through microaspiration or leakage of secretions around the endotracheal tube. Sometimes they enter through inhalation, direct inoculation or hematogenous spread and bacterial translocation from gastrointestinal tract lumen. The infected biofilm in the artificial airway with subsequent embolization is also important in the pathogenesis of VAP. The stomach and sinuses are important reservoirs for pathogens which lead to colonization of oropharynx but their role in pathogenesis of VAP is controversial.

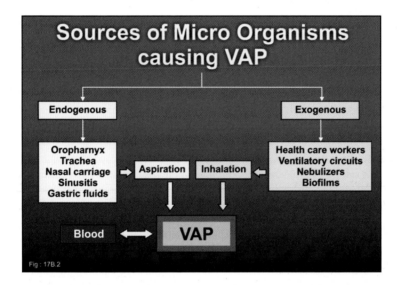

VAP diagnosis (Fig 17B.3)

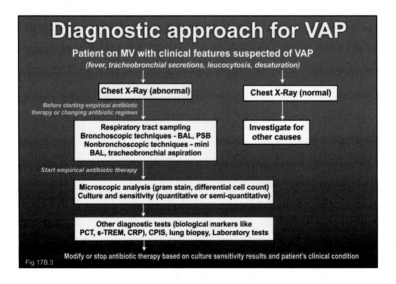

The diagnosis of VAP is challenging. Bedside evaluation using clinical and radiographic criteria is neither specific nor sensitive. Gold standard for the diagnosis of VAP is the histopathologic examination and culture of lung tissue obtained by biopsy or at autopsy.

This also has some inherent problems. Both invasive (bronchoscopic) and noninvasive (endotracheal aspirates) techniques to obtain samples for microbiological cultures are used in clinical practice, without consensus as to which technique is superior.

Clinical features

The presence of a new or progressive radiographic infiltrate plus at least two of three clinical features like
- Fever greater than 38 °C
- Leukocytosis or leukopenia
- Purulent tracheobronchial secretions, represents the most accurate combination of criteria for starting empiric antibiotic therapy.

Tachypnea, decreased tidal volume, increased minute ventilation, and desaturation are some important additional signs.

If only one criterion is used the sensitivity is high but specificity comes down. Other common causes for fever and radiographic infiltrates should be ruled out. Diagnostic evaluation is required whenever VAP is clinically suspected. The goal is to confirm the diagnosis of VAP and to correctly identify the likely pathogen so that unnecessary and inappropriate antibiotics are not administered.

The diagnostic evaluation begins with a chest X-ray. If chest X-ray shows opacities then lower respiratory tract samples should be taken and sent for microscopic analysis, culture and, sensitivity studies. The sample should be taken preferably before initiating the antibiotic therapy or changing the antibiotic regimen, if patient is already on antibiotic therapy because it decreases the sensitivity of microscopic analysis and culture studies. Immediately after samples are obtained empirical antibiotic therapy should be started as per local sensitivity pattern and patient's condition unless there is very low clinical suspicion for VAP. But if for some reason samples cannot be taken immediately and patient is very sick and there is high clinical suspicion of VAP empirical antibiotic therapy should be started because delay in antibiotic therapy increases mortality.

Chest X-ray

It should be done in all patients suspected of VAP. Normal chest X-ray rules out VAP. But abnormal chest X-ray is alone not sufficient to diagnose VAP because it can be caused by many other causes. So, lower respiratory tract samples should be taken.

Respiratory tract sampling

	Nonbronchoscopic Methods	Bronchoscopic Methods
1.	Tracheobronchial aspiration It is performed by passing sterile suction catheter through the endotracheal tube until resistance is met and applying suction to collect the secretions.	Bronchalveolar lavage (BAL) It involves passing a flexible bronchoscope through endo-tracheal tube and wedging over affected bronchial segmental orifice and infusing and aspirating sterile saline.
2.	Mini-BAL It is done by passing sterile suction catheter through endotracheal tube till resistance is met and infusing sterile saline before applying suction to collect the specimen.	Protected specimen Brush (PSB) In this technique a protected specimen brush is used which is contained within a protective sheath. This minimizes the chances of contamination of sample with upper respiratory tract micro-organisms. The bronchoscope tip is placed next to the affected bronchial segmental orifice, and the sheath is passed through the bronchoscope. Then the brush is pushed out of the sheath and into the airway. Samples are collected by brushing the airway wall, withdrawing the brush into the sheath, and then pulling out the sheath from the bronchoscope.
3.	Advantages Less invasiveness, less compromise of oxygenation, ventilation, arrhythmias and respiratory mechanics during the procedure, samples can be obtained even if there is no bronchoscopist and also in patients with small endotracheal tubes, samples can be immediately obtained at lower cost.	Advantages Certainly reduce contamination of the samples (greater specificity) which results in narrower antibiotic regimen and rapid de-escalation and in effect decreasing antibiotic resistance.
4.	Disadvantages More chance of cross contamination of samples and false positive results leading to unnecessary antibiotic therapy.	Disadvantages Invasive, complications during procedure, costly, requires technical expertise and specialized equipment, may not be available in all centers, may lead to delay in collection of samples and initiating empirical antibiotic therapy etc.

Fig 17B.4

It should be taken in all patients who are clinically suspected to have VAP and have abnormal chest X-ray. Lower respiratory tract samples can be taken by various methods (Fig 17B.4).

Both bronchoscopic and non bronchoscopic techniques have been compared in various studies. Bronchoscopic sampling techniques have not been able to reduce mortality, length of hospital stay, duration of mechanical ventilation, or length of intensive care unit stay. The choice of method depends on local expertise, experience, availability, and cost.

Microscopic analysis

Gram stain is the common microscopic analysis. It can also be used to semi-quantitate polymorphonuclear leukocytes and other cell types and to identify the morphology of bacteria. If abundant neutrophils are present then it is more in favor of the diagnosis of VAP and the bacterial morphology may give a clue regarding likely pathogen. A differential count can also be performed on a BAL specimen. A low percentage of neutrophils mean less chance of VAP.

Respiratory tract sample culture

Culture can be done by both quantitative and semiquantitative methods on samples obtained by both bronchoscopic and non-bronchoscopic methods. Both quantitative and semiquantitative cultures are comparable in terms of clinical outcomes and are acceptable depending on local availability. Quantitative cultures are preferred whenever available.

Other diagnostic tests

Various biological markers like procalcitonin, C-reactive protein (CRP) and soluble triggering receptor expressed on myeloid cells-1 (sTREM-1), are used as markers in VAP diagnosis. Procalcitonin is used to decide to de-escalate antibiotics and as a prognostic marker. Clinical pulmonary infection score (CPIS) combines clinical, radiographic, physiologic, and microbiologic data into a numerical result. A CPIS score greater than six correlates with VAP. But the evidence to date does not support widespread use of the CPIS as a diagnostic, prognostic, or therapeutic decision tool, because it is not an adequate surrogate for the diagnosis of VAP. Lung biopsy is an invasive procedure and its reliability and reproducibility is not certain. Therefore, not commonly used for the diagnosis of VAP.

Diagnostic criteria

When a patient who has been on ventilator for ≥48 hours develops a new or progressive infiltrate and the respiratory specimens are positive (i.e., increased neutrophils are seen in the microscopic analysis and growth of a pathogen in culture exceeds a predefined threshold) then it is diagnosed as VAP.

When the culture and sensitivity results are back which usually takes 2 to 3 days, the patient should be reassessed to determine if additional diagnostic evaluation or changes in management are required. These decisions are based upon the culture results and clinical response to empiric therapy

- If there is no clinical improvement and cultures are also negative then patient may not have VAP. So, look for other infection sites or a different diagnosis.
- If there is clinical improvement but cultures are negative then the patient may not have VAP. So, discontinue antibiotic therapy.
- If there is no clinical improvement but cultures are positive then patient has VAP but receiving inadequate antibiotic therapy or has developed VAP complication like abscess or empyema, or has another source of infection. So, antibiotic therapy should be modified and other causes for non-improvement should be sought and addressed.

- If there is clinical improvement and cultures are also positive then patient has VAP which has responded to initial antibiotic therapy. So, antibiotic therapy should be narrowed according to culture results.

Recommendations for VAP prevention (Fig 17B.5)

Prevention of VAP is important because once VAP develops the mortality even with treatment is high. This is more so in late VAP due to multi drug resistant organisms. Invasive mechanical ventilation should be avoided if possible. Use of NPPV especially in COPD, acute cardiogenic pulmonary edema and immuno-compromized patients should be standard of care.

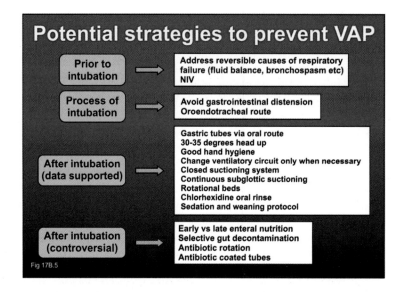

Fig 17B.5

Physical strategies (Fig 17B.6)

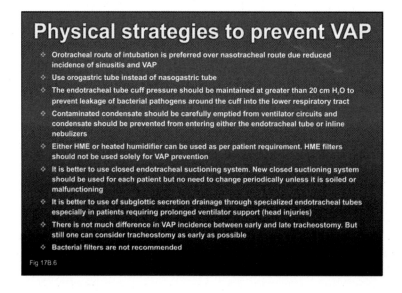

Fig 17B.6

Hazards of Mechanical Ventilation

Positional strategies

- The use of rotating beds should be considered.
- It is advisable that the head of the bed be elevated to 45° (Semi-recumbent positioning). Where this is not possible, attempt to raise the head of the bed as much as possible.
- Prone positioning is associated with a reduction in incidence of VAP, but for safety and feasibility reasons it may not be possible to implement in every patient unless indicated for other reasons like refractory hypoxemia.

Pharmacological strategies

Prophylactic antibiotics

- No recommendation can be made for aerosolized antibiotics, nasal antibiotics, intravenous antibiotics either alone or in combination with oral antibiotics (selective decontamination of the digestive tract) for routine use to prevent VAP because of inconsistent effect on mortality, ICU and hospital length of stay and increased risk of antibiotic resistance
- The use of the oral antiseptic chlorhexidine should be considered.
- The use of the oral antiseptic povidone-iodione should be considered in patients with severe head injury.

Other strategies

- Avoid unnecessary stress ulcer prophylaxis with H_2 receptor antagonists.
- Hand hygiene should be practiced. Wash hands with soap and water when visibly dirty or visibly soiled with blood or other body fluids or after using the toilet or exposure to potential spore-forming pathogens. Use an alcohol-based handrub as the preferred means for routine hand antisepsis, if hands are not visibly soiled in all other clinical situations like, before and after touching the patient, before handling an invasive device for patient care, after contact with body fluids or excretions, mucous membranes, non-intact skin, or wound dressings, if moving from a contaminated body site to another body site during care of the same patient, after contact with inanimate surfaces and objects (including medical equipment) in the immediate vicinity of the patient, after removing sterile or non-sterile gloves, before handling medication or preparing food.
- Use sedation protocols and weaning protocols to decrease the time the patient spends on ventilator.
- Transfusion of red blood cell and other allogeneic blood products should follow a restricted transfusion trigger policy; leukocyte-depleted red blood cell transfusions can help to reduce HAP in selected patient populations
- Patients on EN should be periodically assessed and steps should be taken to reduce risk of aspiration. These are listed below:
- Head end should be elevated to 30°– 45°
- EN should be switched to continuous infusion in high risk patients, if they are intolerant to gastric feeding
- Prokinetic drugs or narcotic antagonists should be used, if feasible
- Small bowel feeding must be considered
- Intensive insulin therapy is recommended to maintain serum glucose levels between 150 and 160 mg/dl in ICU patients to reduce nosocomial blood stream infections, duration of mechanical ventilation, ICU stay, morbidity, and mortality

Treatment

Prompt initiation of antibiotic therapy is a cornerstone of treatment of VAP. Even relatively short delays in administering adequate antibiotic therapy are associated with an increased mortality rate.

Algorithm for initiating empiric antibiotic therapy for VAP (Fig 17B.7)

It is advisable to start empirical antibiotic therapy in all patients with clinical features suggestive of VAP and abnormal chest X-ray once lower respiratory tract samples have been taken using the algorithm described in the figure below. It is important to de-escalate from broad spectrum initial empirical antibiotic therapy to narrow spectrum, reduce the duration and stop antibiotics in selected patients by regular clinical assessment and culture sensitivity reports.

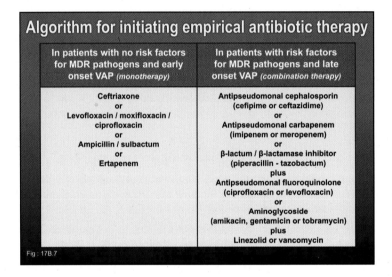

Fig: 17B.7

The risk factors for MDR pathogens are summarised in Fig 17B.8

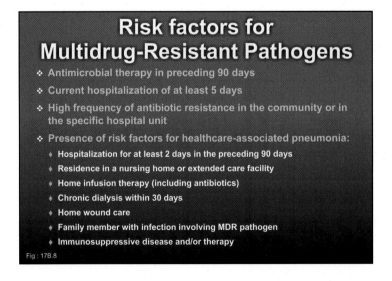

Fig: 17B.8

Hazards of Mechanical Ventilation

Recommendations for initial antibiotic therapy

Patients with increased risk of developing multi drug resistant pathogens should be started on empirical antibiotics. Factors that should be considered when initiating empirical antibiotic therapy are commonly grown local micro organisms, culture sensitivity pattern, and patient related factors like hepatic or renal dysfunction.

Use appropriate antibiotic, in correct dosage and preferentially by intravenous route to avoid excess mortality and morbidity especially in patients with VAP who are likely to be infected with multi drug resistant organisms. If patient has recently been treated with antibiotic it is better to use antibiotic from different class to avoid resistance. Aerosolized antibiotics are not routinely advised but may be considered in selected patients with MDR pathogens who are not responding to systemic therapy.

It is better to start with combination therapy and then switch over to monotherapy once culture sensitivity results are available. It is not necessary to give antibiotic therapy if the patient is improving for 14-21 days in every patient, unless the patient has confirmed *Pseudomonas aeruginosa* infection. Antibiotic therapy of 5-7 days is sufficient in most cases.

Summary of the management strategies for a patient with suspected VAP (Fig 17B.9)

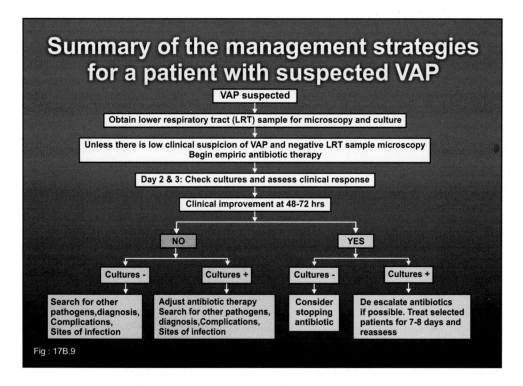

Fig : 17B.9

Possible causes for lack of clinical response to initial antibiotic therapy (Fig 17B.10)

Patient may fail to respond to initial antibiotic therapy if diagnosis is wrong or antibiotic therapy is inappropriate or inadequate or patient might have developed complication of VAP/antibiotic therapy like empyema/lung abscess etc which requires surgical intervention.

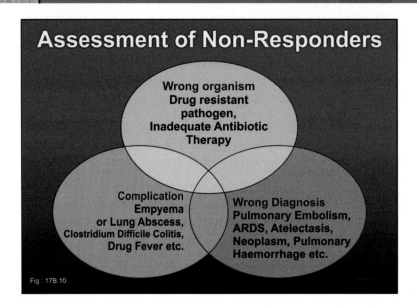

Fig: 17B.10

Assessing response to therapy

Patient's response to therapy should be serially assessed clinically like reducing fever, total leucocyte counts, improving hemodynamics, oxygenation etc. Based on this and culture sensitivity data, antibiotic therapy should be de-escalated and narrowed or stopped. Any improvement in patient's condition usually takes 2-3 days. So antibiotic should not be changed immediately unless there is rapid deterioration in patient's condition. If the patient is not responding to treatment it is better to look for other causes, infectious or noninfectious including extrapulmonary sites, complications of pneumonia like empyema and abscess etc. Procalcitonin can be used to assist in the decision whether to discontinue antibiotics and as a prognostic marker.

Conclusion

An integrated approach should be followed in diagnosing and treating patients with VAP, including early antibiotic therapy and subsequent rectification according to clinical response and results of bacteriologic cultures. It is better to adopt preventive measures for VAP and decrease the incidence because it is difficult to treat VAP.

References

1. Comprehensive evidence-based clinical practice guidelines for ventilator-associated pneumonia: Prevention : John Muscedere, Peter Dodek, Sean Keenan et al. Journal of Critical Care 2008; 23; 126–137
2. Comprehensive evidence-based clinical practice guidelines for ventilator-associated pneumonia: Diagnosis and treatment: John Muscedere, Peter Dodek, Sean Keenan et al. Journal of Critical Care 2008; 23; 138–147
3. American Thoracic Society Documents; Guidelines for the Management of Adults with Hospital acquired, Ventilator-associated, and Healthcare-associated Pneumonia. Am J Respir Crit Care Med 2005 vol 171; pp 388–416

★★★

NEWER MODES OF MECHANICAL VENTILATION

In the dynamic world of ventilation medicine, new modes of mechanical ventilation are being introduced into clinical practice at regular intervals. Advanced close loop systems have seen rapid advances. Many more are in the pipe line and will be introduced in near future. These modes could assume a greater role in supporting critically ill patients in intensive care units (ICUs) for several reasons:

1. Deliver assisted ventilation proportional to the patient's effort, thereby improving patient–ventilator synchrony and patient comfort
2. Automate the medical reasoning
3. Provide a partial solution by reducing ICU-related costs, time spent on mechanical ventilation, and staff workload, especially in a scenario of looming clinician shortage

All the ventilatory modes currently used during mechanical ventilation, function with closed loops. Even a 'simple' mode such as pressure support ventilation uses rules to initiate the pressurization, determine pressurization slope, and end pressurization, regulate flow within the cycle and open the expiratory valve. These rules work in a closed loop based on airway pressure and flow signals. The rules used in newer closed loops are however, more advanced and patient specific.

Dual control modes

Dual modes combine the advantage of pressure and volume ventilation to maintain a set volume by altering pressure assist. This can happen in the course of few breaths or the assist can change from pressure to volume in the same breath (volume assured pressure support). These modes employ a more sophisticated feedback from the patient to the ventilator. The only change from conventional modes is that a set volume is achieved by altering pressure irrespective of changes in lung characteristics (Resistance and Compliance). The target for the ventilator is volume. The target (volume) is not derived in proportion to any part of neuro-ventilatory coupling cascade. Volume is set by clinician. Therefore, dual mode output is not proportional to patients need. Some examples for dual modes include pressure regulated volume control (PRVC); volume assured pressure support (VAPS) and volume support (VS). Dual modes have been dealt in this book as a separate chapter.

Advanced closed loop ventilation

Advances in microchip technology have enabled the development of advanced closed-loop systems that allow 'the ventilator', as opposed to 'the clinician' to manipulate the ventilator variables based on feedback from patient characteristics frequently. These innovations have been possible because of the technological advances in computing and in the field of artificial intelligence. Proportional assist ventilation (PAV+, Puritan–Bennett), neurally adjusted ventilatory assist (NAVA, Maquet), adaptive support ventilation (ASV, Hamilton), Smartcare or Neoganesh (Drager) are some of the commonly used and studied advanced closed loop modes. These modes will be discussed in detail in this chapter. They provide supports according to the lung characteristics and are thus most physiological for a pathological situation.

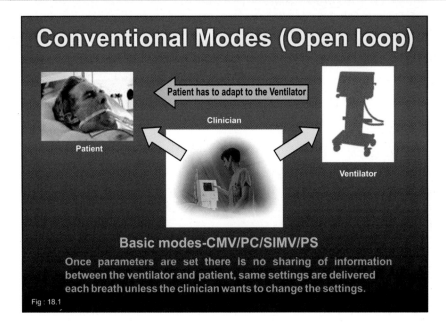

Fig: 18.1

Why do we require newer modes?

Conventional modes (Fig 18.1) have many disadvantages such as

1. Trigger related problems like delayed triggering and missed breaths. These are exaggerated in presence of auto PEEP and leaks
2. Ventilatory assist may not be proportional to patient needs with resultant patient - ventilator dyssynchrony
3. Higher doses of sedation and neuro-muscular blockers are required in these modes leading to ventilator associated pneumonia (VAP), ICU acquired weakness (ICU-AW) and ventilator induced diaphragmatic dysfunction (VIDD)
4. Delayed weaning
5. Hemodynamic compromise

Newer modes have solved some of these problems but the solution to all these problems have not been achieved by a single mode. The quest for ideal mode is still on. The advances that solve the problems of conventional modes are discussed below:

Trigger

Triggering occurs when the patient generates a negative pressure with the movement of chest wall and diaphragm. This is the last part of the neuro-ventilatory coupling (Fig 18.2). The negative pressure drop is identified and relayed back to the machine which initiates the inspiratory flow. The time interval between respiratory center signal output and the ventilator triggered inspiratory flow is around 60 to 80 milliseconds. Trigger delay is an inbuilt problem in conventional modes. Delayed initiation of ventilatory support leads to issues in triggering, pressurization phase and cycling off of inspiration to expiration. This has been solved by NAVA which uses Electrical activity of diaphragm (EAdi) to initiate inspiratory flow which starts when the patient starts his inspiration and ends when the patient wants. The end result is improved patient–ventilator synchrony (Fig 18.3).

Newer Modes of Mechanical Ventilation

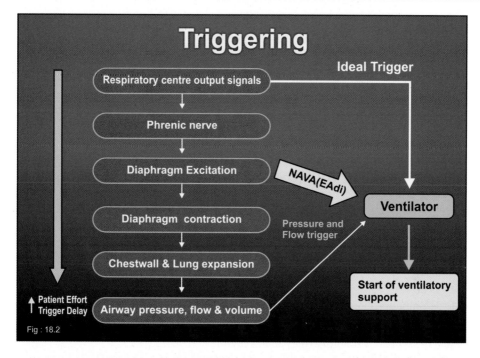

Fig: 18.2

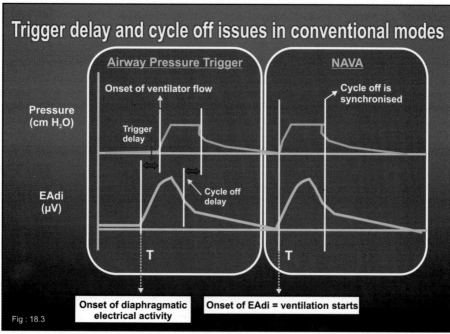

Fig: 18.3

Pneumatic triggering in the presence of auto PEEP leads to missed breaths and increased work of breathing (WOB). These problems are solved by electrical triggering of NAVA (Fig 18.4).

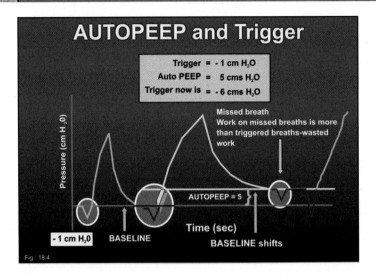
Fig: 18.4

What does proportional support mean?
1. Neural Inspiratory time = Ventilator Inspiratory time
2. Neural Expiratory time = Ventilator Expiratory time
3. Ventilatory support is as much as the patient requires

"Ventilatory assist starts, ends and is as much as the patient wants"

How does the ventilator assess the patient's requirements?

To understand this we have to learn about

1) Neuroventilator coupling mechanism and

2) How the ventilator loops the information derived from part or parts of this cascade to produce a support that is proportional to patient's needs.

Respiratory center output propagation to alveolar ventilation constitutes neuroventilator coupling cascade. Respiratory center output signals are produced after analyzing the inputs derived from chemoreceptors, respiratory muscle efferents, lung and airway reflexes (18.5).

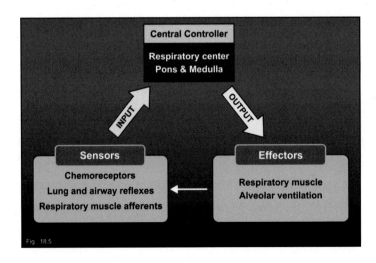
Fig: 18.5

Newer Modes of Mechanical Ventilation

Respiratory output signals propagate as phrenic nerve transmission leading diaphragmatic muscle electrical activity (EAdi). The resultant diaphragmatic contraction and lung distension (respiratory resistance and compliance) cause alveolar ventilation and blood gases stabilization.

Each component along the neuroventilatory coupling chain (Fig18.6) is separately in proportion to physiologically determined respiratory center output. When the ventilator uses information from some parts of this coupling cascade, the ventilatory assist will be proportional to the patient's requirement.

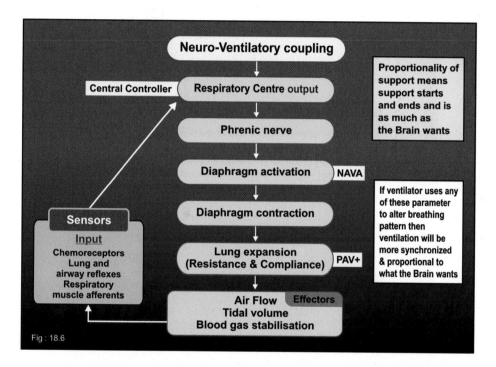

Fig : 18.6

Neuro-ventilator coupling cascade information used by various modes:

1. Nava uses electrical activity of diaphragm (EAdi) to provide ventilator support
2. ASV uses the dead space and expiratory time constant to provide ventilator support
3. PAV+ utilizes airway resistance and compliance measurements to deliver either flow assist (for resistance changes) or volume assist (for compliance changes) to provide ventilator support.

Proportionality of support is vital to prevent suppression of diaphragmatic activity, trigger and cycle dyssynchrony. With better patient-ventilator synchrony, sedation requirements decrease and patients can be weaned faster.

Figures 18.7 and 18.8 show how pressure support and control modes provide a constant ventilatory assist even when the patient requirements change. This may under or over assist the patient.

In case of NAVA and PAV+ the support is in proportion to patient's requirements. Simply put, inspiration starts and cycles to expiration as per patient's requirement and delivers ventilation proportional to the patient's effort.

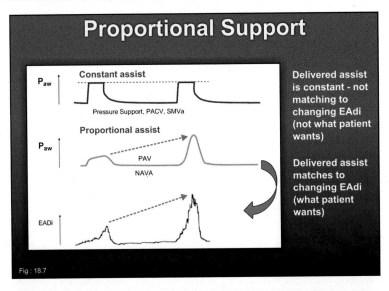

Fig: 18.7

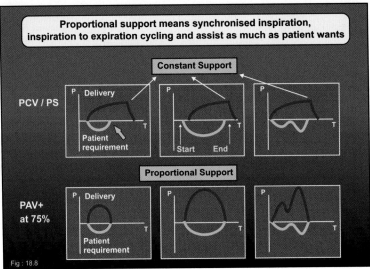

Fig: 18.8

Smartcare's automated medical reasoning is a different closed loop mode which hastens weaning. A clinical protocol is stored in the microchip memory of the ventilator. Clinical knowledge is made use to classify the ventilatory situation into specific diagnoses and to apply therapeutic measures appropriate to the specific diagnosis.

For most new modes to function properly and provide proportional support the neuroventilatory coupling cascade has to be intact. In critically ill patients this may not be the case. Organic issues affecting brain, pulmonary inflammation, other pathologic insults and sedative usage question the assumption that respiratory center output matches the ventilatory needs of the patient. The feedback mechanisms linking the respiratory system (bellows, gas exchange units, and chemoreceptors) with the respiratory centers may not be intact. Sensitivity of the mechanical and chemical receptor responsible for monitoring respiratory function may not be functioning properly. These limitations have to be kept in mind in situations where the newer modes may not work well.

Newer Modes of Mechanical Ventilation

Is breath delivery from the ventilator different in newer modes?

The answer is no.

The ventilator will either deliver flow or pressures at any one point of time. The difference is that the delivery is proportional to the patient's effort. In simple terms, the newer modes deliver same pressure support or pressure control or SIMV breaths looped to patient's neuroventilatory coupling cascade.

Ventilator assist used in newer modes:

1. NAVA- Pressure Support
2. ASV- Pressure support/Pressure Control /SIMV/CPAP
3. Smartcare - Pressure Support
4. PAV-Patient-triggered and pressure-controlled mode with inspiratory flow or volume assistance
5. BI-Level/ APRV- PC and PEEP with spontaneous breaths at both levels

Newer modes are useful only in patients having reasonably intact respiratory output and drive. The exceptions are ASV, BI-level and APRV. These work in passive patients also but work as conventional modes.

Clinical Classification of Modes

1. Modes which adapt to lung characteristics and provide proportional support: PAV+, ASV, NAVA
2. Knowledge based weaning modes: Smartcare, ASV
3. Inverse ratio ventilation with spontaneous breathing: BI-Level, APRV

Evidence basis of newer modes

Although studies have shown that newer modes provide better oxygenation, faster weaning, lesser sedation, less asynchrony and better patient comfort, mortality benefit has not been proved.

Our take on newer modes:

These modes are primarily used when the respiratory drive is intact and patient has reduced sedation requirements. Some primary disease resolution must have also occurred. Better oxygenation, faster weaning, less sedation, patient comfort and decreased hospital stay are the end points hoped to be achieved by using newer modes and not reduced mortality.

Good protocol based weaning, sedation and lung protective ventilation provided in conventional mode will match the ventilation provided by the newer modes because the breath delivery is essentially same. Therefore, any mortality benefit of newer modes over conventional modes may be difficult to prove in an adequately powered RCT.

What then is the place of newer modes in ICU?

Conventional modes with fixed settings require frequent changes. In a study by Donchin et al., it was seen that errors related to ventilatory settings was the second most frequent cause of mortality and morbidity (after errors related to data entry).

Frequent need for change in settings in conventional mode causes high workload and 'burnout syndrome' among physicians, respiratory therapists and nurses working in ICUs. Added to this, the shortage of personnel, high frequency of staff turnover, raising medical costs and budgetary cuts in medical funding necessitate use of newer modes in present day practice.

The verdict is out

a. Closed loop MV = Less work in ICU
b. Quick weaning = Short stay in ICU
c. More automation = Less need for specialists
d. Lower costs and high patient safety.

"Innovation and Automation is the way forward"

Conclusion

Older modes and ventilators are passive, operator-dependant tools. New modes in new generation ventilators are adaptively interactive to patient, are goal oriented and have lower operator activity. It is important to understand that no mode of mechanical ventilation is inherently safer than another. All modes can be safely used (or not) depending on lung protective settings the clinician chooses, the alarms that place the limits on the process and the alacrity with which the care giver makes appropriate adjustments in response to the changing nature of the problem. No new ventilator mode can, at this point in time, claim to improve patient outcome compared to older mode with lung protective ventilation.

The modes most commonly used and studied will be discussed:

1. Adaptive Support Ventilation- ASV (Hamilton)
2. Proportional assist ventilation-PAV+ (Puritan Bennett)
3. Neurally adjusted ventilator assist-NAVA (Maquet)
4. Airway pressure release ventilation - APRV and BI-Level ventilation
5. Smartcare/Neoganesh-SC (Drager)

Adaptive Support Ventilation (ASV)

ASV (Fig 18.9) is based on a complicated mathematical derivation called Otis equation which calculates a breathing pattern requiring least amount of total energy expenditure (WOB). This holds well in different pathological conditions also.

Minimum minute ventilation is the only specific setting that must be chosen by the clinician. It is based on patient's body weight. When starting ventilation in ASV, the ventilator provides three pressure controlled - time cycled inspirations. Expiratory time constant is estimated from the tidal volume curve during each expiration. Then, using Otis's formula, a target respiratory rate is calculated. Target tidal volume is computed from minimum minute ventilation and target respiratory rate. Thereafter, target values are calculated cycle by cycle depending on patient's spontaneous respiratory rate.

ASV can work as

a. PCV- if there is no spontaneous breathing
b. Pressure SIMV- when patient's respiratory rate is smaller than target
c. PSV- if patient's respiratory rate is greater

Pressure level is then adapted to attain the target tidal volume (within limits imposed by pressure alarms). Cycling off criteria is flow based in case of assisted ventilation and time based for mandatory inspiration. ASV applies lung-protective rules and promotes weaning from the first minute. It works in COPD patients but not in patients with very high auto PEEP levels.

Newer Modes of Mechanical Ventilation

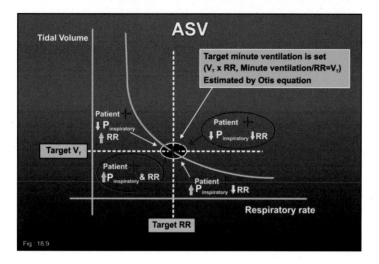
Fig: 18.9

Conclusion

ASV is the only approach that unifies all modes into one mode and thus has the potential to be clinically useful.

Proportional assist ventilation (PAV+)

PAV+ is a mode based on equation of motion (Fig 18.10) for mechanical ventilation. Ventilatory assist is delivered proportional to the patient's inspiratory effort based on the defined level of unloading in order to relieve the resistive and elastic burden of the respiratory system. Pressure assistance is instantaneously adapted to the patient's needs breath by breath. Applied airway pressures develop as a function of volume to overcome respiratory system elastance (elastic unloading, volume assist) or a function of flow to overcome respiratory system resistance (resistive unloading, flow assist). Flow and volume assist are able to unload the resistive and elastic components of total work of breathing separately.

The clinician does not set a rate, tidal volume, flow or target pressure. Instead, the clinician simply sets the percentage of work that the ventilator should do. Start patients at 80% and wean back to stabilize.

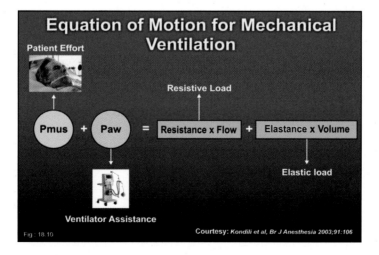
Fig: 18.10

PAV+ uses compliance and resistance information collected every 4-10 breaths to know what it is fighting against. The flow and volume information collected every 5 milliseconds tells what the patient wants. This data along with the percentage of support input given by the clinician determines how much pressure is supplied to the system by the ventilator.

PAV+ has many potential benefits like patient comfort, lower peak airway pressure, decreased need for paralysis and/or sedation and less likelihood for overventilation. Preservation and enhancement of patient's own control mechanisms such as metabolic ABG control and Hering-Breuer reflex is present.

High rate on PAV+ may or may not reflect distress, as some patients have a high rate due to underlying disease process. Check other signs before increasing assist to see if the rate goes down. Respiratory rate may increase when switching from other modes.

PAV+ and NPPV

Some investigators have evaluated the utility of PAV+ over prolonged periods during noninvasive mechanical ventilation. Data suggested that it might be better tolerated without major side effects. Fewer refusals to continue mask assistance were observed with PAV+ in a randomized control study.

PAV+ limitations

Elastance and resistance must be known by the ventilator to work correctly. This may be difficult during assisted ventilation (in PAV resistance and elastance measurements were done using flow interruption method which had some drawbacks, but in PAV+ least square fitting (LSF) method was utilized which is more accurate). Ventilator can overassist with high percentage of assistance, if incorrect high values are introduced. This results in failure to recognize the end of patient breath. This situation is known as "runaway." Under these circumstances, the ventilator inspiration finishes when peak pressure alarm is attained or when patient expiratory effort is strong enough to correct the mistake. Although runaways may not jeopardize patients if alarms are correctly set, it may create major phase asynchronies and discomfort. PAV+ is not advised in patients with low respiratory drive, abnormal breathing pattern, extreme air trapping, large mechanical leaks (small leaks are acceptable) and in children. External nebulizers which add flow into the circuit cannot be used with PAV+.

Conclusion

In PAV+ mode, the ventilator is continuously sensitive to the instantaneous respiratory effort, adjusting the assist pressure in a proportionate and ongoing fashion. This may achieve near-perfect synchrony between the ventilator and spontaneous breathing patient with relief from disease-related increased mechanical work of breathing.

Neurally adjusted ventilatory assist-(NAVA)

NAVA (Fig 18.11) is a new exciting tool that has been recently introduced in clinical practice. The diaphragm is the principal respiratory muscle. The electrical activity generated by the diaphragm, as captured by the EAdi signal (as an expression of the neuronal activity of the respiratory center) is used to trigger the respiratory cycle. NAVA delivers proportional assist in harmony with the patient's neural drive on a breath-to-breath basis. NAVA works like ventilator is "connected," to the patient's own respiratory center. NAVA offers better patient-ventilator synchrony than other available modes of assisted ventilation. Electric trigger of NAVA is not affected by leaks and auto PEEP.

Newer Modes of Mechanical Ventilation

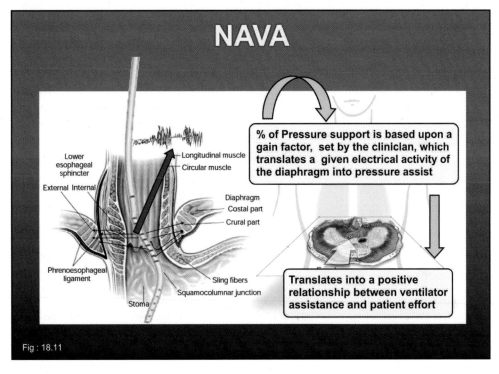

Fig: 18.11

The Electrical Signal from the Diaphragm

The EAdi signal is the sum of the electrical activity of the diaphragm, is expressed in microvolts (µV). The EAdi signal is measured transesophageally by means of an EAdi catheter (doubles as RT tube), which has 8 bipolar microelectrodes mounted on the tip of a gastric tube. It is positioned near the crural diaphragm, where the EAdi signal can be measured.

For NAVA to work properly EAdi catheter should be properly placed to obtain an accurate EAdi signal. EAdi signal capture can be affected in major anatomical defect (diaphragmatic hernia), central apnea without respiratory drive (sedation, brain damage) or in the absence of electrical diaphragmatic activity (phrenic nerve damage, muscle relaxants). NAVA catheter is not approved for MRI environment.

NAVA respiratory cycle in assisted spontaneous ventilation

Mechanical inflation starts when the ventilator detects a deflection of the EAdi signal greater than the set threshold (mostly 0.5 µV). During the inspiratory phase of the respiratory cycle the mechanical assist is adapted to the instantaneous EAdi signal, which is measured every 16 ms and amplified by a set NAVA level.

The NAVA level (set on the ventilator) dictates the amplification of the EAdi signal when delivering assist to the patient. For example, if the NAVA level is set to 0.5 µV/cm of H_2O and the Edi for a specific breath is 20 µV, the maximum level of support for that breath is 10 cm H_2O (0.5 × 20=10 cm of H_2O) (Fig 18.12).

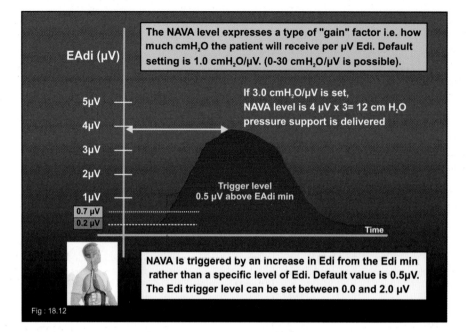
Fig: 18.12

Reduce actual NAVA level by 0.2 µV/cm of H_2O and evaluate after approximately 20 seconds whether or not the patient is still comfortable. If so, a further reduction in NAVA level can be made. If the patient becomes uncomfortable, return to the previous NAVA level. The usual NAVA level is between 0.5 and 3.0 µV/cm of H_2O. In ARDS patients, the tidal volume should be taken into account (generally below 6 ml/kg the predicted body weight). Expiratory phase starts if any one of the following three parameters is reached:

1. EAdi signal reaches 40%–70% of the peak EAdi signal
2. Pressure increases 3 cm of H_2O above the inspiratory target pressure
3. Upper pressure limit is exceeded.

The maximum time for inspiration in adults is 2.5 seconds and in infants 1.5 seconds.

Triggering in NAVA

EAdi signal and pneumatic trigger both operate in combination on first come-first-serve basis. We have found when using NAVA about 20%-30% of breaths are pneumatically triggered. The manufactures are trying to solve this problem with improvements in catheter resulting in better EAdi signals. If there is no EAdi signal but patient has spontaneous breathing efforts, then NAVA works like pressure support. Ventilator can switch to pressure-controlled mechanical ventilation, if spontaneous breathing efforts disappear.

The NAVA Level

The NAVA level is empirically set with stepwise increase of the ventilatory assist. During this titration procedure of the ventilatory assist NAVA patient will sequentially go through, a phase of under-assist, a rapid shallow breathing pattern with high EAdi signals denotes respiratory distress. Then, phase of adequate assist or "comfort zone". In comfort zone the tidal volume is determined by the patient himself. The patient chooses a tidal volume, breathing frequency that meets his respiratory demand resulting in maximal unloading of the respiratory muscles.

Experience has shown that patients who are ventilated with NAVA are able to produce a more variable (noisy), natural breathing pattern as compared to pressure support ventilation. Lastly, in phase of over assist the amplitude of the EAdi signal will decline, but in conjunction with an increase of the tidal volume. The patient is then in a zone of overassist. High pressures lead to lung overdistention and VILI.

NAVA for NPPV

The use of a pneumatic cycle-on in noninvasive ventilation is prone to air leakage, commonly occurring around the face mask. Such leakage may induce patient-ventilator asynchrony and failure of the noninvasive ventilation. The EAdi signal is an electrical cycle-on criterion which is not affected by air leakage. This ensures better patient-ventilator synchrony.

Monitoring of the Diaphragm Signal during Mechanical Ventilation and Weaning

Arguably the most important purpose of EAdi signal monitoring is the assessing the diaphragmatic activity. EAdi monitoring helps in preventing development of diaphragmatic atrophy and avoid ventilator-induced diaphragm dysfunction. EAdi monitoring helps to determine the appropriate depth of sedation, sedation titration and mechanical ventilation strategy. Critical increase in the EAdi signal may serve as a predictive factor for weaning failure. Normalization of the EAdi signal might be predictive of successful weaning and extubation.

Conclusion

NAVA represents true assertion of brain over machine. NAVA's electrical trigger overcomes problems associated with auto PEEP and leaks. NAVA delivers proportional support and improves patient-ventilator synchrony. NAVA results in noisy, natural breathing pattern.

Airway Pressure Release Ventilation (APRV) and BI-Level Ventilation (BI-Level) (Fig 18.13)

Both modes work by prolonging inspiratory time (inverse ratio ventilation modes). These modes work by using long T_i to recruit lung units having increased inspiratory time constants. Short T_e is used to prevent easily de-recruitable lung units with short expiratory time constants. The resultant intrinsic PEEP can have the same effect as applied PEEP but the distribution of intrinsic PEEP (most pronounced in lung units with long time constants) may be different from that of applied PEEP and the resultant V/Q effects may also be different. Spontaneous breathing is possible during both phases of ventilation and these results in better hemodynamics.

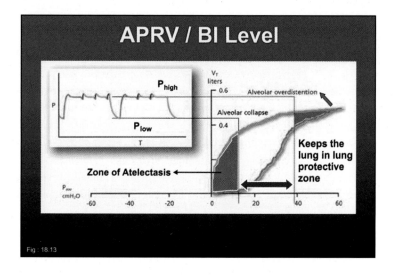

Fig: 18.13

Advantages of APRV and BI-Level modes:

a. Maintain high FRC and better oxygenation

b. Lung is in safe zone. There is less de-recruitment which prevents VILI

Advantages of spontaneous breathing:

a. Keeps diaphragm active

b. Reduces ventilator induced diaphragmatic dysfunction

c. Results in increased venous return, decreased left ventricular transmural pressure and decreased left ventricular afterload. These lead to better hemodynamics

d. Better ventilation of dependent areas, higher glomerular filtration rate and better small-bowel perfusion

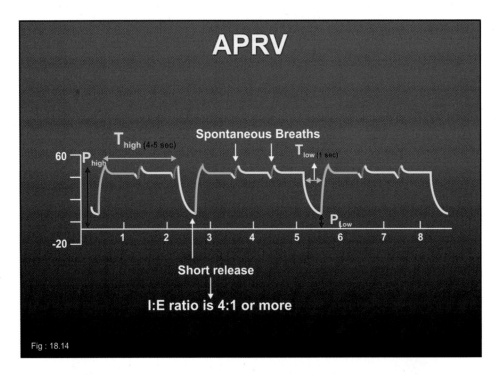

Fig : 18.14

There are some studies claiming a decreased requirement of sedation and analgesia in these modes. However, there have been studies to the contrary also. Both these modes use two pressure levels, pressure high (P_{high}) with a goal of improving oxygenation and pressure low (P_{low}) which facilitates ventilation or CO_2 clearance. Two time periods $T_{inspiratory}$ and $T_{expiratory}$, with synchronized patient triggering and cycling to change phases. Spontaneous breathing is allowed at both levels. APRV (Fig 18.14) uses very short expiratory time (I–E ratio 4:1or more) than Bi-Level which has a I–E ratio of 1:1 or more. Very short expiratory time in APRV leads to patient ventilator dyssynchrony. BI-Level has less synchrony problems.

In BI-level ventilation (Fig 18.15), spontaneous effort at upper pressure are provide with pressure support if pressure support is set higher than $PEEP_{high}$, otherwise only at lower level.

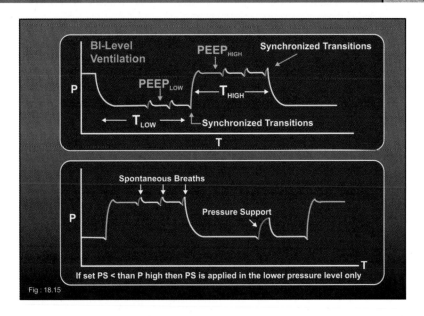

Fig: 18.15

Spontaneous breaths in assisted ventilation increases transpulmonary pressure (Fig 18.16) which is the main determinant of VILI. But studies have shown that it may not cause VILI as anticipated. The reasons may include,

a. Recruitment of dependent atelectatic lung regions
b. Reducing shear stress forces
c. More homogeneous distribution of regional transpulmonary pressures
d. Variability of breathing pattern
e. Redistribution of perfusion towards non-atelectatic injured areas and improved lymphatic drainage.

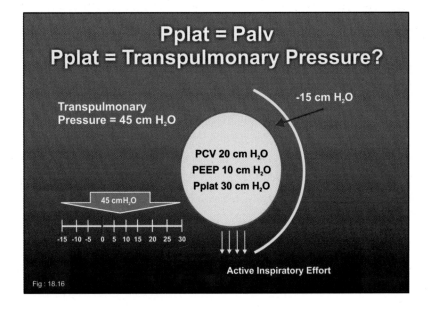

Fig: 18.16

Benefits of APRV/BI-level are based on the spontaneous breathing component. Unfortunately, patients who need heavy sedation or neuromuscular paralysis lack spontaneous breathing efforts.

They may lose the physiological advantages of this mode. Possible contraindications to APRV include conditions that may worsen with the elevation of the mean airway pressure such as unmanaged increase of intracranial pressure and large bronchopleural fistulas.

Conclusions

This mode may be appropriate in ARDS patients as they provide lung protective ventilation and preserved spontaneous breathing resulting in better hemodynamics.

Smartcare/Neoganesh (SC)

SC is a mode of ventilation specifically designed to expedite the weaning process. It utilizes only pressure support breaths, with varying levels of inspiratory pressure with an automated system.

SC controls the ventilator in order to stabilize a patient's spontaneous breathing in a comfortable zone and to reduce inspiratory support until the patient can be extubated. Zone of comfort is based on three parameters:

a. Spontaneous breathing frequency (f_{spn})

I. 15-30 cycles/min

ii. up to 34 in patients with neurologic disease

b. Spontaneous tidal volume (V_T)

I. $V_T > 300$ ml

ii. 250 ml, if weight < 55 kg

c. Endtidal CO_2 (etCO_2)

I. PetCO_2 < 55 mm Hg

ii. 65 mm Hg, if COPD

The system is based on clinical knowledge to classify the ventilatory situation into specific diagnoses and to apply therapeutic measures appropriate to the specific diagnosis (Fig 18.17).

Weaning Steps with Smartcare

"**Step 1:** Stabilizing the patient within a respiratory comfort zone by regulating the level of pressure support based on three parameters: breathing rate, tidal volume and end tidal CO_2."

"**Step 2:** Reducing invasiveness by testing whether the patient can tolerate a lower pressure support level without leaving the comfort zone."

"**Step 3:** Testing readiness for extubation by maintaining the patient at the lowest limit of support"

These therapeutic measures are based on a clinical protocol that has been tested and verified during several years of development (Fig 18.18).

Newer Modes of Mechanical Ventilation

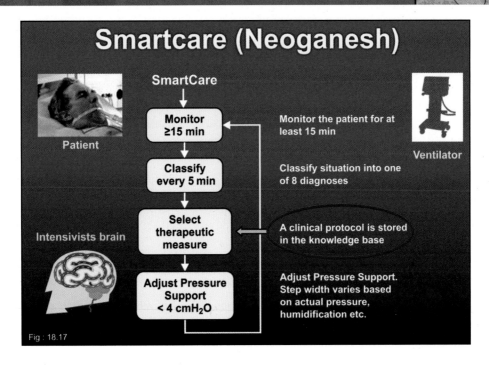

Fig: 18.17

Smartcare/Neoganesh

Smartcare

Classification	f_{spn}	VT	$etCO_2$	SC response
Normal Ventilation	OK	OK	OK	↓PS by 2 or 4
Insufficient Ventilation	OK	↓	OK	↑PS by 2 or 4
	OK	OK	↑	
Hypoventilation	↓	OK	↑	↑PS by 4
Central Hypoventilation	↓	↓	↑	ALARM
Tachypnea	↑	OK	OK	↑PS by 2 or 4
		If 3 X		ALARM
Severe Tachypnea	↑↑	OK	OK	↑PS by 4
		If 3 X		ALARM
Hyperventilation	↓	OK	OK	↓PS by 4
Unexplained Hyperventilation	↑	OK	↓	ALARM

Fig: 18.18

Smartcare

The level of pressure support is periodically adapted by the system in steps of 2 to 4 cm of H_2O. The system automatically tries to reduce the pressure level to a minimal value. At this value, a trial of "spontaneous breathing" with the minimal low-pressure support is performed. When successful, a message on the screen recommends separation from the ventilator.

SC can be used in patients with spontaneous activity, respiratory stability, body weight range of 5 kg to 200 kg. SC is contraindicated in neonates, patients with significant shunting, V/Q mismatch and patients who require high PEEP more than 20 cm of H_2O.

Conclusion

SC should be used for faster weaning with protocol based sedation in all patients without respiratory instability.

References

1) Mechanical ventilation: changing concepts. Pablo Rodriguez, Michel Dojat, Laurent Brochard. Indian J Crit Care Med 2005;9:235-43

2) Advanced closed loops during mechanical ventilation (PAV, NAVA, ASV, Smartcare). F. Lellouche, L. Brochard. Best Practice & Research Clinical Anaesthesiology 2009; 23: 81-93

3) New Modes of Ventilation. Do We Need Them? Bob Kacmarek

4) What Is the Evidence Base for the Newer Ventilation Modes? Richard D Branson and Jay A Johannigman. Respiratory care. July 2004; vol 49: no 7

5) Neurally Adjusted Ventilatory Assist: A Ventilation Tool or a Ventilation Toy? Walter Verbrugghe and Philippe G Jorens. Respir Care 2011; 56(3):327-335. © 2011

★ ★ ★

SEDATION, ANALGESICS AND NEUROMUSCULAR BLOCKERS IN MECHANICALLY VENTILATED PATIENTS

ICU is a foreign environment for patients. It is an environment which they have not chosen and they do not have family members around them continuously for comfort. These patients frequently experience pain and physical discomfort from obvious factors such as pre-existing diseases, invasive procedures or trauma.

Pain and discomfort also can be caused by monitoring and therapeutic devices such as catheters, drains and endotracheal tubes. Performing routine nursing care such as airway suctioning, physical therapy, dressing changes, patient mobilization can be painful at times. Prolonged immobility by itself can cause severe discomfort and pain.

One third of all patients in intensive care units (ICUs) worldwide are mechanically ventilated and require sedation and analgesia frequently to enhance comfort. Assessment of the problem, sound knowledge of medications used and an understanding of disease pathology help in preventing the adverse effects of over- or under-sedation (Fig 19.1)

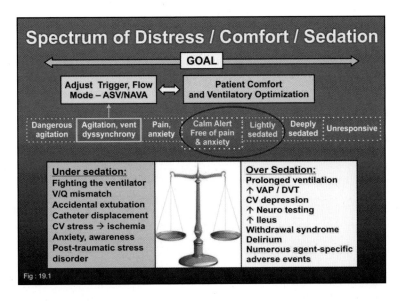

Fig : 19.1

The term "Sedation" in a mechanically ventilated patient first encompasses the component of adequate pain management. Studies in agitated patients in ICU have found that after analgesic was given, more than half the patients did not require sedation. Analgesics have to be administered first to agitated patients (Analgesic first (A-1) strategy). This should be based on patient-centered assessment enabling patients to be comfortable, calm, co-operative and communicative. 'Optimum sedation' has to be tailored to individual patient's needs.

Sedation and analgesics in mechanically ventilated patients helps in:

a. Prevention of pain and anxiety

b. Amnesia during neuromuscular blockade

c. Decreased oxygen consumption
d. Reduced response to stimulation resulting in decreased metabolic consumption
e. Control of delusional agitation and delirium
e. Patient-ventilator synchrony
f. To control behavior
h. Avoid adverse neuro-cognitive sequelae like depression and posttraumatic stress disorder (PTSD)

Pain and anxiety lead to stimulation of the autonomic nervous system and release of humoral factors. This leads to increased heart rate, increased blood pressure and increased myocardial oxygen consumption resulting in myocardial ischemia or infarction. Altered humoral response can lead to hypercoagulability as a result of increased levels of clotting factors, fibrinogen, platelet activity and inhibition of fibrinolysis. Stress hormones produce insulin resistance, increase metabolic rate and cause protein catabolism. Decreased gastric and bowel motility and increased risk of bacterial transgression of bowel wall are seen in these patients. Pain and anxiety result in immunosuppression with reduction in number and function of lymphocytes and granulocytes.

Clinical approach to sedation and analgesic use in mechanically ventilated patient

Agitation and restlessness on ventilator may be due to various reasons like pain, anxiety, delirium, fever and patient-ventilator dyssynchrony. Approach to such patients involves evaluating the cause-effect of the problem, quantifying it and formulating a protocol for its management.

New guidelines for pain, analgesics and delirium (PAD) management are expected to be published by end of 2012. The reader is advised to refer to these guidelines for any changes. The author has tried to incorporate the information already available on these guidelines. The new PAD guidelines will be more patient-centered, integrated and interdisciplinary. Far less emphasis will be placed on specific across-the-board pharmacological recommendations (Fig 19.2).

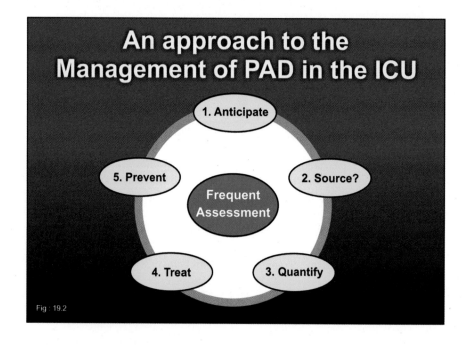

Fig: 19.2

Analgesic first (A-1) strategy

Pain is defined as an unpleasant sensory and emotional experience associated with actual or potential tissue damage, or described in terms of such damage. For a clinician 'pain is what and when the patient says'.

- Usually, simple non-pharmacological interventions decrease or even alleviate the need for drugs. A sympathetic and thorough explanation, perhaps combined with a visit from a family member, may be all that is required.

Non-pharmacological interventions that must tried before drug therapy is initiated

- In comatose patients, flexed elbows and scheduled passive mobilization with change of position
- Careless discussion in front of an awake patient can cause anxiety and should be avoided
- Full bladder, distended bowels and other irritants such as an itch from a plaster cast are all causes of discomfort in the critically ill patients. These are best relieved by dealing with the cause rather than giving sedative drugs
- Efforts to maintain physiological circadian rhythm (room with a window, normal environmental light) may improve quality of sleep. A quiet darkened room combined with ear-plugs and eye-shade will sometimes provide the patient with a better night's sleep than a hypnotic

Assessment of pain in mechanically ventilated patient

No patient should be allowed to 'fight' the ventilator in the ICU. An optimal sedation protocol in mechanically ventilated patients can prevent this. Although modern ventilators that allow synchronized spontaneous breathing have reduced the need for sedation, some is usually needed, particularly following initiation of assisted ventilation.

Guidelines suggest that vital signs alone be not used for pain assessment in adult ICU patients. Vital signs (increased heart rate, blood pressure and sweating) may be used as a cue to begin further assessment of pain in these patients.

Patients on ventilators can either be communicative or they may be drowsy and unable to communicate pain. Hence assessment in these two categories of patients is different and is discussed below:

Pain assessment

Communication is the best way of assessing pain in patients who can self report. A simple question answer interaction can solve the problem. A writing board can be used in patients who are able to write. Many patients in ICU are too weak to write.

In such cases an alphabetical chart in the language understood by the patient can be used by nurses to construct what the patient is trying to communicate. New guidelines recommend that pain be routinely monitored in all ICU patients.

Communicative patients

Numerical rating scale (NPS)

The numeric pain scale (NPS) employs a verbal rating of pain on a scale from 0 to 10, with 10 being the worst pain ever experienced. This is broadly used in a variety of clinical settings. Self-reported pain is considered to be the standard and NPS is recommended by PAD guidelines (Fig 19.3).

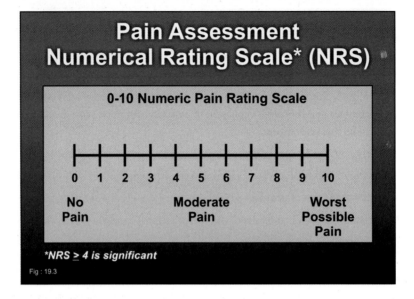
Fig: 19.3

Non-communicative patients

Behavioral pain scale (BPS) and critical-care pain observation tool (CPOT) are the most valid and reliable behavioral pain scales for monitoring pain in medical, postoperative or trauma cases (except in head injury). These tools are used in patients who are unable to self report, in whom motor function is intact and behaviors are observable.

Behavioral pain scale (BPS) is based on a sum score of three components:
1. Facial expression
2. Movements of upper limbs and
3. Compliance with mechanical ventilation.

Based upon the assumption that a relationship exists between the score and pain intensity, each pain indicator is scored from 1 (no response) to 4 (full response), with a maximum score of 12. A BPS score of more than 6 is considered significant. One limitation of BPS is that responsiveness of the patient decreases substantially with deepening levels of sedation. Compliance with mechanical ventilation may be considered to be a separate parameter from other behaviors. Some intensivists therefore only score facial expression and movements of upper limbs in order to assess the individual pain state.

A recently developed behavior pain tool, critical care pain observation tool (CPOT), has four components:
1. Facial expression
2. Body movement
3. Muscle tension and
4. Compliance with the ventilator for intubated patients or vocalization for extubated patients.

Each of these behaviors is assigned a rating of 0 to 2 (CPOT range = 0 to 8, CPOT > 3 is significant). Current practice for adult ICU patients commonly includes a combination of NPS or a similar self-reported pain quantification tool plus an instrument designed to identify pain using behavior and physiologic parameters in the non-communicative patient (e.g. the CPOT).

Sedation, Analgesics and Neuromuscular Blockers

Behavioral Pain Scale (BPS) 3-12

Item	Description	Score
Facial expression	Relaxed	1
	Partially tightened (eg.: brow lowering)	2
	Fully tightened (eg.: eyelid closing)	3
	Grimacing	4
Upper Limbs	No movement	1
	Partially bent	2
	Fully bent with finger flexion	3
	Permanently retracted	4
Compliance with ventilation	Tolerating movement	1
	Coughing but tolerating ventilation for most of the time	2
	Fighting ventilator	3
	Unable to control ventilation	4

Fig: 19.4

BPS is illustrated in Fig 19.4: BPS range = 3-12, BPS > 6 is significant

Yet to be released 2012 PAD guidelines recommend that pre-emptive analgesia and / or non-pharmacologic interventions (e.g. relaxation) should be administered to alleviate pain prior to chest tube removal and for other types of invasive and potentially painful procedures (placement of lines, drainage of pus etc). Guidelines recommend that IV opioids should be considered as the first-line drug of choice to treat non-neuropathic pain in critically ill patients. All available intravenous opioids, when titrated to similar pain intensity endpoints, are equally effective.

It is recommended that either enterally administered gabapentin or carbamazepine, in addition to intravenous opioids, should be considered for treatment of neuropathic pain. Nonopioid analgesics (NSAIDS) should be considered to decrease the total quantity of opioids administered (or to eliminate the need for IV opioids altogether). This decreases opioid-related side effects. Thoracic epidural anesthesia or analgesia should be considered in patients with rib fracture and for postoperative analgesia in patients undergoing aneurysmal abdominal aortic surgery.

Pain management is summarized below (Fig 19.5).

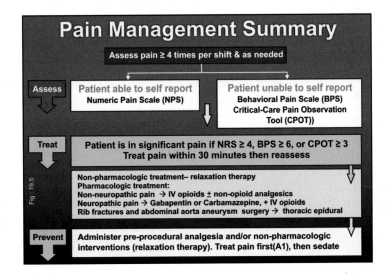

Fig: 19.5

Commonly used analgesic doses and side effects are given below (Fig 19.6):

Commonly used analgesic doses and side effects

Opioid drug	Approximate Equivalent Single IV Dose	Typical Infusion Rate	Onset to Peak Effect	Duration
Fentanyl	100 - 200 mcg	50 - 200 mcg/hr	2 - 5 min	0.5 - 2 hours
Morphine	10 mg	2 - 10 mg/hr	20 - 30 min	3 - 4 hours
Hydromorphone	1.5 mg	7 - 15 mcg/kg/hr	30 - 60 min	2 - 3 hours
Remifentanil	Bolus doses are not usually recommended	0.05 - 0.2 mcg/kg/hr	1 - 2 min	10 - 20 min

Fig : 19.6

Sedation in mechanically ventilated patients

Although the importance of non-pharmacologic approaches such as comfortable positioning in bed and verbal reassurance may be adequate at times, anxiety is common in mechanically ventilated patients and sedation to a point of coma may seem like an attractive option for some patients. Although amnesia is important during surgical procedures, its importance in mechanically ventilated patients during critical illness is far less certain. Indeed, complete amnesia for extended periods during mechanical ventilation in the ICU has never been proven to confer benefit and there is data to suggest that prolonged ICU amnesia may be detrimental.

A scoring scale that assesses level of sedation should be used in the management of all mechanically ventilated ICU patients. The Richmond agitation-sedation scale (RASS) and Sedation Agitation Scale are most extensively evaluated. RASS has been shown to have excellent inter-rater reliability. It is the first scale to be validated to detect changing levels of sedation and correlate it to level of consciousness and delirium over consecutive days of ICU care (Figs 19.7 and 19.8).

Richmond Agitation Sedation Scale (RASS)

Score	State		
+ 4	Combative		
+ 3	Very Agitated		
+ 2	Agitated		
+ 1	Restless		
0	Alert and Calm		
- 1	Drowsy	Eye contact > 10 sec	Verbal Stimulus
- 2	Light Sedation	Eye contact > 10 sec	
- 3	Moderate Sedation	No eye contact	
- 4	Deep Sedation	Physical stimulation	Physical Stimulus
- 5	Unarousable	No response even with physical	

RASS range = -5 to +4, target RASS = 0 to -2

Fig : 19.7

Sedation-Agitation Scale (SAS)

Score	State	Behaviors
7	Very Agitated	Pulling at ET tube, climbing over bedrail, striking at staff, thrashing side-to-side
6	Very Agitated	Does not calm despite frequent verbal reminding, requires physical restraints
5	Agitated	Anxious or mildly agitated, attempting to sit up, calms down to verbal instructions
4	Calm and Co-operative	Calm, awakens easily, follows commands
3	Sedated	Difficult to arouse, awakens to verbal stimuli or gentle shaking but drifts off
2	Very Sedated	Arouses to physical stimuli but does not communicate or follow commands
1	Unarousable	Minimal or no response to noxious stimuli, does not communicate or follow commands

Fig: 19.8 SAS range = 1 to 7, target SAS = 3 to 4

New PAD guidelines recommend maintaining light levels of sedation in adult ICU patients. It is associated with improved clinical outcomes (e.g. shorter duration of mechanical ventilation and a shorter length of ICU stay). Maintaining light levels of sedation increases the physiologic stress response but is not associated with an increased incidence of myocardial ischemia.

The association between depth of sedation and psychological stress in these patients remains unclear. Subjective sedation scoring systems are better than objective measures such as auditory evoked potentials (AEP), bispectral index (BIS), narcotrend index (NI), patient state index (PSI), state entropy (SE) etc. in monitoring depth of sedation in non-comatose, non-paralyzed critically ill adult patients.

The objective measures of brain function may be used as an adjuvant to subjective sedation assessment in patients receiving neuromuscular blocking agents as subjective sedation assessments may be unobtainable. It is recommended that EEG monitoring be used to monitor non-convulsive seizure activity in patients with either known or suspected seizures. EEG may be used in patients with increased intracranial pressure to titrate electrosuppressive medication and achieve burst suppression.

Sedation strategies using non-benzodiazepine sedatives (either propofol or dexmedetomidine) is preferred over sedation with benzodiazepines (either midazolam or lorazepam) to improve clinical outcome. In general, the choice of sedative agent used in ICU patients should be driven by

1) Indications for sedation
2) Goal of sedation
3) Effect and side effects of the drug
4) Cost of medication

Sedation management summary (Fig 19.9)

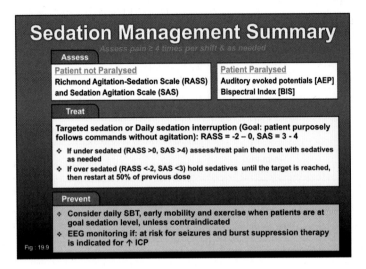

Fig : 19.9

Dexmedetomidine offers a cost advantage over midazolam infusions especially in healthcare institutions that are efficient in transferring patients out of the ICU. In spite of some apparent advantages in using either propofol or dexmedetomidine over benzodiazepines for ICU sedation, benzodiazepines remain important for the management of agitation in ICU patients, especially for the treatment of anxiety, seizures, alcohol or benzodiazepine withdrawal. It is also useful when deep sedation and amnesia are required. In scenarios where combination therapy with other sedative or analgesic agents is required, benzodiazepines are preferred.

It is advised to have institution specific sedation and weaning algorithm to achieve shorter duration of mechanical ventilation and / or shorter ICU length of stay. Other benefits include more 'on-target' sedation, less pain, reduced direct costs, less patient–ventilator asynchrony and decreased incidence of ventilator associated pneumonia.

Commonly used sedatives and their doses are given below (Fig 19.10)

Commonly used Sedatives and their doses

Drug	Typical IV Bolus Dose	Typical Infusion Rate	Onset to Peak	Duration
Propofol	0.03-0.15 mg/kg (max 20 mg)	5-80 mcg/kg/min	1-2 min	< 20 min
Midazolam	1-6 mg	1-10 mg/hr	5-10 min	1.5-2 hours
Lorazepam	1-3 mg	1-5 mg/hr	15-20 min	2-4 hours
Dexmedetomidine	Not recommended	0.2-1.5 mcg/kg/hr	30 min	2-4 hours

Fig : 19.10

A patient's need for sedation will vary from time to time. Factors responsible for this change are:
a. Variation in severity of illness
b. Need for surgical interventions
c. Changes in the mode of ventilatory support
d. Tolerance to drugs
e. Changes in renal and liver function resulting in altered drug elimination and volume of distribution
f. Toxicity of the sedative agent or its solvent
g. Need for patient transfer (e.g. MRI scan)

Delirium in mechanically ventilated patient

Delirium is defined as a change in cognition or the development of a perceptual disturbance that is not accounted for pre-existing established or evolving dementia.

It is a disturbance of consciousness with reduced ability to focus. It develops over a short period of time and tends to fluctuate over the course of the day. Delirium is important because it has serious adverse outcomes.

Causes of delirium (Fig 19.11):

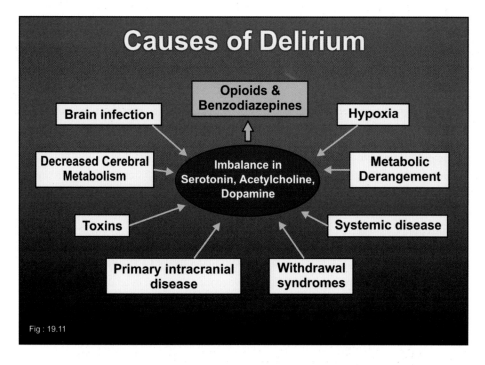

Fig: 19.11

The confusion assessment method for the ICU (CAM-ICU) and the intensive care delirium screening checklist (ICDSC) are the most valid and reliable delirium monitoring tools in adult ICU patients (Fig 19.12).

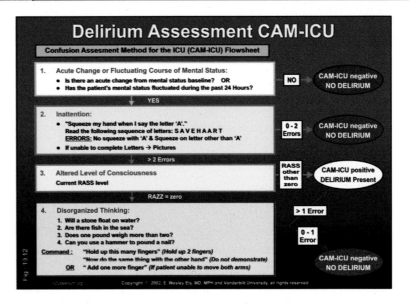

Fig. 19.12

Non-pharmacologic Interventions in Delirium management

Pain, if any, should be monitored and managed using an objective scale. Patient should be orientated to date, place and reason for hospitalization.

Whiteboards should be updated with care giver names. Clocks and calendars should be provided in the room. Current events should be discussed with the patients. Need for hearing aids and/or eye glasses should be ascertained. Good quality sleep should be assured. Patient - ventilator synchrony should be maintained. Promote comfort and relaxation (e.g. back care, oral care, washing face/hands and daytime bath, massage).

ABCDE bundle for management of delirium

There is conflicting data surrounding the relationship between the use of opioids and the development of delirium in patients. Benzodiazepines may be a risk factor in development of delirium in patients. There is insufficient data to determine the relationship between the use of propofol and the development of delirium.

Dexmedetomidine may be associated with a lower prevalence of delirium compared to benzodiazepines in mechanically ventilated patients. Guidelines recommend that early mobilization of adult ICU patients should be performed whenever feasible to reduce the incidence and duration of delirium. Guidelines provide no recommendation for the use of a combined non-pharmacological and pharmacological delirium prevention protocol in adult ICU patients, as this has not been shown to reduce the incidence of delirium.

Although guidelines do not recommend either haloperidol or atypical antipsychotics, many centers in the world use haloperidol with starting dose of 2-10 mg (5 mg over 5-10 minutes) in treating delirium. This is repeated every 20 minutes till end-point is achieved. Guidelines do not recommend administering rivastigmine and dexmedetomidine to reduce the duration of delirium in ICU patients. Sleep should be promoted by optimizing patient's environment, using strategies to control light and noise, clustering patient care activities and to decreasing stimuli (disturbances) at night.

Summary of delirium management (Fig 19.13)

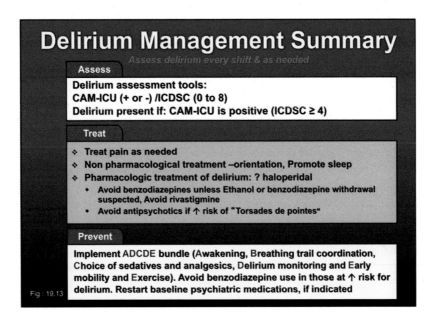

Fig: 19.13

Conclusion

Routinely and separately assess pain, sedation, agitation and delirium using validated tools. Avoid deep sedation. Let patients be interactive. Integrate PAD management with SBT, early mobility and environmental sleep management. Implement the PAD care bundle using an interdisciplinary, team-based approach. Continuously re-evaluate what you are doing and keeping innovating to improve performance.

Use of neuromuscular blockers in mechanically ventilated patients

Better understanding of hazards associated with the use of neuromuscular blockers (NMB) has lead to substantial decline in the use of these drugs in patients on ventilator support. An occasional scenario still demands the use of NMB. Hence, a sound knowledge of these drugs is essential. It should be emphasized that all other modalities to improve the clinical situation must be tried before using NMBs as a last resort. In the rare patient where NMBs are used, patients should be adequately sedated before initiation of neuromuscular blockade.

Indications for the use of NMBs include:

1. Tracheal intubation
2. Ventilatory modes that are difficult for the patient to tolerate (such as high PEEP, prolonged I–E ratio)
3. Extreme hypoxia/hypercarbia
4. To treat muscle spasms as a last resort when all other means have failed
5. To decrease oxygen consumption
6. Raised intracranial pressure
7. Ventilator/patient dyssynchrony, where appropriate sedation and analgesia has failed
8. To facilitate short procedures

Sometimes boluses of NMBs before and during transportation might increase safety. The use of neuromuscular blockers in mechanically ventilated patients is sometimes inevitable as there is an increased respiratory drive secondary to low tidal volume ventilation and resulting permissible hypoxia and hypercapnia. Studies have shown mortality benefit when NMBs are used in the early management of ARDS.

NMB drugs

NMBs are structurally related to acetylcholine (ACh) and act by interfering with the binding of ACh to the motor endplate. They are divided into depolarizing (succinylcholine used only for securing the airway) or non-depolarizing (pancuronium, cisatracurium, pipecuronium, rocuronium, and vecuronium) agents based upon their mechanism of action. Succinylcholine is the only available depolarizing neuromuscular blocker. It is characterized by rapid onset of effect and ultra short duration of action because of its rapid hydrolysis by butyrylcholinesterase.

Non-depolarizing neuromuscular blockers available can be classified according to chemical class (steroidal, benzylisoquinolinium, or other compounds) or, alternatively, according to onset or duration of action (long, intermediate, and short-acting drugs) for equipotent doses. The ideal NMB agents for use in intensive care produces an early, titratable paralysis and has a moderately rapid offset of action (less than 15 minutes) to allow for repeated neurologic assessment. No adverse hemodynamic or other adverse physiologic effects should exist. Elimination should be independent of hepatic or renal function. Metabolites produced should be inactive. There should be no propensity to accumulate. It should be stable over 24 hours to allow for continuous infusion. Cost should be modest.

Doses of commonly used NMB (Fig 19.14)

Doses of commonly used NMB

Drug	Intubating Dose (mg/kg)	Time to Maximum Block (min)	Clinical Duration (min)	Maintenance dose
Succinylcholine	1	1 - 2		
Rocuronium	0.6	1.7	25 - 30 min	0.2-0.5 mg/kg/ hour
Vecuronium	0.1	2.4	25 - 40 min	0.05-0.1 mg/kg/ hour
Pancuronium	0.1	2.4	40 - 60 min	0.03-0.1 mg/kg/ hour
Atracurium	0.5	3.2	20 - 40 min	0.3-1.0 mg/kg/ hour
Cisatracurium	0.2	7.7	25 - 35 min	0.03-0.2 mg/kg/ hour
Mivacurium	0.15	3.3	10 - 20 min	9 - 10 µg/kg/min

Fig : 19.14

Suxamethonium produces a large increase in plasma potassium to levels that could produce cardiac arrest and hence should be used with caution in certain situations. Suxamethonium is contraindicated in patients with renal failure, neuromuscular disease, paraplegia and in those with muscular atrophy due to long-term ICU or hospital stay. Suxamethonium induced fasciculations may lead to increased intracranial pressure and should therefore be avoided in patients with pre-existing raised ICP. Rarely, suxamethonium may cause malignant hyperthermia. In all such circumstances, use of a rapid onset non-depolarising agent such as rocuronium is preferred. The usual dose of suxamethonium is 75–100 mg. Potassium levels up to 6 mEq/L is considered safe for single dose administration.

The majority of patients in an ICU who are prescribed an NMB agent can be managed effectively with pancuronium. For patients for whom vagolysis is contraindicated (e.g. those with cardiovascular disease), NMB agents other than pancuronium may be used. Because of their unique metabolism, cisatracurium or atracurium is recommended for patients with significant hepatic/renal disease.

For patients on corticosteroids, every effort should be made to discontinue NMBs as soon as possible.

Drugs which may potentiate/antagonize the action of non-depolarizing NMB are listed below (Fig 19.15):

Drugs which may potentiate/antagonize the action of NMB

Drugs that Potentiate the Action of Non-depolarizing NMB agents
Local anesthetics- Lidocaine
Antimicrobials - Minoglycosides, Polymyxin B, Clindamycin, Tetracycline
Antiarrhythmics - Procainamide, Quinidine, Magnesium
Calcium channel blockers
B - Adrenergic blockers
Immunosuppressive agents - Cyclophosphamide, Cyclosporine
Dantrolene
Diuretics
Lithium carbonate
Drugs that Antagonize the Actions of Non-depolarizing NMB agents
Phenytoin
Carbamazepine
Theophylline
Ranitidine

Fig: 19.15

Hazards of using neuromuscular blockers

There will be life-threatening hypoxia in the event of accidental tracheal airway extubation. Neuromuscular blockers contribute to ICU induced weakness in some patients. Steroid-based neuromuscular blocking agents (pancuronium and vecuronium especially) are most commonly implicated. Protective reflexes are reduced resulting in increased risk of micro-aspirations and development of ventilator associated pneumonia (VAP). Measures to prevent corneal abrasion like artificial tears should be instilled every two to four hours and eyelids should be taped shut. Neuromuscular blockers exacerbate complications related to immobility. There is probably an increased risk of deep vein thrombosis (DVT), muscle wasting and peripheral nerve injury.

All paralyzed patients require the following precautions to prevent complication. Ensure adequate sedation and analgesia prior to paralyzing the patient. Back up ventilation rate and settings have to be properly set. Supervise patients closely, as interruption of ventilator circuit can be fatal.

Patients require frequent turning and dry, wrinkle-free bedding in order to prevent skin breakdown and decubitus ulcers. Prophylactic deep venous thrombosis therapy with either low dose subcutaneous heparin or mechanical compression devices is mandatory. Head end of the bed should be elevated to 450 to reduce the risk of aspiration, particularly during enteral feeding. Pupillary reflexes should be closely monitored to assess neurologic status (unreliable if pancuronium is used as it has antimuscarinic effects).

Monitoring NMB

Excessive muscle relaxation is unnecessary and potentially dangerous. For example, prolonged overuse of muscle relaxants can be complicated by persistent residual weakness. A simple method of measurement is to discontinue administration of the agent until movement is observed. Patients receiving NMBs should be assessed both clinically and by train of four (TOF) monitoring, with the goal being to adjust the degree of neuromuscular blockade to achieve one or two twitches.

Conclusion

NMB use in mechanically ventilated patients has substantially declined over a period of time. Rarely some situations do require the use of NMB. Hence, clinicians should know the NMBs available and hazards associated with their use. Institution based protocol for sedation, NMB use and weaning should be in place to minimize the use of NMB.

References

1. Highlights of the 2012 SCCM Pain, Agitation and Sedation Guidelines
2. PACT Sedation and analgesia update
3. Sedation and Analgesia in the Mechanically Ventilated Patient. Shruti B. Patel and John P. Kress. Am J Respir Crit Care Med Mar 1, 2012; vol 185: Iss. 5, pp 486–497.
4. ICU Pain, Agitation, & Delirium Care Bundle Metrics. Juliana Barr, MD, FCCM, Chair, ACCM PAD Guideline Task Force.
5. Clinical practice guidelines for sustained neuromuscular blockade in the adult, critically ill patients. Murray MJ, Cowen J, DeBlock H, et al. Crit Care Med 2002; 30:142–156.
6. ICUdelirium.org

★★★

NUTRITIONAL ASSESSMENT AND MANAGEMENT IN MECHANICALLY VENTILATED PATIENT

Proper nutrition is an important aspect of management in critically ill. The benefits of nutritional support include improved wound healing, decreased catabolic response to illness and improved gastrointestinal tract integrity and function. Increased metabolic requirements arise from increased protein breakdown and synthesis and changed substrate turnover. It varies depending on the clinical scenario. The catabolic depletion of protein reserves is one of the most striking features of the critically ill (Fig 20.1).

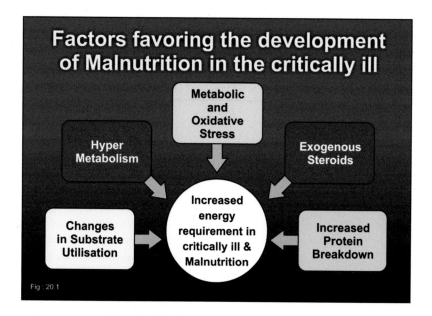

Fig: 20.1

Nutritional support had three main objectives:
1. To preserve lean body mass
2. To maintain immune function
3. To avoid metabolic complications

Of late, the goal has changed from supportive to "Therapeutic". Goals are more focused on nutrition therapy targeted towards attenuating metabolic stress response, oxidative stress and favorably modulating the immune response.

Nutritional modulation of the stress response to critical illness includes early enteral nutrition (EN), appropriate macronutrient and micronutrient delivery and tight glycemic control. Delivering early nutrition support therapy, primarily using the enteral route results in maintenance of peristalsis, blood flow to the gut and gut integrity. It is seen as a proactive therapeutic strategy that may reduce disease severity, decrease complications, reduce length of stay in the ICU and favorably impact on patient outcome.

Assessment of nutritional requirement in mechanically ventilated patients

Prior to initiation of feeding, one should assess weight loss, nutrient intake before admission, level of disease severity, co-morbid conditions, function of the gastrointestinal tract, any history of surgery and patient activity levels.

Determination of a patient's energy requirement is what guides the practice of providing energy to the patient. Methods of estimating resting energy requirement (RER) fall into three categories:

1. Indirect calorimetry
2. Predictive equations
3. Traditional assessment tools and laboratory methods

Medical history, simple anthropometric measurements, physical examination and a few simple laboratory tests if used along with predictive equations are generally adequate for evaluation of nutritional status.

Derived Anthropometric Measures: Ideal body weight (IBW) is a practical estimate of lean body weight discounting the effects of excessive fat, edema or third-space fluid collections (common in critically ill patients). Other anthropometric tools used are body fat estimation, triceps skin fold thickness and arm muscle circumference. Somatic protein stores can be evaluated on physical examination by gross assessment of muscle mass (e.g. quadriceps, intrinsic hand muscles, and temporalis muscle mass) or testing voluntary grip strength. These tools are not validated in ICU population.

Laboratory Measurements: Albumin, prealbumin, transferrin and serum electrolytes (especially phosphate and magnesium) have been used in estimating patient's nutritional status. Nitrogen balance studies provide a means to assess the degree of protein turnover and to titrate nitrogen administration (i.e., protein, peptides, or amino acids). Nitrogen balance is the difference between nitrogen intake and nitrogen excretion. All these measures are affected by critical illness and hence are not accurate measures to estimate patients' energy requirements.

Indirect calorimetry: Although not widely available, indirect calorimetry is the Gold Standard for estimating energy requirement in mechanically ventilated patients. It uses the ratio of CO_2 produced to O_2 consumed which reflects cellular metabolic process. Conditions where indirect calorimetry is inaccurate in mechanically ventilated patients are listed below (Fig 20.2).

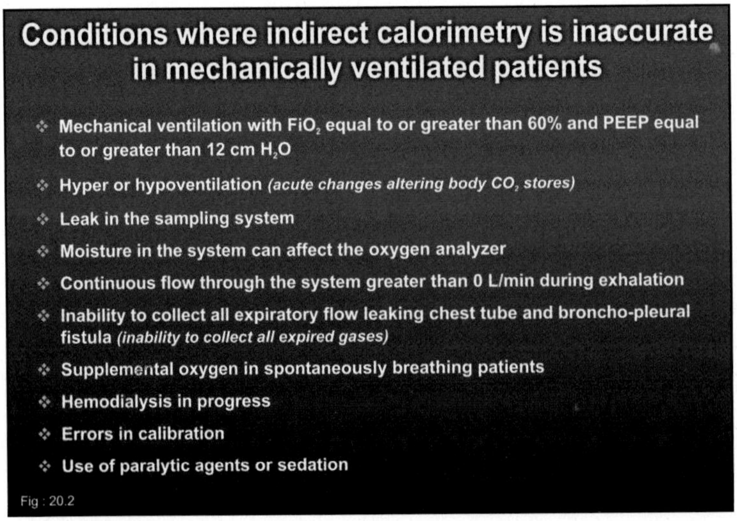

Conditions where indirect calorimetry is inaccurate in mechanically ventilated patients

- Mechanical ventilation with FiO_2 equal to or greater than 60% and PEEP equal to or greater than 12 cm H_2O
- Hyper or hypoventilation *(acute changes altering body CO_2 stores)*
- Leak in the sampling system
- Moisture in the system can affect the oxygen analyzer
- Continuous flow through the system greater than 0 L/min during exhalation
- Inability to collect all expiratory flow leaking chest tube and broncho-pleural fistula *(inability to collect all expired gases)*
- Supplemental oxygen in spontaneously breathing patients
- Hemodialysis in progress
- Errors in calibration
- Use of paralytic agents or sedation

Fig : 20.2

Nutritional Assessment and Management

Predictive equations for energy requirement assessment

Predictive equations should be used with caution as they are less accurate than indirect calorimetry. In obese patients, predictive equations are even more problematic without the availability of indirect calorimetry. Total energy expenditure (TEE) is the energy required by the organism daily and it is determined by the sum of 3 components:

1. Basal metabolic rate (BMR)
2. Diet induced thermogenesis (DIT)
3. Physical activity (PA)

Resting metabolic rate (RMR) is almost similar to BMR but depends on many factors like body composition, age, gender, body temperature, medications and medical condition.

There are essentially two types of predictive equations. The first involves calculating basal metabolic rate by equations like Harris–Benedict which are previously derived in healthy subjects. A stress or correction factor is added to account for the illness or injury.

If the estimated stress factor is within a reasonable range, then the accuracy of the energy estimation is accurate. Typically, stress factors between 1.2 and 1.6 have been used for mechanically ventilated ICU populations. The second type of predictive formulae is multivariate regression equations. These include an estimate of healthy resting energy expenditure or parameters associated with resting energy expenditure plus clinical variables that relate to the degree of hypermetabolism. Studies suggest REE estimated on the basis of body weight, height, minute ventilation and body temperature is clinically more relevant. An alternative and simpler method of estimating energy expenditure is to use a 'calorie per kilogram' approach.

The American college of chest physicians (ACCP) recommends using 25 kcal/kg as the energy requirements for ICU patients. There are more than 200 equations to estimate energy requirements. Penn state equation and Harris–Benedict equation are commonly used and are discussed below:

Penn State equation: RMR = 0.85(BEE by Harris–Benedict equation) + 33(VE) + $175(T_{max})$ – 6433 (VE minute ventilation, T_{max} is the maximum temperature in degree centigrade).

Harris-Benedict equation: Men = $66.5 + (13.75 \times kg) + (5.003 \times cm) - (6.775 \times age)$

Women = $655.1 + (9.563 \times kg) + (1.850 \times cm) - (4.676 \times age)$

Ventilators with inbuilt calorimeters are being developed and if successfully introduced to clinical practice, they would be of much help.

Clinical management of enteral nutrition (EN)

Enteral feeding access

Nasogastric (NG) tube is simple to place and is the most preferred method for enteral feeding. Patients on NG tube who cannot be put in head up position and are not tolerating enteral feeds even after using prokinetics and continuous feeding regimes are at high risk for aspiration. In these patients, small bowel feeding methods should be used. Another indication for small bowel feeding is if EN is required for more than 4-6 weeks.

Nasojejunal tube (NJ), percutaneous endoscopic gastrostomy (PEG), percutaneous endoscopic jejunostomy (PEJ), surgical gastrostomy or jejunostomy are some of the alternate routes for enteral feeding. Normal daily nutritional requirements are mentioned in Fig 20.3.

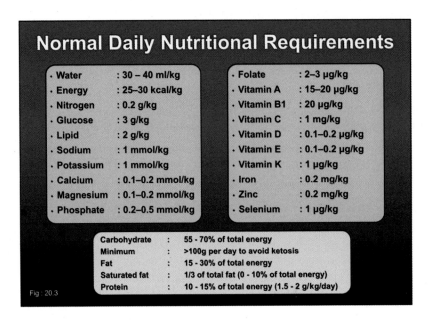

Fig : 20.3

Enteral feeding

"If the gut works – use it". Nutrition support therapy in the form of EN should be initiated only if patient is unable to maintain oral intake. Gut is the motor for sepsis. As enteral feeding preserves gut barrier function and prevents MODS, it is the method for nutritional support and should be preferred over parenteral nutrition (PN).

Early enteral feeding should be started within the first 24–48 hours of admission and advanced towards estimated patient requirement over the next 48–72 hours (target is 60% of estimated calories). In critically ill patients, strategies to optimize delivery of nutrients starting at target rate, accepting a higher threshold of gastric residual volumes, use of prokinetics and small bowel feedings should be considered.

Continuous feeding regimes are better tolerated than bolus intermittent feeding. Closed feeding systems are better than open systems.

EN should be withheld in patients requiring significant hemodynamic support, including high-dose catecholamine agents (alone or in combination with large volume fluid) and blood product resuscitation to maintain cellular perfusion until the patient is fully resuscitated. Neither presence/absence of bowel sounds nor evidence of passage of flatus, stool is required for the initiation of enteral feeding in ICU patients. Initiating supplemental PN should be considered after 7–10 days if energy requirements (100% of target goal calories) cannot be met by enteral route alone. Initiating supplemental PN before this 7–10 days period does not improve outcome and may be detrimental to the patient.

In patients with body mass index (BMI) less than 30, protein requirements should be in the range of 1.2–2 g/kg actual body weight per day, and may likely be even higher in patients with burns or polytrauma. In the critically ill obese patients, permissive underfeeding or hypocaloric feeding with EN is recommended. Across classes of obesity with BMI more than 30, goal of the EN regimen is not to exceed 60% to 70% of target energy requirements or 11–14 kcal/kg actual body weight/day (or 22–25 kcal/kg ideal body weight/day). Protein should be provided in a range more than 2 g/kg ideal body weight/day for (BMI 30 to 40), more than 2.5 g/kg ideal body weight/day (BMI more than 40).

Monitoring Tolerance and Adequacy of EN

Evidence of bowel motility (resolution of clinical ileus) is not required to initiate EN in the ICU. Patients should be monitored for tolerance of EN. One should look for symptoms of pain and/or distention and passage of flatus / stool. Physical examination and abdominal radiographs should be done when indicated. Inappropriate cessation of EN should be avoided. EN should not be withheld if gastric residual volume (GRV) is less than 500 ml as long as there are no other signs of intolerance. There is little to no data that monitoring GRV prevents the development of aspiration pneumonia. On the other hand, it may lead to a reduction in the daily delivery of enteral nutrition.

Impaired motility in ICU patients can be due to medications (narcotics), metabolic abnormalities, electrolyte imbalance and underlying disease. The resulting dysmotility is linked to decreased tolerance of EN and increased infection through gastro-pulmonary route.

It is advisable to use agents to promote motility such as prokinetic drugs or narcotic antagonists prophylactically. Paralytic ileus is prolonged if patients are not fed orally.

Keeping the patients nil orally for prolonged periods of time before and after diagnostic tests or therapeutic procedures is counterproductive and should be minimized.

Enteral feeding protocols help in achieving caloric targets. Patients on EN should be periodically assessed and steps (Fig 20.4) taken to reduce risk of aspiration.

Steps taken to reduce risk of aspiration

- Head end should be elevated to 30°– 45°
- EN should be switched to continuous infusion in high risk patients if they are intolerant to gastric feeding
- Prokinetic drugs (metoclopramide and erythromycin) or narcotic antagonists (naloxone and alvimopan) should be used if feasible
- Small bowel feeding must be considered

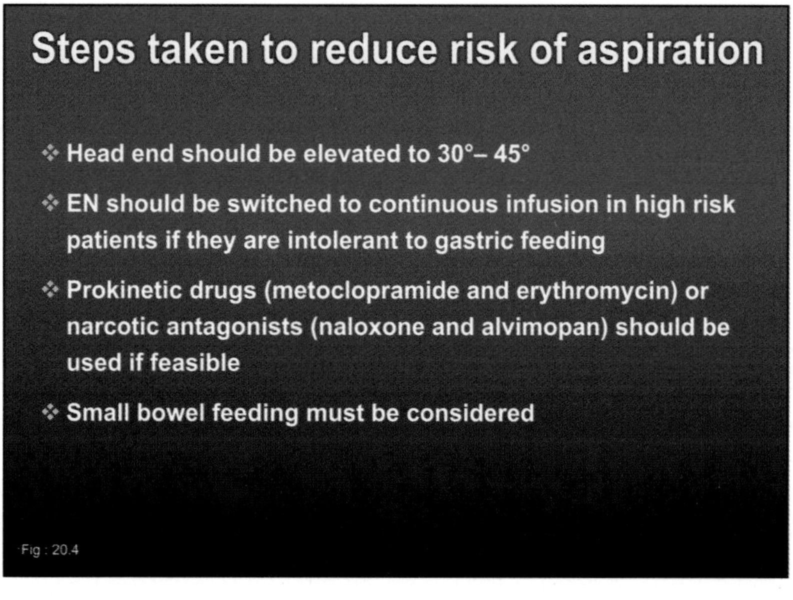

Fig : 20.4

Surrogate markers for aspiration like blue food coloring and glucose oxidase strips should not be used in the critical care setting.

Bowel disturbances associated with EN

Diarrhoea: Development of diarrhea associated with enteral tube feedings warrants further evaluation for the cause. Causes of diarrhea in critically ill are:
- Medications with high osmolarity or containing sorbitol
- Antibiotics
- Infection due to clostridium difficile or other gastrointestinal (GI) bacteria
- Disease states like inflammatory bowel disease, short bowel syndrome
- Fecal impaction which may lead to stool leaking around the impaction
- Intolerance to a specific component of EN e.g. fat or osmolarity

Soluble fiber-containing or small peptide formulations may be used in patients having diarrhea.

Constipation: The common causes of constipation in patients on EN are immobility, dehydration, lack of fiber and certain medications.

Treatment includes increased provision of fluid or fiber, stool softeners, laxatives, enemas or manual evacuation when necessary. Regular bowel regimens are helpful in treating and preventing constipation.

Gastrointestinal bleeding and enteral feeding

Enteral nutrition is probably the best way to prevent GI bleeding in ICU patients. EN is not contraindicated in patients with coffee ground aspiration and non-haemorrhagic oesophageal varices.

EN should be withheld for 48 hr if acute upper gastrointestinal bleeding occurs due to ulcer with high risk of re-bleeding or with variceal bleeding. Upper GI endoscopy should be performed and a decision to restart EN should be taken.

Pulmonary Failure and EN

Specialty high-lipid, low-carbohydrate formulations designed to manipulate the respiratory quotient and reduce CO_2 production are not recommended for routine use in acute respiratory failure. Fluid-restricted calorically dense formulations should be considered in these patients. Serum phosphate levels should be monitored closely and replaced appropriately.

Contraindications for Enteral feeds

Absolute
- Nonfunctional gut: anatomic disruption, obstruction and gut ischemia
- Generalized peritonitis
- Severe shock states

Relative
- Expected short period of fast except in severely injured patients
- Abdominal distension during EN
- Localized peritonitis, intra-abdominal abscess, severe pancreatitis

Nutritional Assessment and Management

Adjunctive Therapy

Administration of probiotic agents has been shown to improve outcome (most consistently by decreasing infection) in specific critically ill patient populations involving transplantation, major abdominal surgery and severe trauma. No recommendation can currently be made for use of probiotics in the general ICU population because of a lack of consistent outcome reports.

It seems that each species may have different effects and variable impact on patient outcome, making it difficult to make broad categorical recommendations.

Similarly, no recommendation can currently be made for use of probiotics in patients with severe acute necrotizing pancreatitis, as there is disparity of evidence in the literature. Insoluble fiber should be avoided in all critically ill patients. Both soluble and insoluble fiber should be avoided in patients at high risk for bowel ischemia or severe dysmotility.

When to Use Parental Nutrition

In the patients who were previously healthy before critical illness with no evidence of protein calorie malnutrition, use of PN should be reserved and initiated only after the first 7 days of hospitalization (if EN is not available). If there is evidence of protein-calorie malnutrition at admission and EN is not feasible, it is appropriate to initiate PN as soon as possible, following admission and adequate resuscitation.

In previously well nourished patients expected to undergo major upper gastrointestinal surgery, PN need not be initiated in the immediate postoperative period and can be delayed by 5 to 7 days. In malnourished patients, PN should be initiated 5 to 7 days preoperatively and continued in the immediate postoperative period.

PN therapy provided for less than 5–7 days has no beneficial effect and may result in increased risk to the patient and it should be initiated only if the duration of therapy is anticipated to be ≥7 days.

Some recent studies have shown that combined feeding can be used as a second-line tool around day 4 in patients not achieving their targets.

When indicated, maximize efficacy of PN

Need for PN therapy should be evaluated if EN is not available or feasible. If the patient is deemed to be a candidate for PN, steps should be taken to maximize efficacy by adjusting the dose, content, choice of supplemental additives and monitoring the results.

In patients on PN, permissive underfeeding should be considered initially. As the patient stabilizes, PN may be increased to meet energy requirements. 80% of the energy required is the ultimate goal of parenteral feeding. Patients should be given a parenteral formulation without soy-based lipids during first week of ICU stay.

Protocol based moderately strict control of serum glucose should be implemented. A range of 150-160 mg/dL may be most appropriate. When PN is used in the critical care setting, consideration should be given to supplementation with parenteral glutamine.

In patients stabilized on PN, periodic repeat efforts should be made to initiate EN. PN calories supplied should be reduced as tolerance improves and the volume of EN calories delivered increases. PN should not be terminated until more than 60% of target energy requirements are being delivered by EN.

The complications of enteral nutrition and parenteral nutrition are summarized in Fig 20.5.

Complications of EN	Complications of PN
❖ Tube misplacement, mucosal ulceration, nasopharyngeal or oesophageal perforation	❖ Catheter-related problems (infection, thrombosis, catheter misplacement)
❖ Diarrhoea	❖ Metabolic derangement (hyperglycaemia, electrolyte disturbances)
❖ Nausea and vomiting	
❖ Abdominal discomfort	❖ Acute fatty liver; hepatic dysfunction (cholestasis)
❖ Reflux	
❖ Pulmonary aspiration	❖ Fluid excess
	❖ Acid–base disturbance
	❖ Gut mucosal Atrophy
	❖ Overfeeding

Fig : 20.5

Pharmaconutrition

Immuno nutrition refers to nutrition supplemented with immune enhancing nutrients. The term pharmaconutrition is more appropriate as it alludes to the pharmacologic effects also. Nutritional deficits produce significant atrophy of lymphoid organs and lead to impaired function. Pharmaconutrients (including arginine, glutamine, nucleotides and ω-3 fatty acids) exert immune enhancing effects independent of their energy/protein value. Three potential targets exist for pharmaconutrition. They are

1. mucosal barrier function
2. cellular defense and
3. local or systemic inflammation.

Individual components of pharmaconutrition have been reported to preserve or augment various aspects of cellular immune function and to modify the production of inflammatory mediators.

Use of pharmaconutrition in ICU population

ICU patients not meeting criteria for immune- modulating formulations should receive standard enteral formulations. Patients with acute respiratory distress syndrome and severe acute lung injury should be placed on an enteral formulation containing an anti-inflammatory lipid profile (i.e., omega- 3 fish oils) and antioxidants. At least 50% to 65% of goal energy requirements should be delivered to receive optimal therapeutic benefit from the immune-modulating formulations. A combination of antioxidant vitamins and trace minerals (specifically including selenium) should be provided to all patients receiving specialized nutrition therapy. The addition of enteral glutamine to an EN regimen (not already containing supplemental glutamine) should be considered in burns, trauma, and mixed ICU patients.

Nutritional Assessment and Management

Summary of pharmaconutrition use in ICU (Fig 20.6)

Nutrients and Specific Underlying Causes in ICU
What Nutrient for What Population?

Nutrients	Critically Ill				
	General	Septic	Trauma	Burns	Acute Lung Injury
Arginine	Not recommended	Harm	Not recommended	Not recommended	Not recommended
Glutamine	PN Beneficial (? receiving EN)	---	EN Possibly Beneficial	EN Possibly Beneficial	---
Omega-3 FA	---	---	---	---	Recommended
Antioxidants Vitamins and trace elements	Should be considered	Should be considered	Should be considered	Should be considered	Should be considered

Fig : 20.6

Summary of selected immune-modulating nutrients (Fig 20.7)

Summary of selected immune-modulating nutrients, including their probable mechanisms and beneficial effects in critically ill patients

Nutrient	Effects	Mechanisms
Omega-3 fatty acids	Reduce inflammation Lead to production of less inflammatory prostaglandins and leukotrienes	Enhance immunity- Effect signal transduction and gene translation through incorporation into cells
Glutamine	Enhances wound healing	Fuel for enterocytes and lymphocytes
Arginine	Enhances wound healing	Precursor to collagen and nitric oxide
Antioxidants	Reduce oxidative stress	Neutralize reactive oxygen species and reactive nitrogen species

Fig : 20.7

Conclusion

Nutrition is a very important aspect of patient care in critical illness. Use of appropriate nutritional support is cost effective as it reduces complication rates and duration of stay. Optimal nutritional support to prevent and treat nutritional deficiencies should become part of routine management.

Nutrition is a part of multitude of treatments and therapies that are optimally applied by a multi-disciplinary team of professionals. Supplementation of specialized nutrients in pharmacologic amounts may lead to beneficial outcomes in selected critically ill patients. Once thought of only as nutritional support, these supplements have now come to be regarded as important therapeutic interventions. Don't miss feeding as it becomes harder to catch up on later.

References

1. Guidelines for the provision and assessment of nutrition support therapy in the adult critically ill patient. Society of Critical Care Medicine and American Society for Parenteral and Enteral Nutrition. Crit Care Med 2009: vol. 37, No. 5
2. Nutritional support in the intensive care unit. James A. Kruse. Multiprofessional Critical Care Review Course - 2005
3. Canadian Clinical Practice Guidelines. May 28th, 2009
4. Gastric residual volume during enteral nutrition in ICU patients: the REGANE study. Intensive Care Med 2010: 36:1386–1393
5. Indirect Calorimetry: Applications in Practice. Jennifer A. Wooley. Respir Care Clin 2006: 12 619–633.
6. Pharmaconutrition: a new emerging paradigm. Naomi E. Jonesa and Daren K. Heyland. Current Opinion in Gastroenterology 2008: 24:215–222
7. www.criticalcarenutrition.com

★★★

21 AEROSOL THERAPY AND HUMIDIFICATION

A : AEROSOL THERAPY

More and more patients with breathing disorders particularly with airway hyperreactivity are requiring mechanical ventilation. These patients require bronchodilators, steroids and other medications for control of their symptoms. Delivery of these drugs in aerosolised form is being used widely. The advantages of aerosol therapy are:
1. Delivery of the medications to target site of action
2. Rapid onset of action
3. Less systemic absorption
4. Less dose is required therefore less side effects

However, there are some disadvantages like the efficacy is dependent on optimal delivery technique. Also due to many varieties of inhalation devices available, there is lot of confusion about the devices and right technique of administration.

An aerosol is defined as airborne suspension of particulate matter. Aerosol droplet size is most commonly characterized by the mass median aerodynamic diameter (MMAD). MMAD is that diameter around which the mass of particles is equally distributed. The drug deposition in the lower respiratory tract of mechanically ventilated patients is more efficient with devices generating aerosols with a MMAD of 1–3μ. Optimal technique of administration, lead to deposition of the drug in the lower respiratory tract of ventilated patients. Pressurized metered dose inhalers (pMDIs) with spacer result in deposition of around 10% to 11% of nominal dose and 6% to 10% of nominal dose for nebulizer. Efficiency of drug deposition in the lower respiratory tract of ventilated patients is lower with nebulizers than with pMDIs. This is offset by the higher drug dose used by the nebulizers.

There are some fundamental differences in aerosol delivery in spontaneously breathing and mechanically ventilated patients which are mentioned below in Fig 21A.1. These differences can

Aerosol delivery in spontaneously breathing versus Mechanically Ventilated Patients

	Spontaneously breathing patient	Mechanically Ventilated Patient
Position of the patient	Sitting or standing	Supine or semi-recumbent
Aerosol device	PMDI / PMDI and spacer / nebulizer / dry powder inhaler	PMDI and spacer/nebulizer
Mode of delivery	By mouthpiece or facemask	Connected to endotracheal tube or inspiratory limb of ventilator circuit
Humidity	Ambient humidity	Humidified (approximately 96% to 97% relative humidity)
Temperature	Room or ambient	Warmed to approximately 35°C
Inspiratory airflow	Sinusoidal	Constant or ramp flow
Breath configuration	Patient controlled	Ventilator controlled (in assisted mode it is influenced by patient)
Aerosol administration	Administered by patient	Administered by staff or respiratory therapist
Airway	Oral or nasal cavity and upper airway	Endotracheal or tracheostomy tube

Fig : 21A.1

have impact on amount of drug deposited at the target site of action. Most of the discussion in this chapter will be about aerosol therapy in mechanically ventilated patients.

Types of aerosol delivery devices

There are three classes of aerosol delivery devices

1. Nebulizers:
    a. Jet nebulizers [also known as small volume (SVN) or pneumatic nebulizers]
    b. Ultrasonic nebulizers
    c. Vibrating mesh nebulizers
2. Metered dose inhalers
3. Dry powder inhalers

Metered dose inhalers (MDIs), nebulizers, and dry powder inhalers (DPIs) are the aerosol-generating devices of choice in ambulatory patients. In mechanically ventilated patients pressurized MDIs and nebulizers are preferred for inhalation therapy. Vibrating mesh nebulizer (expensive and requires disassembly and thorough cleaning) and dry powder inhalers (not very suitable for mechanically ventilated patients) are not commonly used. Therefore it will not be discussed in detail.

Nebulizers

SVN uses the Bernoulli principle to produce an aerosol. It produces a broad range of particle size, from 0.5 to 15µm MMAD. Usually, more than 50% of the drug volume is not released from the nebulizer and is trapped on the baffles and internal walls at the completion of nebulization. This quantity of residual drug is referred to as dead volume. Jet nebulizers are placed in the inspiratory limb of the ventilator circuit during mechanical ventilation and may be run continuously by pressurized gas from outside source or intermittently by using a separate line to provide driving pressure and gas flow from the ventilator. The nebulizer generates aerosol only during the inspiratory phase during intermittent operation, and the ventilator compensates for the flow to the nebulizer to maintain a constant tidal volume. It is important to know whether the ventilator takes

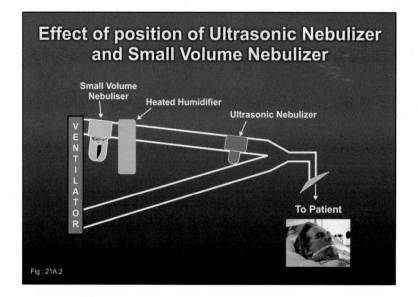

Fig: 21A.2

Aerosol Therapy and Humidification

into account the extra volume of gas used to drive the nebulizer otherwise it can result in lung injury due to excess tidal volume and pressure. Intermittent operation is more efficient for aerosol delivery than continuous aerosol generation because drug is deposited only in the lower respiratory tract only during inspiration. Some ventilators provide driving pressure which is lower compared to the external source (compressed air or oxygen sources) which could change aerosol characteristics and affect the efficiency of the nebulizer.

SVN- position in the ventilator circuit

The SVN position in the ventilator circuit significantly influences the efficiency of aerosol delivery. It is found to be least effective when it is placed proximal to the patient, between the ventilator circuit and the endotracheal tube.

Aerosol delivery is most effective

- When placed at a distance of at least 30 cm from the endotracheal tube in the inspiratory limb
- Between the ventilator and heated humidifier (refer Fig 21A.2). This is because the inspiratory limb of the ventilator circuit acts as a reservoir for aerosol produced late in the inspiratory phase and during exhalation, which increases the amount of aerosol available with subsequent inspiration. Also a smaller more stable aerosol particle is produced in a cool dry atmosphere before entering the humidifier resulting in better deposition to the lung.

The advantages and disadvantages of SVN are summarized in Fig 21A.3:

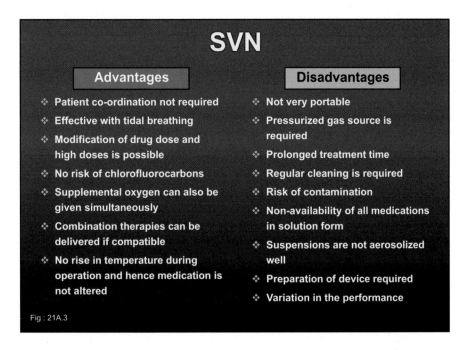

Fig : 21A.3

Ultrasonic nebulizer: Uses a piezoelectric crystal to convert electrical energy to high-frequency sound waves. These sound waves cause disruption of the solution surface resulting in aerosol formation. The aerosol particle size and drug output are influenced by the frequency and amplitude of vibration of the piezoelectric crystal, respectively.

Ultrasonic nebulizers (USN) - position in the ventilator circuit

When the USN is placed in the inspiratory limb of the ventilator circuit, close to the patient wye, it delivers significantly more medication to the airway than SVN and it is less efficient when placed closer to the ventilator (refer Fig 21A.2).

The advantages and disadvantages of USN are summarized in Fig 21A.4:

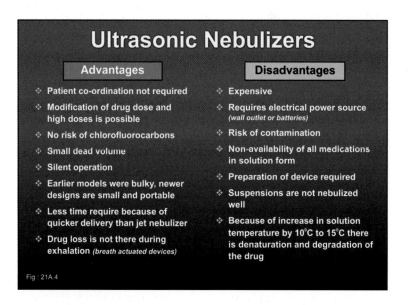

Fig : 21A.4

Metered dose inhalers (MDI)

Pressured MDIs contain the drug in the form of micronized crystals, suspended with a surfactant in a mixture of two or three chlorofluorocarbon (CFC) propellants. Preservatives and antioxidants are added to improve the shelf-life of the inhaler. Aerosol suspension is released from the tip of the canister at a very high velocity (around 60 mph) when MDI is actuated.

The aerosol may exceed 30-40 μm MMAD initially, but as the particles slow down and the propellants evaporate, size of the aerosol particles decrease to around 2-5 μm. Previously, most pMDIs used chlorofluorocarbon (CFC) propellants. Due to environmental concerns CFC (causes damage to ozone layer) are being phased out and being replaced by hydrofluoroalkane (HFA) propellants.

MDI-position in the ventilator circuit

Immediately after MDI actuation the MMAD of aerosol is large but decrease rapidly as the propellant evaporates. The larger particles which are traveling at high speed are lost by impaction when MDI is directly connected to the endotracheal tube.

On the contrary, if MDI is actuated into a spacer device placed at a distance from endotracheal tube the particle size decreases as a result of propellant evaporation which in turn increases the delivery of aerosol into the patient's lungs. Therefore, it is advisable to actuate MDI into a spacer device with a chamber placed at a distance (around 15 cm) from the endotracheal tube for optimum aerosol delivery in mechanically ventilated patients.

The advantages and disadvantages of MDI are summarized in Fig 21A.5.

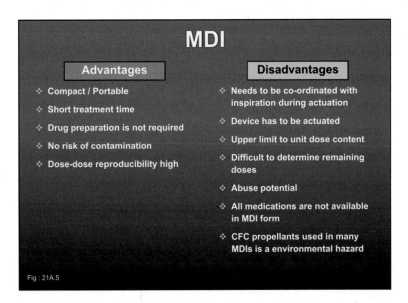
Fig : 21A.5

Spacer or adapter devices

Many commercially available adapters or actuators (Fig 21A.6) are used to connect the pMDI canister to the ventilator circuit. The efficiency of drug delivery is greatly affected by the type of adapter used. Many varieties of adapters are available for clinical use like elbow adapters, inline devices that may be unidirectional or bidirectional, and chamber or reservoir (collapsible and non collapsible) adapters. A chamber spacer with a pMDI in a ventilator circuit results in better aerosol drug delivery, compared with either an elbow adapter or a unidirectional inline spacer.

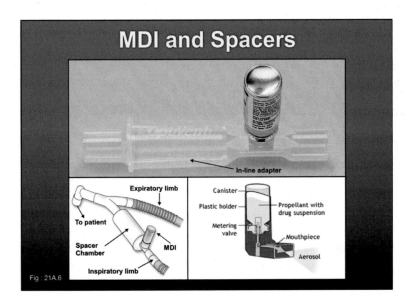
Fig : 21A.6

Factors effecting aerosol therapy during mechanical ventilation (Fig 21A.7)

Aerosol particle size

The deposition of aerosol particles is determined by three mechanisms:

1. Inertial impaction
2. Sedimentation
3. Diffusion - having little therapeutic effect

The ventilator circuit and endotracheal tube in mechanically ventilated patients, act as baffles that trap particles with larger diameter *en route* to the bronchi. The MMAD of aerosols produced by different brands of nebulizer vary widely. Nebulizers producing <2 μm aerosols are more likely to result in greater deposition in the lower respiratory tract of ventilated patients. When MDI is actuated into a spacer at the beginning of inspiration, a sizeable proportion of aerosol emerging from the distal end of the endotracheal tube was in the respirable range, with a MMAD of 1–2μm. Hence, deposition in the lower respiratory tract of mechanically ventilated patients is more likely with devices that generate aerosols with a MMAD of 1–3 μm.

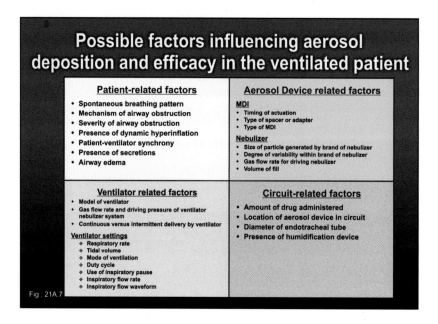

Fig : 21A.7

Heating and humidification

Due to increased particle loss in the ventilator circuit, humidification of inspired gas decreases aerosol deposition with MDIs and nebulizers by approximately 40%. When MDI (four puffs at 20-30 second intervals) is used to deliver aerosol therapy, the absence of humidification during that brief period does not cause much problem. Some nebulizers take a very long time sometimes up to 30-40 minutes to deliver the medication and inhalation of dry air for such long time causes damage to the airway. Therefore, it is not advisable to switch off the humidifier for aerosol therapy. Also disconnection of the ventilator circuit interferes with the ventilation sometimes resulting in de-recruitment, fatal hypoxemia (ARDS) and accidental disconnection later.

If HME is being used it should be removed before administering aerosol therapy because drug gets trapped in HMEs. If a patient requires multiple or continuous aerosol therapy (status asthmaticus or severe COPD), it is better to use MDI with spacer or nebulizer with heated humidifier in a ventilator circuit.

Density of the inhaled gas

Because of the turbulence in the airway during high inspiratory flows, the impaction of aerosol particles is increased. This loss of aerosol particles due to impaction can be reduced by preserving the laminar flow by decreasing the density of inspired gas (i.e. helium–oxygen). Therefore, breathing helium–oxygen may improve aerosol deposition.

Studies in ambulatory patients with airway obstruction have revealed higher lower respiratory tract aerosol delivery when breathing helium–oxygen compared with air. Helium–oxygen mixtures improved aerosol deposition during *in vitro* studies from a MDI during continuous mandatory ventilation (CMV) of a simulated adult patient.

On the contrary, helium–oxygen with pneumatic nebulizer produces less respirable mass of drug per liter of operating flow compared to when air or oxygen is used necessitating increased flow rate to produce similar nebulizer output.

Endotracheal tube size

Endotracheal tube reduces aerosol delivery in mechanically ventilated patients due to aerosol impaction and is inversely related to the airway diameter. However, no difference in drug deposition has been shown between endotracheal tubes with 9.0–7.0 mm internal diameter (ID). As airway ID gets smaller (6.0–3.0 mm ID) aerosol delivery to the lower respiratory tract is reduced. With an adult-sized endotracheal tube, ≥ 7.0 mm, the loss of aerosol during mechanical ventilation appears to be more in the ventilator circuit, between the aerosol generator and the artificial airway, than in the endotracheal tube itself.

Ventilator mode and settings

The characteristics of the breath used to deliver aerosol therapy in mechanically ventilated patients, is influenced by mode, tidal volume, inspiratory flow rate and respiratory rate. Actuation of an MDI into a spacer needs to be synchronized with the precise onset of inspiration for optimal aerosol delivery.

The tidal volume of the ventilator-delivered breath must be more than the volume of the ventilator tubing and endotracheal tube for better efficiency of aerosol delivery to patient's lungs. Tidal volumes of 500 ml or more in adults are associated with satisfactory aerosol delivery. But, at the same time one should keep in mind that higher airway pressures associated with higher tidal volume can worsen lung injury. Aerosol delivery is better with lower inspiratory flows and higher inspiratory time (higher duty cycle).

Aerosol delivery is affected by flow patterns, with decelerating flow pattern delivering around 20% more drug to the lower respiratory tract than square wave patterns. The significance of inspiratory hold on aerosol deposition has not been determined.

Aerosol delivery from nebulizers has been shown to decrease by as much as 80% by continuous flow through the ventilator circuit, whereas reductions in delivery from MDIs were not statistically significant.

The technique for using nebulisers and MDIs in ventilated patients has been summarized in Figs 21A.8 and 21A.9.

Technique for using Nebulizers in Mechanically Ventilated Patients

1. Place drug solution in nebulizer to optimal fill volume (2–6 mL)*
2. Place nebulizer in inspiratory line at least 30 cm from the patient wye
3. Ensure airflow of 6–8 L/min through the nebulizer
4. Ensure adequate tidal volume (500 mL in adults). Attempt to use duty cycle >0.3, if possible
5. Adjust minute volume to compensate for additional airflow through the nebulizer, if required
6. Turn off flow-by or continuous flow mode on ventilator
7. Observe nebulizer for adequate aerosol generation throughout use
8. Disconnect nebulizer when all medication is nebulized or when no more aerosol is being produced
9. Reconnect ventilator circuit and return to original ventilator setting

*The volume of solution placed in the nebulizer that is associated with maximal efficiency of the nebulizer is variable in different nebulizers and should be known before using any nebulizer

Fig : 21A.8

Technique for using MDIs in Mechanically Ventilated Patients

1. Ensure V_T > 500 mL (in adults) during assisted ventilation
2. Aim for an inspiratory time (excluding the inspiratory pause) > 0.3 of total breath duration
3. Ensure that the ventilator breath is synchronized with the patient's inspiration
4. Shake the MDI vigorously
5. Place canister in actuator of a cylindrical spacer situated in inspiratory limb of ventilator circuit
6. Actuate MDI to synchronize with precise onset of inspiration by the ventilator
7. Allow a breathhold at end-inspiration for 3–5 seconds *
8. Allow passive exhalation
9. Repeat actuations after 20–30 seconds until total dose is delivered

*The effect of a postinspiratory breathhold has not been evaluated in mechanically ventilated patients

Fig : 21A.9

Care of spacers and nebulizers

Contamination of nebulizers placed in-line in the ventilator circuit can result in micro organisms being delivered as microaerosols directly to the lower respiratory tract. Therefore the Centers for Disease Control and Prevention recommended that nebulizers should be sterile at the start of aerosol therapy and should be detached from the ventilator circuit after each use and either replaced or disassembled, cleaned with sterile water, rinsed, and air dried. Also, it is preferable to use single-dose ampoules of drug compared to multidose vials, which can become contaminated easily. Condensate collects inside chamber spacer when it is left in the ventilator circuit between aerosol therapy which can be reduced by using collapsible chamber actuators and the heated wire type of circuits. Even though, no data suggest that contamination in the spacer results in pathogens being delivered by aerosol to the patient, care must be taken to prevent the condensate in the spacer from being drained down into the patient's respiratory tract when the spacer is manipulated during use.

Aerosol Therapy and Humidification

Assessing bronchodilator response

β2-agonists are effective in improving respiratory mechanics in mechanically ventilated patients. Following changes in peak airway pressures, transairway pressure ($P_{ta} = P_{peak} - P_{plat}$) and auto-PEEP are useful in assessing the efficacy of bronchodilator therapy. Improvement in clinical signs and symptoms like reduced wheezing, decreased sensation of dyspnea and work of breathing, improvement in hemodynamics and patient-ventilator synchrony are also important. Bronchodilator therapy could assist weaning in patients with limited cardiopulmonary reserve.

Aerosol delivery during noninvasive positive pressure ventilation (NPPV)

NPPV is being more and more preferred for treatment of patients with acute and chronic respiratory failure. NPPV is often used as a first line mode of ventilatory support in as much as 50% of patients with hypercapnic respiratory failure. If NPPV is successful then it will avert the need for endotracheal intubation and all its associated complications and improve mortality. Inhaled bronchodilators are often being used in patients with acute or acute-on-chronic hypercapnic respiratory failure who are receiving NPPV.

Although it seems that during NPPV, inhaled drugs (e.g. bronchodilators) could be efficiently delivered via either nebulizer or MDI spacer, there is a lacunae in medical knowledge about the ventilator features best suited for this application. Some studies have shown optimum drug delivery is achieved if nebulizer position is between the leak port and patient connection, administering high inspiratory pressure, low expiratory pressure, and a breath rate of 20/min.

Devices used for aerosol therapy during NPPV (Fig 21A.10).

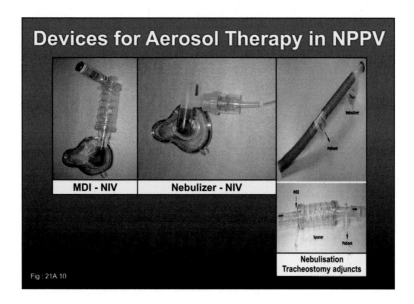

Fig: 21A.10

Aerosolized drugs

Bronchodilators

Aerosolized bronchodilators are one of the most frequently used drugs in ventilator-supported patients with asthma or chronic obstructive pulmonary disease (COPD). The goals of bronchodilator therapy are to reverse bronchoconstriction, decrease tachypnoea and the work of breathing, or alleviate dyspnea. Both aerosolized β-adrenergic or anticholinergic bronchodilators are used for bronchodilator therapy. But, the combination of β-adrenergic and anticholinergic bronchodilators (ipratropium) is found to be more effective than ipratropium alone in a group of ventilator-supported patients with COPD.

In mechanically ventilated patients, considerable bronchodilator effects occur after administration of 2.5 mg of albuterol (or salbutamol) with a standard nebulizer or four puffs (400 µg) with a pMDI. Usually 2.5ml of salbutamol respules contain around 2.5 mg of salbutamol which is diluted with another 2.5 ml of sterile water and used in jet nebulizer. 2.0 ml of ipratropium respules contains 500 µg which is diluted with sterile water to a final volume of 4 to 5 ml and used in the jet nebulizer. Each puff from pMDI (salbutamol) delivers 100µg of salbutamol.

So, around 4 puffs are given at 20 to 30 seconds interval. Each puff from pMDI (ipratropium) delivers 20µg of ipratropium bromide. So, around 2 puffs are given at 20 to 30 seconds interval. Higher doses result in negligible therapeutic advantage, whereas the potential for side-effects was increased. However, in certain clinical settings, higher doses of bronchodilators may be needed in patients especially with severe airway obstruction or if the technique of administration is not optimal. In stable mechanically ventilated patients with COPD the duration of bronchodilator response appears to be shorter than that in ambulatory patients (2–3 hr versus 4–6 hr, respectively). Hence, patients on ventilator support require scheduled administration of short-acting β- agonist bronchodilator (albuterol) every 3–4 hr.

Inhaled steroids are used in conjugation with bronchodilators to suppress inflammation in COPD and asthma.

Toxicity

Administration of very high doses of β- agonists is associated with an increased risk of arrhythmias, tremors, restlessness and hypokalemia. When pMDIs are used in excessive doses or when pMDI aerosol is delivered directly beyond the endotracheal tube by attaching a catheter to the canister nozzle, propellants in the formulation could cause local ulceration.

Surfactant

In surfactant deficiency (ARDS) disease states, surfactant replacement therapy (SRT) has been evaluated. The viscosity of exogenous surfactants makes them difficult to administer in aerosol form and they tend to foam and form stable bubbles during nebulization. Therefore, surfactant delivery to the lower respiratory tract by nebulisation is inefficient and the bulk of the aerosol is lost in the delivery system and the ventilator circuit. It may deposit and get in the way of the functioning of valves and monitoring devices of the ventilator which can be avoided to some extent by placing filters in the expiratory limb of the circuit to trap any aerosol before it reaches the ventilator. Further developments in the design of exogenous surfactants and better delivery systems and studies supporting surfactant therapy in ARDS patients are desirable for aerosolized surfactant to become an effective treatment for ARDS.

Other drugs

Aerosolized antibiotics are used for treatment of cystic fibrosis and multi-drug resistant ventilator associated pneumonia. Prostanoids and mucolytics are not commonly used in ICU. The inhalation route of drug delivery is also being evaluated for a variety of anti-inflammatory, immuno-regulatory agents, and for gene therapy. Some of these therapies may become available for treatment of patients receiving mechanical ventilation in future.

Choice of aerosol-generating device: MDIs vs. Nebulizers

Studies have established that nebulizers and MDIs are equally effective in the treatment of airway obstruction in ambulatory patients and in mechanically ventilated patients. The use of MDIs for aerosol therapy in mechanically ventilated patients is preferred because of numerous problems associated with the use of nebulizers.

- The rate of aerosol production and particle size of aerosol is highly unpredictable, not only in nebulizers of different brands but also in different batches of the same brand. Also the operational efficiency of a nebulizer varies with the pressure of the driving gas and with different fill volumes. Hence, it is essential to characterize the efficiency of nebulizer in a ventilator circuit before using.
- Risk of contamination with bacteria is also possible with nebulizer use unless the nebulizers and solutions are meticulously cleaned and disinfected.
- Tidal volume and inspiratory flow needs to be monitored and adjusted. The additional gas flow driving the nebulizer can lead to lung injury due to excess tidal volume. Additional flow leads to lack of triggering in assisted mode resulting in hypoventilation.

MDIs are easy to administer, portable, require less personnel time, are free from the risk of bacterial contamination and provide a reliable dose of the drug. Also, ventilator circuit need not be disconnected if a spacer is used minimizing the risk of airway contamination and de-recruitment.

Conclusion

Use of MDIs for bronchodilator therapy instead of nebulizers is an economical and time-saving measure especially when cost of medical treatment is going up. There is inadequate evidence to guide the choice of MDI or nebulizer for NPPV support.

References:

1. Inhalation therapy in invasive and noninvasive mechanical ventilation: Rajiv Dhand. Current Opinion in Critical Care 2007: 13:27–38

2. Aerosol Therapy in Mechanically Ventilated Patients: Recent Advances and New Techniques: James B. Fink, and Rajiv Dhand. Seminars in respiratory and critical care medicine 2000: vol. 21, no. 3

3. Bronchodilator Aerosol Delivery in Mechanical Ventilation: Jantz MA, Collop NA. Intensive Care Med 1999: 14: 166-183

4. Device Selection and Outcomes of Aerosol Therapy: Evidence-Based Guidelines, American College of Chest Physicians/ American College of Asthma, Allergy, and Immunology. Myrna B. Dolovich, Richard C. Ahrens, Dean R. Hess et al. Chest 2005; 127:335–371

5. How Best to Deliver Aerosol Medications to Mechanically Ventilated Patients. Rajiv Dhand, Vamsi P. Guntur, Clin Chest Med 2008: 29: 277–296

B : HUMIDIFICATION

Humidification is an essential part of any successful ventilatory strategy. The importance of this strategy and its impact on control of bronchial secretions, gas exchange, weaning and complications such as ventilator-associated pneumonia (VAP), are under-recognized by clinicians. Understanding pathophysiology and techniques of humidification is important for instituting safe mechanical ventilation.

Water in vapour form (gaseous state) is humidity and process of conditioning inspired air to body temperature and 100% relative humidity is termed as humidification. To understand humidification some basic understanding of physical aspects of humidity and process of humidification and various devices of humidification is essential which will be discussed in this chapter.

Basic definitions

Humidity is the amount of water vapor present in the air. It can be expressed in several ways:

- *Relative humidity (RH)* is a ratio of the actual water vapor content of air to the amount of water vapor needed to reach saturation at a particular temperature.
- *Absolute humidity (AH)* is the mass of water vapor contained in a given volume of air. It is commonly expressed in milligrams of water per liter of gas.

Alveolar gas has a temperature of 37° C, relative humidity 100% and contains 43.9 mg H_2O/l of water vapor.

Relationship between gas temperature, absolute humidity and water vapor pressure (Figs 21B.1 and 21B.2)

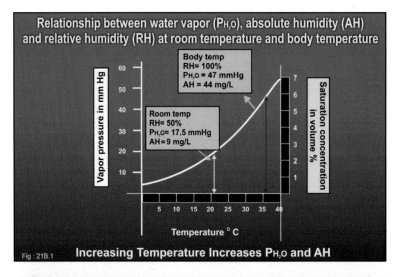

Fig: 21B.1

Gas Temperature °C	Absolute humidity mg H_2O/L	Water vapor pressure P_{H_2O}	
0	4.85	4.6	The relationship of Gas temperature, Absolute Humidity & Water Vapor pressure
5	6.8	6.5	
10	9.4	9.2	
15	12.8	12.8	
20	17.3	17.5	
25	23.0	23.7	
30	30.4	31.7	
32	33.8	35.5	
34	37.6	39.8	
36	41.7	44.4	
37	43.9	46.9	
38	46.2	49.5	
40	51.1	55.1	
42	56.5	61.3	
44	62.5	68.1	

Fig: 21B.2

Hotter gas can hold more amount of water vapor therefore absolute humidity and water vapor pressure increases. As the inspired air leaves the humidifier and moves towards the patient, it cools.

Aerosol Therapy and Humidification

This results in condensation as the capacity to hold the water vapor decreases with the drop in temperature. This can be reduced by using heated wire circuit. A water trap will be necessary to collect the condensed water.

Physiologic and thermodynamic basics:

Usually respiration occurs through nose when inspired air is warmed and humidified by evaporation of water from the surface of mucous membranes. Ambient air at a temperature of 37°C has a moisture content of 10 mg/l. Therefore, 34 mg of water has to be added to each liter of inspired air along with warmth to achieve physiologic saturation condition (100% relative humidity at body temperature). Part of this (around 20% to 30%) is recovered during subsequent expiration by condensation. This exchange of warmth and moisture mainly occurs in the nasopharyngeal region.

Therefore, effective moisture loss from nasopharyngeal region is around 17 mg/l and from the lower respiratory tract it is around 7 mg/l leading to a total water loss of around 24 mg/l. Hence, the process of conditioning the inspired gas is an active one (Figs 21B.3 and 21B.4)

Humidity of Medical Gas and Ambient Air

	Medical Gases	Ambient Air	Lungs
Temperature	15 °C	22 °C	37 °C
Relative humidity	2%	35%	100%
Absolute humidity	0.3 mg/L	7 mg/L	44 mg/L

Fig: 21B.3

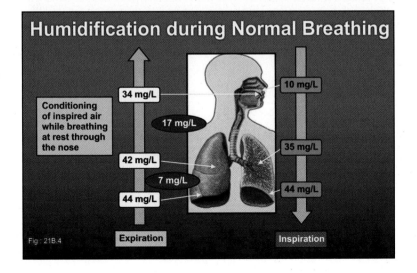

Fig: 21B.4

Intubation bypasses the nasopharyngeal region which results in isothermic saturation boundary (point in the respiratory tract at which inspired air attains 100% relative humidity at 37°C and this is normally at or just below the carina) being shifted down towards the lung's periphery. The process of humidification of inspired air is now shifted to lower respiratory tract which is exposed to dry air for long periods. This problem is further worsened by the fact that medical gases are drier when compared to ambient air. Increased water loss from the lower respiratory tract is around 32 g/l (Fig 21B.5). This results in impaired function of the mucociliary elevator.

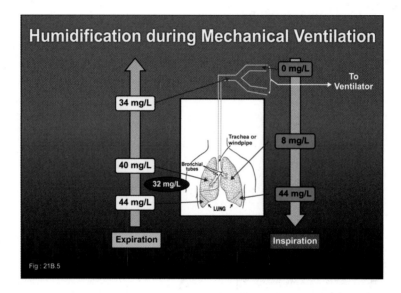

Fig : 21B.5

Mucociliary elevator (Fig 21B.6)

Respiratory mucous consists of a thick superficial (gel) layer and a deep watery (sol) layer. This allows the tips of the cilia to 'grip' mucous and push it cranially on a forward stroke, yet pass back through it on the recovery stroke. This is the basic unit of the mucociliary elevator. Loss of water leads to lowering

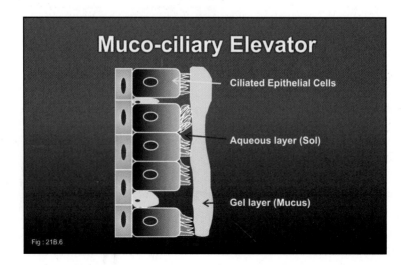

Fig : 21B.6

of the liquid sol layer, which does not allow cilia to function optimally. Therefore, micro-organisms are not cleared which predisposes the patient for respiratory infections. The relationship between the mucociliary transport system's performance and the humidity of the inspired gas has been studied extensively. At any given level of temperature and humidity, mucosal dysfunction is expected to worsen serially through four steps as listed below:

- Thickened mucus (or thinned mucus, in the case of overhydration)
- Slowed mucociliary transport
- Mucociliary stasis
- Cell damage

The rate of worsening through these steps is proportional to the humidity deficit. Humidity-related mucosal dysfunction may be further compromised by the presence of lung disease.

Complications of mechanical ventilation with suboptimal humidification

Due to dry medical gases and shifting of ISB downward towards the periphery of lungs, mechanical ventilation without appropriate humidification results in various complications, as discussed below in Fig 21B.7.

Complications of Mechanical Ventilation with Sub-optimal Humidification

Morphological changes in airway epithelium:
- Inflammation of respiratory tract epithelium
- Loss of cilia, ulceration and necrosis of the epithelium
- Sol phase depth reduction
- Increased viscosity of airway secretions

Functional changes in the airway:
- Transfer of ISB downwards towards the lung periphery
- Modification of ciliary function, ciliary paralysis
- Reduction in mucous transportation velocity, retention of secretions
- Increase in airway resistance and airway obstruction
- Decrease in threshold of bronchospasm

Changes in pulmonary and mechanical function:
- Respiratory tract infection
- Reduction in functional residual capacity (FRC) and compliance
- Atelectasis and Increase in intrapulmonary shunt and V/Q mismatch resulting in Hypoxemia

Fig: 21B.7

Types of humidifiers

Humidification of respired gases during mechanical ventilation is a standard of care. The humidification of respiratory gases should be started as early as possible and should not be dispensed with, even during short-term postoperative mechanical ventilation, patient transport or other emergency room situations.

Two systems are commonly used to humidify and warm inspired gases:

1. Heated humidifiers (HHs) also known as active humidifiers and
2. Heat and moisture exchangers (HMEs) also known as passive humidifiers

There is one more type of humidifier which tries to combine the features of both heated humidifiers and HME's known as active heat moisture exchanger (not commonly used).

Passive humidifiers/Heat moisture exchangers (HME)

In passive humidifiers (Fig 21B.8), the heat and moisture in expired air is trapped and transferred to inspired air during subsequent respiratory cycle. There is no external source for addition of heat and moisture. These are provided by the patient.

Types of HMEs

1. Condenser humidifier which is unsuitable for mechanical ventilation
2. Hygroscopic condenser humidifier
3. Hydrophobic condenser humidifier
4. Hygroscopic condenser humidifier filters (provide both humidification and filtration)
5. Hydrophobic condenser humidifier filters (provide both humidification and filtration)

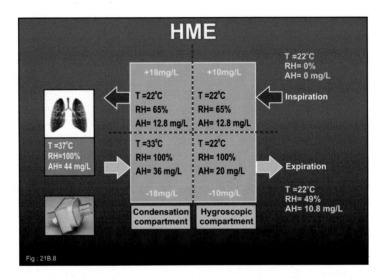

Fig : 21B.8

Mechanism

Heat and moisture in the expired air are absorbed by the hygroscopic or hydrophobic material in HME, trapped, stored and transferred to the dry gas during subsequent inspiration. The efficiency of each device varies. HMEs that provide an AH <26 mg/l should not be used. The use of HMEs that deliver an AH of at least 30 mg H_2O/l are recommended, as they are associated with a lower incidence of endotracheal tube (ETT) blockage.

Usage

- It should visible and accessible in order to detect contamination or disconnection
- It should be positioned next to the tracheal tube, mask or supra-glottic airway device
- If a nebulizer or metered dose inhaler is used to deliver medication, it should be inserted in between the HME and the patient or preferably the HME should be removed from the circuit during aerosol therapy.

Contraindications

There are no contraindications to providing humidification of inspired gas during mechanical ventilation. But HME is contraindicated under some circumstances.

- In patients with frank bloody or thick, copious secretions as HME can get blocked and the resistance is increased.

Aerosol Therapy and Humidification

- In patients with an expired tidal volume less than 70% of inspired tidal volume (e.g. large broncho-pleural fistula, endotracheal tube cuff defect etc.) as HME uses heat and moisture in expired air to humidify inspired air.
- In ARDS/ALI and obstructive airway disease, because HMEs add additional dead space, resistance and cause increased work of breathing and $PaCO_2$
- In patients with body temperatures <32°C because HMEs use patients own body heat to warm inspired gas
- In patients with high spontaneous minute volumes (>10 l/min)
- It should be removed from the ventilator circuit during aerosol therapy or should be bypassed

Heated humidifiers (HH)

In heated humidifiers, heat and moisture is added to inspired gas from an external source by active process.

Types of heated humidifiers:

1. Cascade humidifier
2. Bubble through humidifier
3. Surface-contact humidifier
4. Wick humidifier

Mechanism

Heated humidifiers add moisture and heat to the inspired air from temperature-regulated water reservoirs. Based on the mode of temperature control there are two types servo controlled unit and non-servo controlled unit. A servo controlled unit automatically controls power to the heating element in the humidifier in response to the temperature sensed by a probe near the patient connection or the humidifier outlet. A non-servo controlled unit provides power to the heating element according to the setting of a control, irrespective of the delivered temperature (Fig 21B.9)

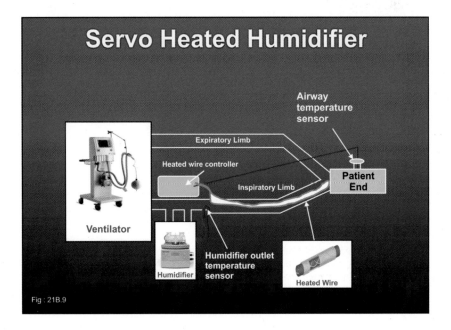

Fig: 21B.9

Usage

- It should be placed in the inspiratory limb
- To avoid the risk of water entering into patient's airway it should be at a lower level than the patient
- Periodically the condensate must be drained or a water trap must be inserted in the most dependent part of the tubing to prevent blockage or aspiration. Since condensate is considered as infectious waste, it should not be drained back into humidifier reservoir.
- The heater wire in the ventilator circuit should not be bunched, but strung evenly along the length of the circuit.
- One should not fill the chamber above the maximum level as liquid could enter the ventilator circuit and then the patient's airway, if the chamber is overfilled.

Contraindications

Heated humidifiers have no contraindications and can be used on any patient requiring ventilatory assistance or supplemental oxygen.

Advantages and disadvantages of various humidification devices (Fig 21B.10)

Advantages and Disadvantages of Humidification devices

	Advantages	Disadvantages
HH with heated wire circuit	• Wide range of temperatures • Universal application • Reliable • Temperature monitoring • Alarms • Elimination of condensate	• Potential for reduced relative humidity and airway obstruction • Cost if used <48 hrs • Lack of portability • Complexity
HME	• Passive operation • Portable • Lightweight • Simple • Low cost	• Net water loss from respiratory tract • Not suitable for all patients • Dead space • Resistance • Potential for occlusion • Must remove to administer aerosol therapy
Active HME	• Universal application • Low water consumption • Elimination of condensate • Temperature monitoring • Alarms • Continued passive operation if water or electricity is lost • Elimination of water traps / heated wires	• Dead space • Weight • Potential for occlusion • Limited temperature range • Heat source near patient • Must remove to administer aerosols

Fig : 21B.10

Complications of humidification devices:

Complications of HME

- Hypothermia
- Hypercapnia due to hypoventilation caused by the increase in dead space
- Low-pressure alarm may become ineffective during disconnection, due to resistance through the HME

Complications of Heated Humidifiers

- Potential for electrical shock
- Hyperthermia
- Risk of burns to the patient and health staff, thermal injury to the airway, and tubing meltdown

- Unintentional tracheal lavage because of overfilling, tilting of the water reservoir or draining of condensate
- The condensation in the circuit may cause patient ventilator dyssynchrony and triggering issues and may affect ventilator performance.
- May cause dehydration of the airway if temperature is set to body temperature, yet the RH is low.
- Risk of over hydration with associated complications like pulmonary edema, hyponatremia etc.

Complications common to both HME and Heated humidifier
- If AH is <26 mg H_2O/l, it can lead to dehydration and thickening and impaction of mucus secretions
- Insufficient AH can lead to mucus plugging of airways resulting in hypoventilation, gas trapping, increase airway resistance causing increase in work of breathing
- Increased resistance through the humidifier (more in HME) could result in elevated airway pressures and possible disconnection
- When humidifier (more so in heated humidifier) is disconnected from the patient, some ventilators generate a high flow through the ventilator circuit that may aerosolize contaminated condensate, increasing risk of nosocomial infection for both the patient and clinician.
- Compressible volume loss (more in heated humidifier) can lead to inaccurate effective tidal volume and possible hypoventilation (if not calculated)

Mechanical effects of Heated humidifier and HME:

There are some mechanical effects due to usage of heated humidifier and HME which are summarized in (Fig 21B.11).

Mechanical Effects of HH and HME

	Heated Humidifier	HME
Compressible volume	+++	+
Dead space	0	++
Inspiratory resistance	±	+
Expiratory resistance	0	++
Intrinsic PEEP	0	+
Ventilatory load	0	++

Fig: 21B.11

Selecting the type of Humidifier (Fig 21B.12)

As HMEs are less expensive, light weight and portable they are preferred for short-term use (≤96 hr) and also during transport. HH should be used for patients who exhibit contraindications for HME use. There is no major difference in the incidence of ventilator-associated pneumonia in patients humidified with HMEs versus HHs.

Assessing the adequacy of humidification

It is difficult to objectively measure humidification. Therefore, humidification should be assessed clinically and it is understood to be appropriate if the patient exhibits none of the complications of under- or over-humidification listed above. The presence of condensate in the ET connector implies that RH is 100%.

Infection Control:

- Heated humidifiers should be thoroughly disinfected. Aseptic technique should be used when filling the water reservoir and only medical grade sterile water should be used.
- The water left over in the water feed reservoir remains sterile and need not be discarded when the ventilator circuit is changed. Nevertheless, the water feed system should be used for single patient only.
- Condensation from the ventilator circuit should be considered infectious waste and disposed of according to hospital policy, using strict universal precautions. Condensate should never be drained back into the humidifier reservoir.
- There is no need to change the circuits on a timely basis. But it should be changed when they are visibly soiled or not functioning properly
- There is no need to change HME daily for reasons of infection control. They should be changed only when they are visibly soiled, blocked or damaged. HME can be safely used for at least 48 hours, and sometimes for up to 1 week.

Recommendations for humidification are summarized in Fig 21B.13

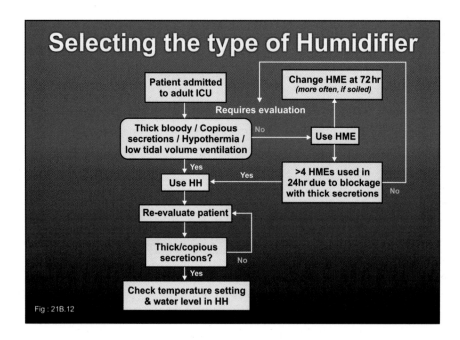

Fig : 21B.12

Aerosol Therapy and Humidification

> **Humidification Recommendations**
>
> - Humidification is recommended for every patient receiving mechanical ventilation
> - For NPPV heated humidification is recommended, as it may improve adherence and comfort
> - For invasively ventilated receiving active humidification, it is suggested that the heated humidifier should provide a humidity level between 33 mg H_2O/L and 44 mg H_2O/L and inspired gas temperature between 34°C and 41°C at the circuit Y-piece, with an RH of 100%
> - HME should provide a minimum of 30 mg H_2O/L
> - Passive humidification is not recommended for NPPV
> - In patients (ARDS) who require low tidal volumes, such as when lung-protective ventilation strategies are used, HMEs are not recommended because they contribute additional dead space, which can increase the ventilation requirement and $PaCO_2$
> - It is suggested that HMEs are not used as a prevention strategy for ventilator-associated pneumonia
>
> Fig : 21B.13

Humidification for NPPV

From a pathophysiological view point, spontaneously breathing patients without an endotracheal tube or tracheostomy tube do not necessarily require additional strategies for conditioning respiratory gases. In NPPV there are large leaks around the mask and high inspiratory flow (sometimes up to 120 l/min) of dry medical gases.

These overwhelm the mucosal humidification capacity. Added to these, there may be worsening of secretions and fluid depletion. It is, therefore, advisable to use active humidifier as they have a large capacity to produce heated and humidified air.

Well humidified air at a temperature between 25-30°C is one of the factors for success in NPPV therapy. This improves both secretion clearance and the tolerance of the NPPV therapy. Passive humidification is not recommended for NPPV.

Conclusion

All mechanically ventilated patients should receive adequate humidification of inspired gases to avoid the hazards of under- and over-humidification. The selection of type of humidifying device depends on many factors like patient's temperature, quantity and quality of secretions, history of chronic lung disease, duration of ventilatory support etc.

In patients requiring short term ventilation considering the cost advantage of HME, it can be preferred over heated humidifier provided there are no contraindications. Humidification should not be considered in isolation but as part of total airway management.

It should be associated with careful fluid balance, physiotherapy, bronchial hygiene therapy and appropriate drug therapy.

References

1. Devices used to humidify respired gases. Dr. Jorg Rathgeber. Respir Care Clin 2006: 12: 165–182
2. Humidification during mechanical ventilation: Current Trends and Controversies. Tim Op't Holt
3. Humidification during invasive and noninvasive mechanical ventilation: 2012, Restrepo RD, Walsh BK. Respir Care 2012 May; 57(5):782-8.

★ ★ ★

HEART–LUNG INTERACTION DURING MECHANICAL VENTILATION

Chandramohan M
Chandrashekar TR

Heart is inside the thorax and surrounded by lungs. It is a pressure chamber within a pressure chamber and interaction between them is inevitable. Interaction can be mechanical, neural and humoral in nature. Delivery of oxygen to tissues being a joint cardio-respiratory function, these interactions have more significant consequences in patients with cardiac and/or respiratory problems. Therefore both systems have to complement each other for maintaining aerobic metabolism. Cardiac failure can impair gas exchange by inducing pulmonary edema and decreasing blood flow to the respiratory muscles. Ventilation can modify cardiovascular function by changing lung volume, intrathoracic pressure (ITP) and by increasing metabolic demands due to increased work of breathing. The differences in the hemodynamic effects between spontaneous and positive pressure ventilation are related to the directionally opposite changes in ITP (Fig 22.1).

Heart Lung Interactions
Spontaneous breathing versus mechanical ventilation

Effects	Spontaneous breathing	Positive pressure ventilation
ITP	Decreases	Increases
Effect on RV preload	Increases	Decreases
Effect on LV afterload	Increases	Decreases
Ventricular interdependence	By parallel interdependence	By series interdependence (mostly)

Fig : 22.1

Ventilation as exercise

Breathing is an active process which involves muscular contraction requiring blood flow, energy, and O_2 producing CO_2 as a byproduct. Under normal conditions, the work cost of breathing is very low, comprising less than 5% of total O_2 (cardiac output) consumption. In patients with lung disease, the work cost of breathing can increase in excess of 25% of total O_2 consumption and it might become the primary limiting factor. The increased demand cannot be met by patients with limited cardiac reserves (due to ischemia, sepsis induced cardiomyopathy, congestive heart failure etc.). This results in cardiac failure, reduced oxygen delivery to tissues, hypoxia, lactic acidosis, progressing to multiorgan dysfunction and death if untreated.

Ventilatory support in such patients reduces the work of breathing and metabolic demand from respiratory muscles resulting in increased blood flow to other hypoperfused tissues. A better knowledge and understanding of the interaction between heart and lungs, in normal health and critical illness, is vital in reducing complications and providing optimum care to patients.

Pertinent basic cardiovascular and respiratory physiology

In order to understand the heart lung interaction, one should know basic physiology. This is discussed below:

Relationship between airway pressure and pleural pressure (or intrathoracic pressure)

$dP_{pl}/dP_{aw} = C_L/(C_L + C_{CW})$

P_{pl} = pleural pressure

P_{aw} = airway pressure

C_L = compliance of the lung, C_{CW} = compliance of the chest wall.

As per the above equation describing the relationship between changes in pleural pressure and changes in airway pressure, the compliance of the lung (C_L) and chest wall (C_{CW}) determines the amount of airway pressure that is transmitted to pleural space. In normal subjects $C_L \approx C_{CW}$ so that the change in intrapleural pressure (P_{pl}) is approximately 1/2 the change in airway pressure (P_{aw}). In patients with decreased lung compliance (and or increased chest wall compliance), this relationship predicts that the pleural pressure will be increased by a lesser proportion (may be $1/3^{rd}$ to $1/5^{th}$) of a change in airway pressure.

In primary ARDS, the chest wall elastance remains normal but in secondary ARDS, chest wall elastance is increased much more than lung elastance. So, higher pleural pressure has significantly more negative effect on cardiac output in secondary ARDS than in primary ARDS.

Relationship between flow and pressure (Figs 22.2 and 22.3)

Fluid always flows from a region with higher pressure (P1) to a region with lower pressure (P2) i.e. when there is a pressure gradient (ΔP). When the pressure gradient is constant, then the flow is inversely proportional to resistance (R) Flow= ΔP/R

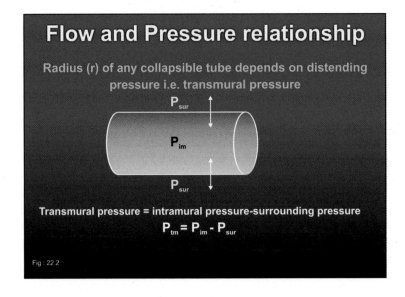

Fig: 22.2

Heart–Lung Interaction During Mechanical Ventilation

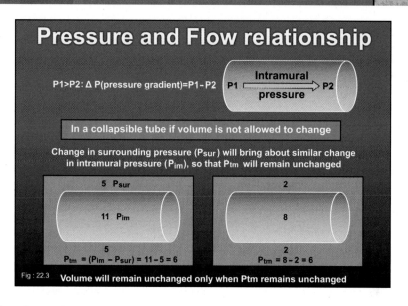

Fig : 22.3 Volume will remain unchanged only when Ptm remains unchanged

When the volume of a collapsible tube is kept constant, then any change in surrounding pressure (P_{sur}) will cause similar change in the intramural pressure (P_{im}) so that the transmural pressure (P_{tm}) which is the difference between intramural pressure and surrounding pressure ($P_{tm}=P_{im}-P_{sur}$) remains the same. Also the radius of any collapsible tube depends on distending pressure which is the transmural pressure.

Various pressures acting on the circulatory system (Fig 22.4)

Changes in the cardiac output during heart lung interaction are due to effects of various pressures like pleural pressure, alveolar pressure, right atrial pressure, pericardial pressure and abdominal pressure on circulatory system. The pleural pressure is not uniform throughout the lungs when lungs are inflating. It is more around the heart and is linearly transmitted to the pericardium which in turn acts on the heart.

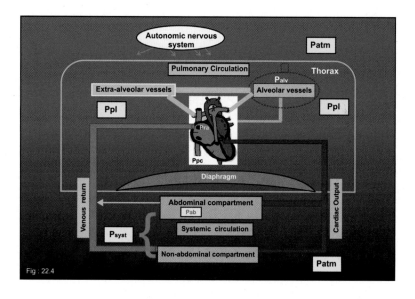

Fig : 22.4

Heart is immediately surrounded by pericardium and is affected by pericardial pressure (P_{pc}). When the heart is not distended and pericardium is not diseased, the pericardial pressure is low and an increase in the juxtacardiac pleural pressure is linearly transmitted to the pericardium which in turn acts on the heart. The pressure in right atrium is known as right atrial pressure (P_{ra}). The pulmonary circulation is composed of alveolar vessels which are affected by alveolar pressure and the extra-alveolar vessels which are affected by pleural pressure. The systemic circulation is divided into abdominal component which is affected by the abdominal pressure (P_{ab}) and the non-abdominal component which is affected by atmospheric pressure (P_{atm}). The average of the pressures throughout the systemic circulation is known as mean systemic filling pressure (MSFP or P_{syst}). The autonomic nervous system also has influence over many components.

Determinants of cardiac performance

Often, left ventricle is thought to be the main cause of ventricular dysfunction. It is also important to comprehend that the same basic principles apply to the right ventricle. The left and right sides of the heart exist in a series, and are thus interdependent. Under normal circumstances, the right heart input and left ventricle output are equal.

Cardiac output is the volume of blood pumped each minute, and is expressed by the following equation:

CO = SV × HR

CO is cardiac output expressed in l/min (normal ~5 l/min)

SV is stroke volume per beat.

It is determined by three factors: preload, afterload, and contractility (Fig 22.5). The preload is the volume of blood that is available to the ventricle to pump. The contractility is the force that the cardiac muscle can generate at the given length, and afterload is the arterial pressure against which the heart will contract. These factors determine the volume of blood pumped with each heart beat.

HR is the number of beats per minute. It is directly proportional to cardiac output. Adult HR is normally around 80-100 beats per minute (bpm). Heart rate is an intrinsic factor of the sino-atrial (SA) (pacemaker) node in the heart and it is affected by autonomic, humoral, and local factors.

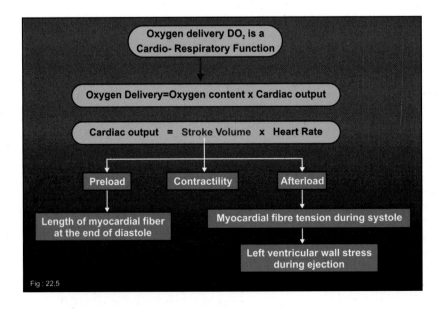

Fig : 22.5

Frank–Starling law (Fig 22.6)

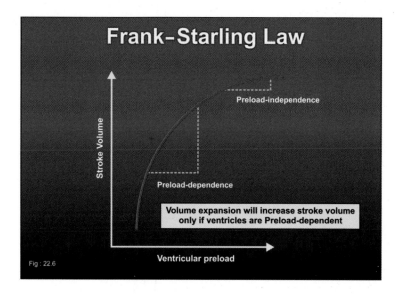

Fig : 22.6

The Frank–Starling law describes the relationship between myocardial muscle fiber length (preload) and the force of contraction (ultimately stroke volume). As per the above law, the greater the initial stretch of the muscle fiber in diastole (or more the end diastolic volume) in the ventricle, the stronger the subsequent contraction will be in systole increasing the stroke volume. But, this phenomenon will occur until a physiological limit has been reached after which the force of contraction will begin to decline, in spite of the increase in amount of fiber stretch. The heart will fail if the volume that comes in is not pumped out.

Heart-lung interactions

Major determinants of cardiovascular response to ventilation are listed below (Fig 22.7):

1. Change in intrathoracic pressures (ITP) leads to change in the right ventricular preload (venous return) and left ventricular afterload.

2. Change in the lung volume affects PVR, produce mechanical compressive effects on heart, and result in humoral effects and changes in autonomic tone.

3. Ventricular interdependence-The right heart preload is the left heart output (series effect). RV and LV share common septum and are surrounded by circumferential fibers (i.e. they are mechanically coupled). Pericardium covers both ventricles hence, affects the expansion of both ventricles (parallel effect).

The purpose of ventilation is to place a volume (tidal volume) in the alveoli. When a volume is placed in a cul-de-sac (alveoli), the pressure (ITP) is increased. For volume to move from mouth to alveoli a pressure gradient has to be established between the two regions. Lung cannot expand by itself. It can only move passively in response to external pressure. The pressure gradient is created by negative pleural pressure in spontaneous ventilation and in positive pressure ventilation increasing airway pressure pushes the air into alveoli. Therefore the changes in intrathoracic pressure (ITP) and hemodynamic effects are directionally opposite and also the energy needed to create these changes. The effects of ventilation on heart are due to lung volume and resulting pressure changes. These are discussed in detail in the following text.

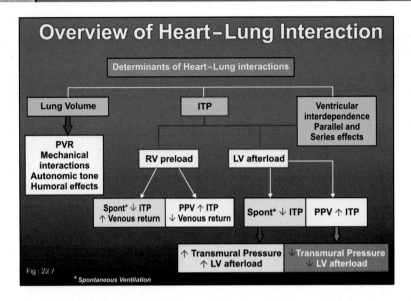

Fig: 22.7
*Spontaneous Ventilation

Cardiovascular effects due to changes in the intrathoracic pressure

a. Effects of ITP on venous return and right heart function (Figs 22.8 and 22.9)

To understand the effects of ITP, the circulatory system can be divided into three compartments thorax, abdomen and periphery. Three important points have to be remembered to understand the effects of ITP on right heart.

1. Right atrial pressure (P_{ra}) changes during inspiration. (P_{ra}) decreases during spontaneous respiration and increases during positive pressure ventilation.

2. Intra-abdominal pressure increases with inspiratory diaphragmatic descent.

3. Peripheral venous pressure is related to atmospheric pressure and not affected by respiratory cycle.

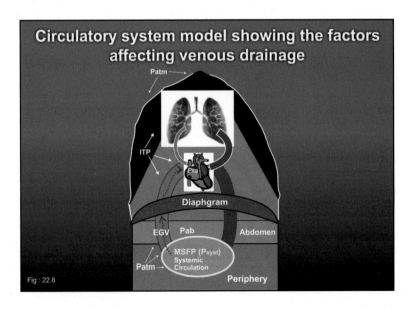

Fig: 22.8

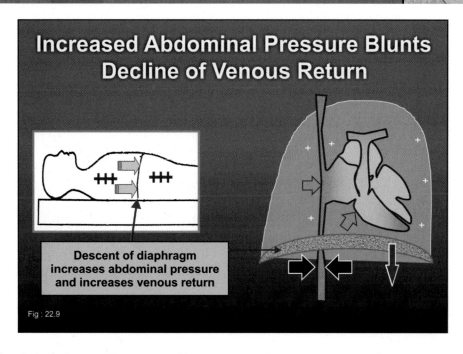

Fig : 22.9

Flow from the heart to the reservoir (the venous system or capacitance vessels) requires cardiac contraction, but venous return occurs passively, driven by the pressure gradient between the extrathoracic great veins (EGV) and right atrium. The components of pressure gradient are mean systemic filling pressure (MSFP) which acts as driving pressure and right atrial pressure (P_{ra}) which acts as back pressure. This is normally around 5 mm Hg.

Patients with acute congestive heart failure might actually benefit from PPV (with intubation or NPPV) because increased ITP decreases venous return, thereby decreasing RV end diastolic volume and improving LV diastolic compliance through ventricular interdependence. Increased ITP also reduces LV afterload. At same time ventilator support offloads respiratory muscles and decreases the O_2 requirement which decreases burden on failing heart. PEEP also improves oxygenation.

b. Effect of changes in intrathoracic pressure on the left ventricle

- **Left ventricular afterload**
- **Intrathoracic aortic transmural pressure**

Left ventricular afterload

Ventricular afterload is defined as the force opposing ejection. LV afterload is a measure of maximal systolic wall tension, which according to Laplace equation, is as follows:

Myocardial systolic wall tension (i.e. LV afterload) $\propto$ Transmural LV pressure × Radius of curvature of LV. Clinically this can be understood by analyzing the following facts:

- LV transmural pressure = Intraventricular pressure – Pleural pressure
- Radius of curvature = LV end diastolic volume

It is obvious that if pleural pressure is negative then the ventricle has to work against increased load. If PEEP (PPV) is applied then the pleural pressure becomes positive and aids ventricular contraction. This is illustrated in Fig 22.10 (The values used in the example are just for illustration purpose).

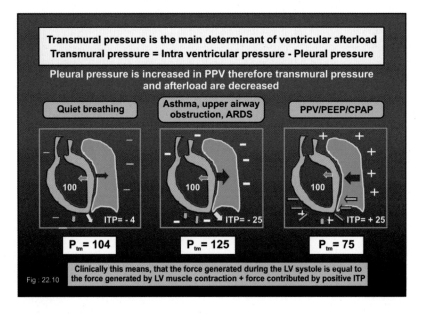

Fig: 22.10

Intrathoracic aortic transmural pressure

The afterload depends on the level of transmural pressure, in the course of systole, within the aortic root (LV afterload). In thorax, great vessels and the heart are exposed to extramural pressure (i.e. ITP) which is not atmospheric pressure, hence the transmural pressure instead of intraluminal pressure should be considered. The transmural pressure (P_{tm}) of the aorta is the difference between the pressure within the aorta and pleural pressure (P_{pl}).

During spontaneous or negative pressure inspiration, there is decrease in both P_{pl} and intravascular aortic pressure, but the decrease in pleural pressure is comparatively greater than the decrease in aortic pressure. Consequently, P_{tm} actually increases, resulting in an increased LV afterload and a drop in LV stroke volume and vice versa in positive pressure ventilation. In positive pressure ventilation the aortic valve (AV) transmural pressure is decreased. The LV transmural pressure required to open AV is reduced. This results in decreased tension generated in ventricular muscle fibers. The net effect of all this is,

- Decreased afterload
- Increased stroke volume
- Decreased work of pumping

This is illustrated in Fig 22.11.

Clinical implication: In patients with acute asthma, airway obstruction etc. the pleural pressure during inspiration is already considerably negative and LV afterload is increased. Any further negative swing in the intrathoracic pressure will acutely increase LV afterload further and result in cardiac failure and pulmonary edema. Patients with limited cardiac reserve are more prone to failure.

The application of positive pressure ventilation increases ITP and thus reduces transmural pressure of the LV besides decreasing LVEDV by direct compression and reduced venous return. This results in reduced afterload and myocardial O_2 consumption. In addition, the work of breathing is reduced, and O_2 demand by respiratory muscles is decreased resulting in increased O_2 delivery to other vital organs. Therefore, increased ITP (PEEP/CPAP) offloads an ischemic and failing left ventricle.

Heart–Lung Interaction During Mechanical Ventilation

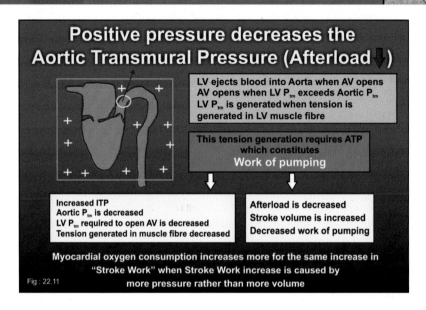

Fig: 22.11

Raised ITP can lessen or overcome "negative inspiratory swings" in intrathoracic pressure, and by decreasing the afterload, potentially restore the hemodynamics to a more favorable position on the Starling curve.

This is also important in patients with LV systolic dysfunction especially during weaning from positive pressure ventilation (PPV) which may induce dramatic changes in ITP swings, from positive to negative (cardiac stress test). This acutely increases afterload and precipitates myocardial ischemia and cardiac failure. Patients with poor cardiac function require gradual weaning and inotrope support e.g. dobutamine infusion during weaning may be required for some time after extubation and then gradually weaned and stopped.

Cardiovascular effects due to changes in lung volume

Effect of changes in lung volume on right ventricular afterload

The right ventricle output is the LV stroke volume. The RV stroke work is ≈25% of that of LV. This is because of the low resistance of the pulmonary vasculature. Therefore the right ventricle is thin walled and compliant. Right ventricular (RV) afterload is nothing but RV systolic wall tension. RV systolic wall tension depends on both systolic right ventricular pressure and end diastolic volume. The right ventricular systolic pressure is in fact equal to the difference between pulmonary artery pressure and ITP (also known as transmural pressure).

RV afterload is mainly determined by pulmonary vascular resistance (PVR). Any increase in PVR increases RV afterload, obstructing RV ejection, reducing RV stroke volume, causing RV dilation, ischemia and infarction and passively causing venous return to decrease. If this is not rapidly addressed, then acute corpulmonale develops.

Elevated ITP related PVR increase is more in following conditions:

1. Pre-existing lung disease
2. Pulmonary hypertension
3. Right heart failure (Corpulmonale)
4. Use of large tidal volumes and
5. Auto PEEP

Mechanical ventilation can affect PVR by changing pulmonary vasomotor tone (hypoxic pulmonary vasoconstriction) or by changing the pulmonary vasculature cross-sectional area. These are discussed in detail below:

Hypoxic pulmonary vasoconstriction (HPV)

Whenever there is hypoxia, systemic vessels dilate, but pulmonary vessels constrict especially once alveolar PO_2 (PAO_2) decreases below 60 mm Hg, or acidemia develops increasing pulmonary vasomotor tone. This is known as hypoxic pulmonary vasoconstriction which reduces the V/Q mismatches caused by local alveolar hypoventilation. When lung volumes are low, the terminal bronchioles collapse and whatever oxygen that is left in the trapped gas is absorbed which leads to alveolar collapse. This is mainly responsible for increased PVR in patients with acute hypoxemic respiratory failure. Therefore instituting mechanical ventilation (CPAP/ NPPV) in such patients may decrease vasomotor tone. This is due to improving PAO_2, recruiting collapsed alveoli, reversing respiratory acidosis and reducing sympathetic output (by decreasing work of breathing).

Volume-dependent changes in pulmonary vascular resistance

The pulmonary circulation is comprised of two components: the alveolar and extra-alveolar vessels. The PVR is determined by the balance in the vascular tone of these components. As shown in Fig 22.12, PVR can be increased at both extremes of lung volume.

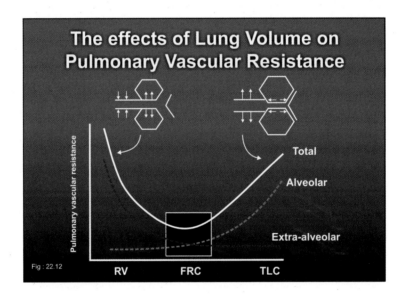

Fig : 22.12

High lung volumes:

PEEP increases PVR if it causes overdistension of the lungs. Alveolar vessels which are affected by alveolar pressure become compressed by alveolar distension when the lung is inflated above FRC. Therefore this increases the PVR.

Low lung volumes:

When the lung volume decreases from FRC towards residual volume, two things can happen:

1. The tortuousity of extra-alveolar vessels is increased and they collapse.
2. Terminal airway collapses at low lung volume which results in HPV. Both these events cause increase in PVR.

On the other hand, as the lung is inflated from residual volume towards FRC there is decrease in vascular resistance of extra-alveolar vessels because of the increase in diameter due to tenting effect of the expanded alveoli on the perivascular sheath. Therefore, PVR is least at FRC and is increased when lung volume increases or decreases from FRC (Figs 22.13 and 22.14).

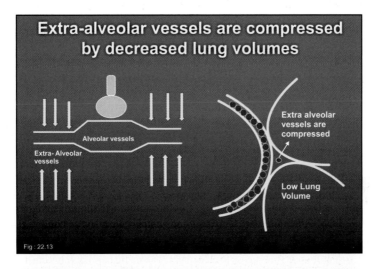

Fig: 22.13

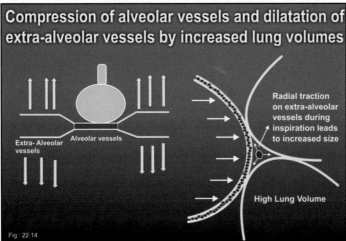

Fig: 22.14

Clinical implication: In patients with normal cardio-respiratory function minimal changes are seen in RV afterload with a PEEP of less than 10 cm H_2O. This may not be the case in patients who have hyperinflated lungs due to asthma or obstructive pulmonary disease, where PPV increases RV afterload and can cause RV failure. This can be prevented by using small tidal volume and avoiding over distension of lungs.

Mechanical compression of the heart due to increased lung volumes

As lung volume increases, the lungs press on against the heart, the chest wall, and diaphragm. Whereas, the chest wall can expand outwards and diaphragm can descend downwards, the heart and pericardium, and the coronary arteries, become compressed by the lungs in the cardiac fossa.

Therefore, at extreme lung volume, or in patients with hyperinflated lungs, ventricular filling can be reduced to produce the clinical picture of cardiac tamponade. Low tidal volume ventilation will avoid this complication.

Autonomic Tone

The lung is abundantly innervated with autonomic nerves that sense lung volume and vascular pressure changes causing bronchomotor and vasomotor shifts and alterations in cardiac inotropy and chronotropy. Small increase in lung volume (<10 ml/kg) increase heart rate by vagal withdrawal and reverse happens during expiration. This phenomenon is referred to as respiratory sinus arrhythmia. It indicates the existence of a normal autonomic state and a responsive cardiovascular system. This arrhythmia is absent in dysautonomic states, such as diabetes mellitus. Lung inflation to larger tidal volumes (>15 ml/kg) results in bradycardia, vasodilatation and decreased cardiac contractility due to sympathetic withdrawal and vagal overstimulation. This problem may lead to deleterious consequences in patient who are on beta blockers, and in patients requiring high dose of sedatives.

Humoral effects

Mechanical ventilation and PEEP cause increase in ITP which decreases intrathoracic blood volume and offloads the right atrium. This reduces plasma levels of atrial natriuretic peptide (ANP, which is released from secretory granules in the atrial myocytes in response to stretch causes natriuresis and diuresis) and causes antidiuresis. In addition to this, there is rise in the levels of vasopressin, renin, aldosterone, and angiotensin II. Consequently there is salt and water retention.

Clinical implication: It lies in the fact that when such patients are weaned from mechanical ventilation and are extubated, this excess fluid can get reabsorbed and precipitate acute LV failure, pulmonary edema and worsen gas exchange leading to extubation failure. Therefore, fluids should be restricted before weaning trials and sometimes forced diuresis and gradual reduction in the level of ventilatory support may be required if obvious fluid overload is present.

Ventricular interdependence and left ventricular diastolic function

The change in right ventricle (RV output, contraction or end diastolic volume) influences the output from left ventricle (LV). This process is known as ventricular interdependence.

They can be series or parallel effects which are described in Fig 22.15.

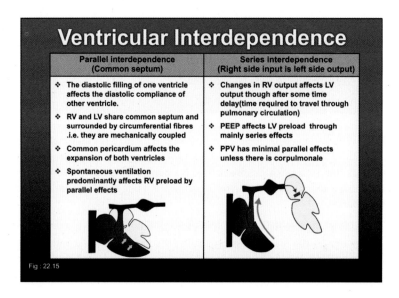

Fig : 22.15

Pulsus paradoxus, which is defined as more than 10 mm Hg inspiratory decrease in systolic arterial pressure is due to ventricular interdependence.

Spontaneous breathing patient

Spontaneous inspiratory efforts lead to reduced right atrial pressure and increased venous return and RV end-diastolic volume. This may affect left ventricle in two ways:

- Increase in RV end-diastolic volume causes intraventricular septal shift into the LV resulting in decreased LV diastolic compliance. This is more pronounced in patients with cardio-respiratory diseases.
- If pericardium is diseased and cannot expand or cardiac fossal volume expansion is restricted then RV dilation increases pericardial pressure which is transferred to left atrium and obstructs pulmonary venous return.

Consequently, left ventricular preload is decreased and cardiac output is decreased (parallel interdependence). This effect is seen immediately.

Patient on PPV

RV volume increase and associated decrease in left ventricular diastolic compliance is not significant during positive pressure ventilation (with normal tidal volume). When there is excessive hyperinflation, such as associated with PEEP levels more than 20 cm H_2O, or when moderate increases of ITP and lung volume are added upon on either an obstructed pulmonary circulation or a failing RV, then RV can dilate due to increase in right ventricular afterload and decrease left ventricular diastolic compliance.

However, increases in ITP during positive pressure ventilation may decrease venous return and right ventricular filling which in turn decreases left ventricular preload and cardiac output. But this effect may not be noticed immediately because right ventricular output has to travel through pulmonary circulation which is approximately 2 seconds, before it reaches left ventricle and affects left ventricular output (series interdependence). So, inspiratory decrease in right ventricular filling causes decreased left ventricular stroke volume only a few heart beats later (usually in the expiratory period). This is illustrated in Fig 22.16

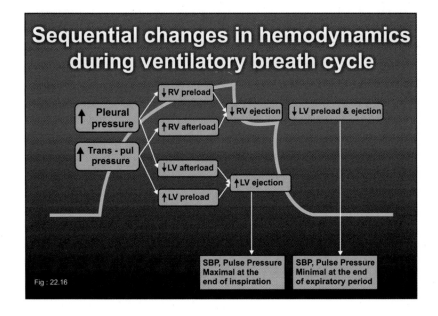

Fig : 22.16

Heart–lung interactions can be used in hemodynamic monitoring to assess fluid responsiveness

Routine indicators of preload like measurements of right atrial pressure, left atrial pressure and RVEDV do not accurately estimate preload responsiveness since preload is not preload responsiveness. In a passive patient on PPV with low tidal volume (<10 ml/kg), the systolic pressure and arterial pulse pressure is determined by vasomotor tone and stroke volume. Since there is no beat to beat variation in vasomotor tone, any change in systolic arterial pressure (ΔSP) and pulse pressure (ΔPP) with positive pressure inspiration is an outcome of change in stroke volume. Positive pressure inspiration reduces venous return, which is further exaggerated in hypovolemic patients. This causes decreased stroke volume resulting decrease in pulse pressure and systolic pressure. The larger the degree of change in systolic and pulse pressure, the larger will be the increase in stroke volume in response to fluid challenge. This has been validated in a study done on septic shock patients.

Pulse pressure variation is calculated as the ratio of the difference between maximum and minimum arterial pulse pressures to the mean of those two pulse pressures (Fig 22.17). If the pulse pressure variation was greater than the threshold value of 15%, then cardiac output will increase, and if it is less than 15%, then cardiac output will not increase in response to fluid loading. This can be used at bed side to assess preload responsiveness.

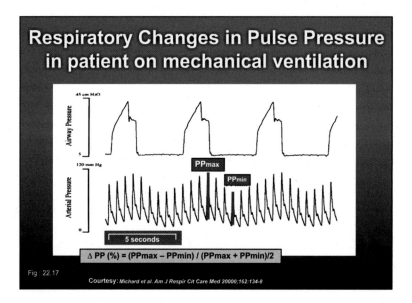

Fig: 22.17 Courtesy: Michard et al. Am J Respir Crit Care Med 20000;162:134-8

Summary and conclusion

Positive pressure ventilation has considerable effects on the hemodynamics of the patient some of which can be beneficial and some deleterious depending on cardiopulmonary and volume status of the patient. The adverse effects predominate if the patient has acute or chronic pulmonary disease, hypovolemia and RV dysfunction. On the other hand PPV can improve cardiac function in patients with impaired LV function. Therefore, in order to minimize the adverse effects and enhance the beneficial effects, appropriate mode of ventilation, optimal ventilatory settings, inotrope support, fluid restriction, fluid resuscitation while initiating PPV etc. are required. These interventions may vary in different patients depending on preexisting pulmonary and cardiac problems. Cardio–respiratory interaction can affect other organ systems.

Heart–Lung Interaction During Mechanical Ventilation

It is not unusual for critically ill patients to have pre existing dysfunction of multiple organ systems. It is important for critical care physician to understand the mechanical ventilation induced effects on multiple organ systems in order to anticipate and minimize the problems by appropriate ventilatory settings and supportive care. These are summarized in Fig 22.18 below:

Summary of the effects of PPV and PEEP on cardiac output

Impairs cardiac function (decreased CO)	Improves cardiac function (increased CO)

• Decreases RV function
  – Decreases venous return
  – Increases PVR
• Decreases LV function
  – Decreases preload
  – Ventricular interdependence
  – Mechanical compression
	• Increases PaO_2 and myocardial DO_2
	• Decreases VO_2 and myocardial demand
	• Decreases preload
	  – Decreases venous return
	• Decreases RV afterload
	  – Decreases PVR
	• Decreases LV afterload

Effect of PPV on haemodynamics depends on cardiorespiratory status	
Haemodynamics adversely affected	Haemodynamics favourably affected
In hypovolaemic patients	LV dysfunction(with hypervolemia)
RV dysfunction	Asthma, obstructive sleep apnea, upper airway obstruction etc

Fig : 22.18

References

1. Cardiovascular Effects of Mechanical Ventilation. G. J. DUKE. Critical Care and Resuscitation 1999: 1: 388-399
2. Clinical use of respiratory changes in arterial pulse pressure to monitor the hemodynamic effects of PEEP. Michard F, Chemla D, Richard C et al. Am J Respir Crit Care Med 1999: 159:935–939.
3. Cardiovascular effects of mechanical ventilation. Lara Shekerdemian, Desmond Bohn. Arch Dis Child 1999: 80:475–480.
4. Hemodynamic Consequences of Heart-Lung Interactions. Jay S. Steingrub, Mark Tidswell et al. J Intensive Care Med. 2003:18:92-99.
5. Heart-lung interactions: applications in the critically ill. H.E. Fessler. Eur Respir J, 1997: 10: 226–237
6. Interactions between respiration and systemic hemodynamics. Part I: basic Intensive Care Med 2009: 35:45–54
7. Using heart–lung interactions to assess fluid responsiveness during mechanical ventilation. Frédéric Michard and Jean-Louis Teboul. Crit Care 2000, 4:282–289
8. The effects of mechanical ventilation on the cardiovascular system. Pinsky MR. Crit Care Clinics. 1990: 6:663–678

★ ★ ★

PATIENT-VENTILATOR ASYNCHRONY

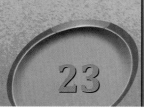

Rajesh Chawla, *MD, FCCM*
Senior Consultant Respiratory Medicine and Critical Care,
Indraprastha Apollo Hospitals, Delhi, India

During mechanical ventilation, the most effective unloading of the inspiratory muscles would occur if the ventilator cycles in synchrony with patient's own respiratory rhythm. Patient-ventilator asynchrony (PVA) can result if mechanical ventilator lacks the simultaneous responsiveness needed for interaction with the constantly changing conditions of patient. PVA is defined as mismatching between the patient's breaths (neural) and ventilator-assisted breaths and the inability of the ventilator's flow delivery to match the patient's flow demand.

Patient-ventilator asynchrony is common and usually not appreciated by treating team. 24% of mechanically ventilated patients exhibit some form of major patient-ventilator asynchrony. The most common clinical feature is agitation and respiratory distress. When it is severe, patients may appear to be fighting the ventilator.

PVA not only causes discomfort, hypoxemia and barotrauma but also prolongs duration of mechanical ventilation and hospital stay in the critically ill patients. Sedation is often used to manage asynchrony, but it is not the best answer for various types of asynchrony. Patient-ventilator synchrony is influenced by factors related to the patient and factors related to the ventilator (ventilator triggering, ventilator cycling off).

Patient Factors

It is very difficult to attain patient-ventilator synchrony during assist control mode (A/C) and synchronized intermittent mandatory ventilation (SIMV) because patients' ventilation is controlled by mechanical, chemical, behavioral, and reflex mechanisms which change with time. Respiratory center output, respiratory mechanics, various disease states, and endotracheal tube type or size all influence patient ventilator interaction.

Factors that may Increase Respiratory Drive

- Hypoxemia, hypercapnia, acidosis states
- Increased ventilatory demand (pain, fever, shivering, overfeeding, metabolic acidosis, sepsis, burns, trauma, hyperthyroidism)
- Underlying lung disease
- Increased workload
- Pain, increased psychogenic stimuli or agitation
- Medications (theophylline, doxapram, acetazolamide

Fig 23.1

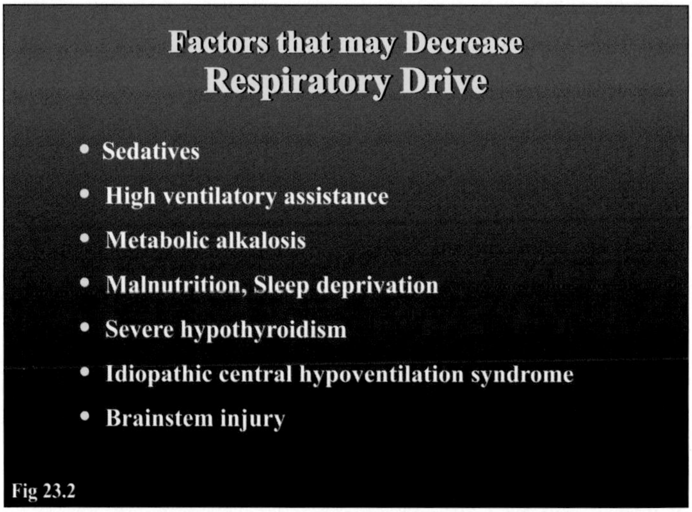

Patient-Ventilator Asynchrony

Factors that may Decrease Respiratory Drive

- Sedatives
- High ventilatory assistance
- Metabolic alkalosis
- Malnutrition, Sleep deprivation
- Severe hypothyroidism
- Idiopathic central hypoventilation syndrome
- Brainstem injury

Fig 23.2

The patient's respiratory center output can vary and it may contribute to the development of PVA. Respiratory drive can decrease or increase under various circumstances. When the respiratory drive is decreased, the ventilator is not able to respond to the reduced effort by the patient especially if the operator has not set the ventilator's sensitivity enough to detect the patient's effort. Respiratory drive can also be reduced by sedatives, opioids, and hypnotics. All these increase the time delay between the start of the patient's inspiratory effort and ventilator triggering and this leads to PVA. Various factors that increase or decrease respiratory drives are mentioned in Figs 23.1 and 23.2.

Respiratory mechanics have an impact on the patient–ventilator synchrony(Fig 23.3). The patient may have a prolonged inspiratory time. If the patient's inspiratory time is longer than the ventilator's preset inspiratory time, the patient takes an additional breath because the need for ventilation has not been met, and it results in the double triggering.

On the other hand, if the patient's exhalation time is shortened it will lead to the development of intrinsic positive pressure at the end of expiration (PEEPi, auto-PEEP) and thereby resulting in dynamic hyperinflation. This will compel patient to breathe with high lung volumes and high elastic recoil pressures.

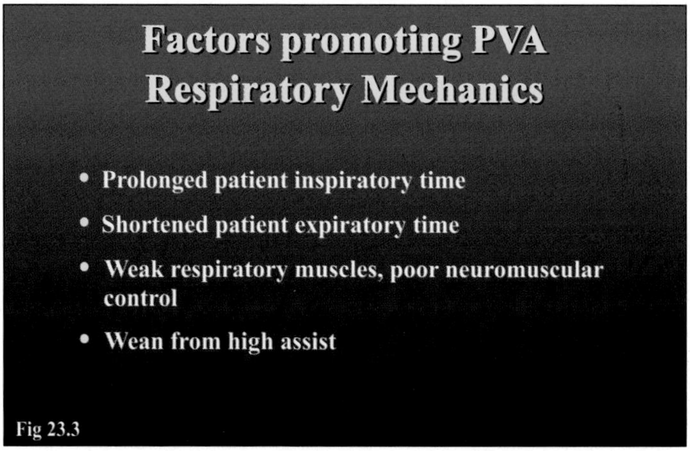

Factors promoting PVA Respiratory Mechanics

- Prolonged patient inspiratory time
- Shortened patient expiratory time
- Weak respiratory muscles, poor neuromuscular control
- Wean from high assist

Fig 23.3

Auto-PEEP will also result in increased workload for the patient's diaphragm and may promote failure-to-trigger, since the patient has to first overcome excess auto-PEEP by decreasing intrathoracic pressure through muscular effort before the ventilator triggers a breath. Factors such as prolonged ventilator assistance, immobility, poor nutrition, and neuromuscular disease can decrease muscular power.

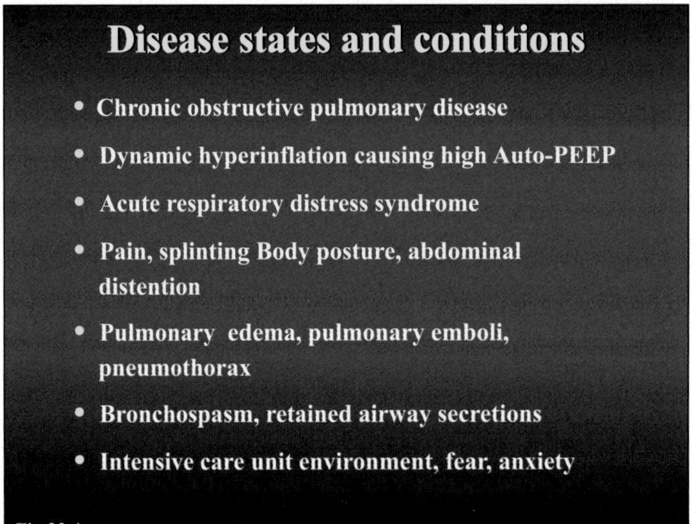

Disease states and conditions

- Chronic obstructive pulmonary disease
- Dynamic hyperinflation causing high Auto-PEEP
- Acute respiratory distress syndrome
- Pain, splinting Body posture, abdominal distention
- Pulmonary edema, pulmonary emboli, pneumothorax
- Bronchospasm, retained airway secretions
- Intensive care unit environment, fear, anxiety

Fig 23.4

Patient's underlying diseases and conditions can also predispose to PVA (Fig. 23.4). Dynamic hyperinflation may exist in patient with chronic obstructive lung disease or ARDS receiving inverse-ratio ventilation or airway pressure release ventilation. Flat diaphragm due to dynamic hyperinflation limits the patient's ability to generate enough force to overcome trigger threshold and results in ineffective trigger.

Restlessness and agitation in patients who are receiving mechanical ventilation are also increased by many factors, such as bronchospasm, pulmonary edema, pulmonary embolism, pneumothorax and secretions.

A narrow endotracheal tube increases resistance and limits flow to a patient with high flow demand. The endotracheal tube is also narrowed by secretions and debris when they get dried up. Cuff leak and disconnection from the circuit can also result in asynchrony.

Ventilator-Related Factors

Patient-ventilator synchrony requires a ventilator to be sensitive to the patient's respiratory efforts and respond to airflow demand of the patient. Two major factors contributing to PVA are ventilator triggering and cycling. Ventilator should respond to a patient's inspiratory effort immediately. The sensitivity trigger is stimulated by pressure, flow, or time. If the sensitivity level is set too low which cannot sense the patient's effort it will not only increase respiratory muscle loading but will also result in ineffective trigger.

The errors in the ventilator's pressure transducer or the ventilator's delay in sensing pressure signals or the time from onset of diaphragm contraction to the drop in airway pressure can prolong the trigger phase. All these result in phase asynchrony.

There is a lag (delay time) between the time when the ventilator senses the trigger and the time when the gas flow starts from the ventilator. When inspiration is triggered by pressure trigger, usually the delay time is 110 -120 milliseconds before the gas flow starts. If the trigger delay time is prolonged the patient may prolong inspiratory effort.

Types of Asynchrony

Four major types of PVA occur within the different phases of a patient's assisted ventilation breath. (Figs 23.5 and 23.6)

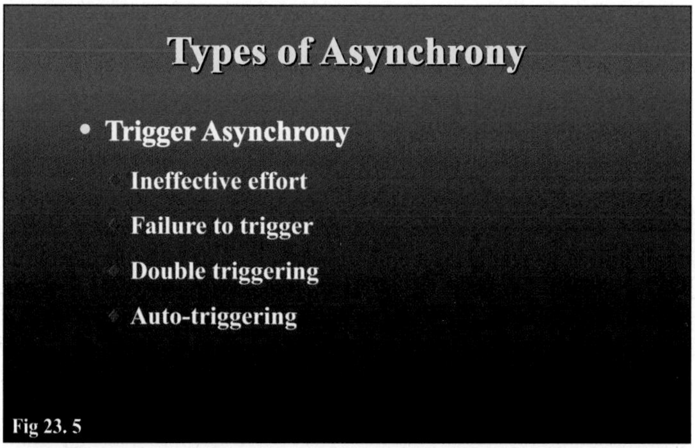

Types of Asynchrony
- Trigger Asynchrony
  - Ineffective effort
  - Failure to trigger
  - Double triggering
  - Auto-triggering

Fig 23. 5

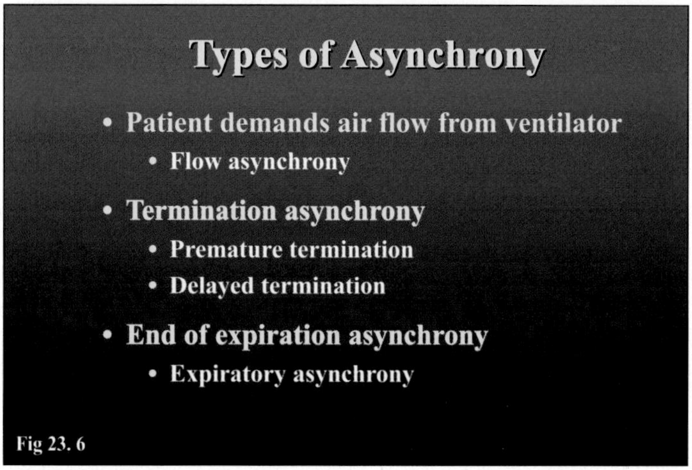

Types of Asynchrony
- Patient demands air flow from ventilator
  - Flow asynchrony
- Termination asynchrony
  - Premature termination
  - Delayed termination
- End of expiration asynchrony
  - Expiratory asynchrony

Fig 23. 6

1. TRIGGER ASYNCHRONY

The first phase of a ventilator-assisted breath is its initiation of breath (trigger phase). It is important for patient to have adequate respiratory drive and effort (patient factors) and ventilator to have adequate response to detect the signal pressure or flow and ability to reach the set pressure (ventilator factors) for patient ventilator synchrony. These factors must be functional to avoid trigger asynchrony, a common form of PVA. Trigger asynchrony can be of various types: failure to trigger, auto triggering and double triggering (Figs 23.5 and 23.6).

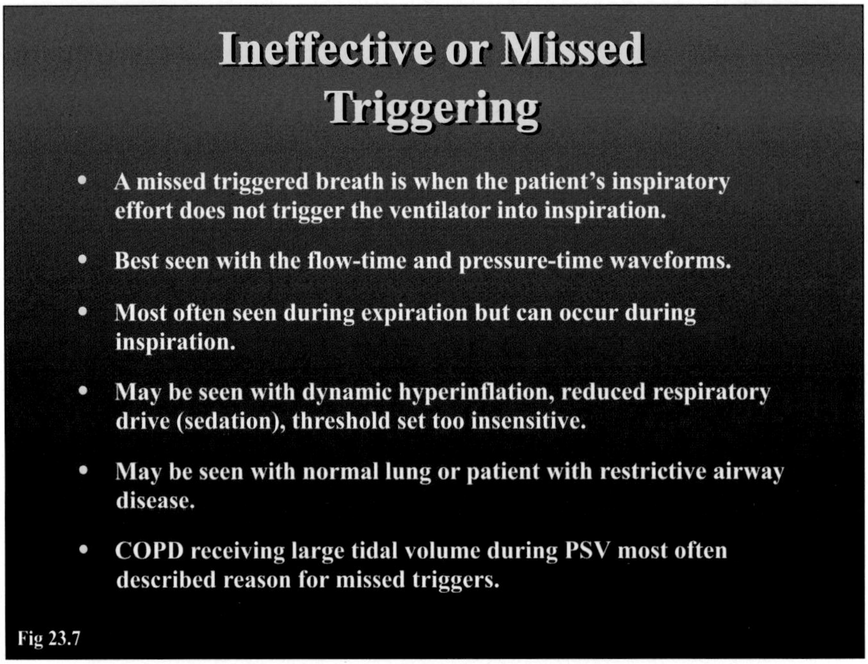

Ineffective or Missed Triggering

- A missed triggered breath is when the patient's inspiratory effort does not trigger the ventilator into inspiration.
- Best seen with the flow-time and pressure-time waveforms.
- Most often seen during expiration but can occur during inspiration.
- May be seen with dynamic hyperinflation, reduced respiratory drive (sedation), threshold set too insensitive.
- May be seen with normal lung or patient with restrictive airway disease.
- COPD receiving large tidal volume during PSV most often described reason for missed triggers.

Fig 23.7

A. Ineffective or Missed Trigger and Delayed Triggering

Ineffective trigger occurs when the ventilator does not sense the pressure or flow generated by the patient. As mentioned above mostly this condition arises as a result of a poor respiratory drive or excessive PEEPi that prevents the patient's effort from being detected by the ventilator's sensor. Dynamic hyperinflation can be caused by high ventilatory demands, increased expiratory resistance and short expiratory time. In the presence of dynamic hyperinflation end-expiratory lung volume is greater than passive FRC determined by set extrinsic PEEP (PEEPe). Under these circumstances elastic recoil pressure at end-expiration is higher than PEEPe.

The difference in elastic recoil pressure and extrinsic PEEP, called auto-PEEP or intrinsic PEEP, represents an elastic threshold load for the patient.

So, patient has to first generate pressure equivalent to auto-PEEP to be able to decrease alveolar pressure below PEEPe and trigger the ventilator in pressure or flow triggering. Part of patient muscular effort is used to counteract intrinsic PEEP. This delays the onset of effective inspiratory effort and hence the triggering. Delayed triggering can result in out of phase ventilator cycle which defeats the purpose of assisted ventilatory support.

When patient cannot decrease the pressure below PEEP either because of auto–PEEP or low muscular effort by patient it results in ineffective trigger or missed trigger (Figs 7 and 8). Ineffective triggering is defined during both A/C and PSV as an abrupt airway pressure drop (≥ 0.5 cm H_2O) with concomitant decrease in flow and not followed by an assisted cycle during the expiratory period. This commonly arises in patients, with chronic obstructive pulmonary disease when the patient cannot usually overcome the trigger threshold or when trigger levels are not adjusted appropriately .This can also occur in normal patient or in restrictive lung disease particularly when sensitivity setting is high.

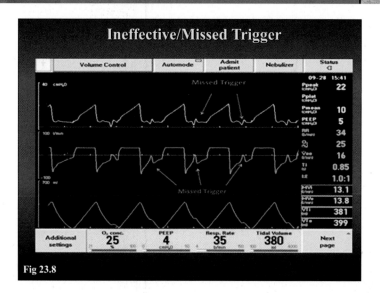

Fig 23.8

Ineffective triggering not only results in patient-ventilator asynchrony and wasted efforts, it may also have serious effects on inspiratory muscle function. Ineffective triggering usually occurs during expiration phase of the last mechanical breath, the inspiratory muscles are contracting when they would normally be relaxing as lung volume decreases. This type of muscle contraction (pilometric contraction) causes ultra-structural damage to the muscles resulting in reduced muscle strength and weaning failure.

Ventilatory parameters associated with high incidence of ineffective triggering are with poorly sensitive trigger, high tidal volume, high peak inspiratory pressure, and high level of pressure support. Triggering sensitivity can be improved by various methods as mentioned in Fig 23.9.

Newer models like neurally adjusted ventilator assist (NAVA) is also being used to overcome trigger delay which is described in the book.

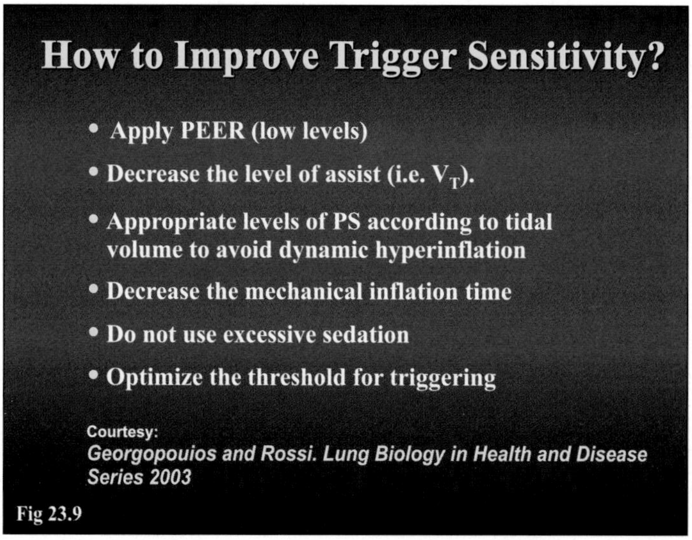

How to Improve Trigger Sensitivity?

- Apply PEER (low levels)
- Decrease the level of assist (i.e. V_T).
- Appropriate levels of PS according to tidal volume to avoid dynamic hyperinflation
- Decrease the mechanical inflation time
- Do not use excessive sedation
- Optimize the threshold for triggering

Courtesy:
Georgopouios and Rossi. Lung Biology in Health and Disease Series 2003

Fig 23.9

B. Double Triggering

Double triggering is present when there are 2 consecutive inspiratory breaths and between each breath the mean inspiratory time is less than half of what is set on the ventilator. If the mean inspiratory time is 1.0 second and the time between each breath drops to 0.5 seconds or less it is considered double triggering.

It may result in higher pressure in the second breath. This commonly occurs with VC continuous mandatory ventilation. Double triggering could result from sighs, coughing with breathing, change in clinical status, or inappropriate ventilator settings. This can also occur with pressure support ventilation with high termination flow criterion, high respiratory drive, and insufficient respiratory support such as low minute ventilation or tidal volume with a high respiratory rate (Figs 23.10 and 23.11).

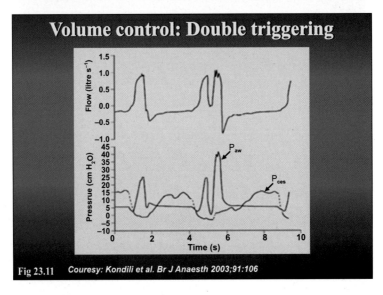

Fig 23.10

Fig 23.11 Couresy: Kondili et al. Br J Anaesth 2003;91:106

Patient-Ventilator Asynchrony

Patient's I time (neural) is different (longer) than the ventilator set I-time. The PaO_2/FiO_2 ratio in these patients is lower and peak inspiratory pressure is higher than in patients without asynchrony, suggesting that double-triggering is associated with greater severity of lung injury and probably with a greater drive to breathe as indicated by a higher respiratory rate. It is important to determine the cause of the double triggering to resolve PVA. If the cause is excessive coughing, one may just disconnect the ventilator for a short duration until the cough subsides. Adjust ventilator flow or volume settings to meet the patient's demand to overcome double triggering. Increase inspiratory time to match patient inspiratory time.

C. Auto-triggering

Auto-triggering results when inappropriate sensitivity level recognizes signals other than the patient's effort and delivers breath. This could be random noise in the circuit like water (increased resistance); air leaks (i.e. circuit leaks, cuff leaks)(Figs 23.12 and 23.13) and cardiogenic oscillations from larger heart and high filling pressures in the ventricle.

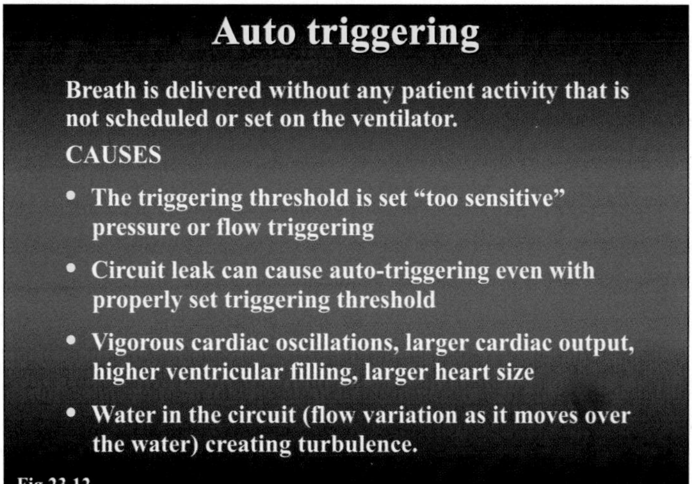

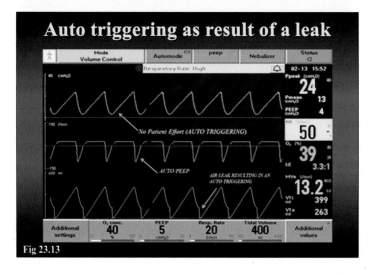

Fig 23.12

Fig 23.13

Auto-triggering is promoted by low respiratory drive, decreased respiratory rate and when dynamic hyperinflation is absent. These factors allow zero flow for some time during expiration and the system becomes vulnerable to triggering from any change in pressure without any inspiratory effort. The risk of auto-triggering also increases with greater sensitivity of the triggering system. It has been seen that decreasing the flow threshold for triggering from 2 to 1 l/min increased the frequency of auto triggering from 15% to 22% (Figs 23.12 and 23.14).

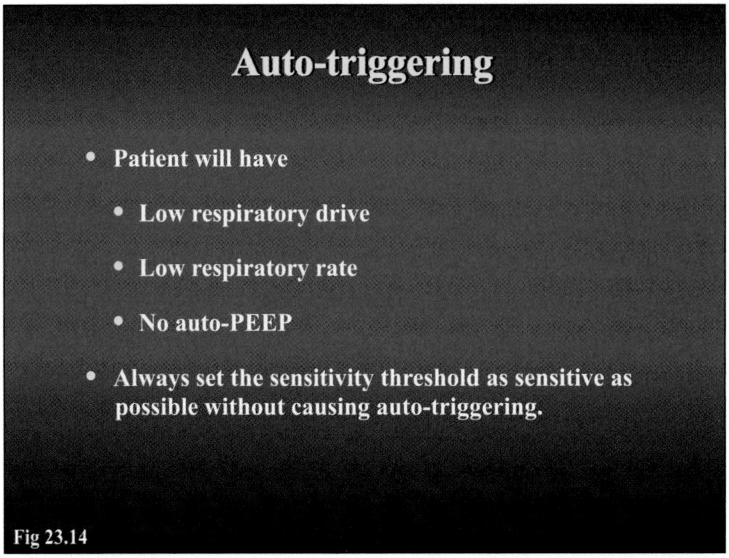

Auto-triggering

- Patient will have
  - Low respiratory drive
  - Low respiratory rate
  - No auto-PEEP
- Always set the sensitivity threshold as sensitive as possible without causing auto-triggering.

Fig 23.14

Auto-triggering can greatly affect patient management; reduce $PaCO_2$ which will decrease patient effort. Auto-triggering can have many serious implications as it can delay declaration of brain dead patient, if not recognized and corrected. It is important to find out the cause of auto triggering and take the appropriate action.

2. FLOW ASYNCHRONY

The second phase of inspiration is the delivery of air flow. Flow asynchrony can occur if the flow rate on the ventilator is set too low and the patient's inspiratory demand is high, it will result in flow asynchrony. Auto-PEEP is created as a consequence of flow asynchrony.

Auto-PEEP is identified on the flow time graphic (refer Fig 11.24). Peak inspiratory pressure will also increase as a consequence of this. Flow asynchrony can occur in both volume- or pressure-cycled ventilation.

In volume ventilation the flow pattern is fixed and flow asynchrony can be identified by comparing the shapes of the pressure-time waveforms during complete passive breathing and patient-triggered breathing. A dished out "deflection" appearance of the pressure wave graphics is suggestive of flow asynchrony (refer Figs 11.31 and 23.16).

A flow-volume loop demonstrates a "notch" on the inspiratory limb of the curve (refer Fig 11.32). This can be corrected by increasing flow rate with rise time (shorter I time) or changing to pressure targeted ventilation or a mode with a variable-flow mode.

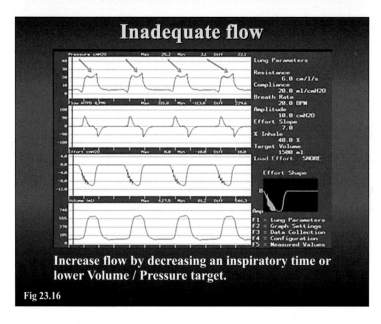

Fig 23.15

Fig 23.16

3. TERMINATION ASYNCHRONY

Cycling from inspiration to expiration on the ventilator is based on volume, pressure, flow, or times which are set by the clinician. These settings to obtain ideal synchrony between the end of inspiration and beginning of expiration are not ideal, so termination of ventilator flow occurs either before or after the patient stops inspiratory effort.

Delayed termination- if the mechanical breath is terminated late after the patient's muscular inspiration is complete, the expiratory time for exhalation is shortened and air trapping will occur. Auto-PEEP will be generated which will result in ineffective trigger as patient may not be able to reach the trigger threshold.

On the contrary, if expiratory valve opens prematurely it will result double triggering as patient's inspiratory effort is still continuing.

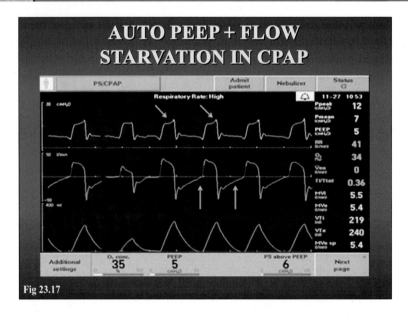

Fig 23.17

Premature termination of ventilator flow will result in excessive inspiratory muscle work during the Expiratory Phase (Fig 23.18) and will overestimate respiratory rate.

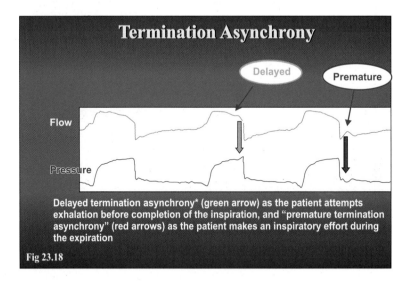

Fig 23.18

4. EXPIRATORY ASYNCHRONY

Expiratory asynchrony will occur if the end of patient expiration does not match with the ventilator end of expiration. As a result, the expiration may be shortened or prolonged. If expiration is shortened it will result in air trapping and ineffective triggering.

Prolonged expiration does not usually cause difficulties for the patient, unless the patient initiates a breath before the completion of the expiration on the ventilator. Hypoventilaion can result from prolonged expiration.

Clinical Intervention

PVA can be recognized on the ventilator with little experience by noting changes in the volume, pressure, and flow waveforms. Although PVA can be detected through waveform analysis, majority of clinicians either don't understand or don't use this information to fine tune ventilation at the bed side.

Instead of using validated pressure/flow waveforms, clinicians often use markers of physiological instability and agitation as well as patient's behaviors to identify PVA. Any patient on ventilator experiencing agitation and distress may be suffering from PVA. Forceful expiration, nasal flaring, use of accessory muscles, intercostal retractions, paradoxical thoraco-abdominal breathing, and use of accessory muscles in the neck may be suggestive of PVA (Fig 23.19).

Physical signs like tachycardia, tachypnea, agitation, coughing, or grimacing, as well as frequent ventilator pressure alarms have often been used by clinicians to suspect PVA (Fig 23.20). Interestingly these have not been validated as reliable marker of PVA.

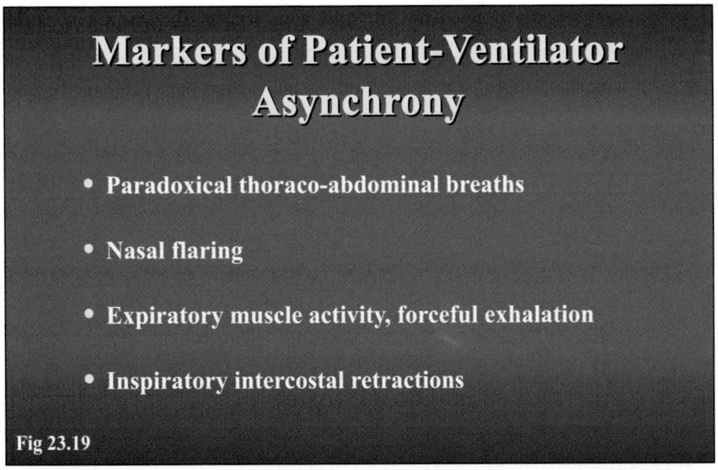

Markers of Patient-Ventilator Asynchrony

- Paradoxical thoraco-abdominal breaths
- Nasal flaring
- Expiratory muscle activity, forceful exhalation
- Inspiratory intercostal retractions

Fig 23.19

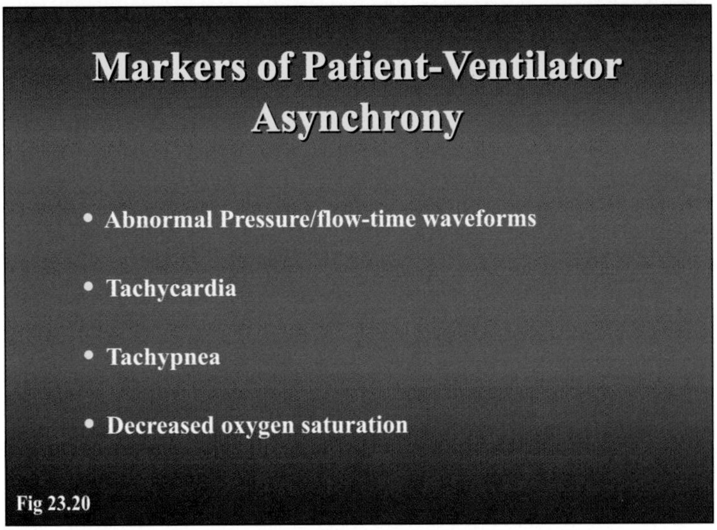

Markers of Patient-Ventilator Asynchrony

- Abnormal Pressure/flow-time waveforms
- Tachycardia
- Tachypnea
- Decreased oxygen saturation

Fig 23.20

When a patient has signs of respiratory distress, examining the ventilator's graphic display will confirm whether patient has patient-ventilator asynchrony. The pressure-time curves of the stable patient are positive and similar. Flow-time curves in the stable patient appear smooth and similar.

Asynchrony is evident when abnormalities in either the pressure and/or flow curves are seen. Typically, these curves will vary significantly and it is extremely important to correct PVA to prevent prolongation of ventilation. Early detection of optimal patient-ventilator synchrony by assessing the patient and ventilator graphics is essential. After making proper adjustments in the ventilator, if needed, sedation can be given. It is important to correct PVA to prevent prolonged time on mechanical ventilation and potential weaning failure.

References:

1. E. Kondili, G. Prinianakis and D. Georgopoulos. Patient-ventilator interaction. Br J Anaesth 2003; 91: 106–19

2. Karen Bosma, Gabriela Ferreyra, Cristina Ambrogio, Daniela Pasero, et al. Patient-ventilator interaction and sleep in mechanically ventilated patients: Pressure support versus proportional assist ventilation. Crit Care Med 2007; 35:1048–1054

3. Karen G. Mellott, Mary Jo Grap, Cindy L. Munro, Curtis N. Sessler and Paul A. Wetzel. Patient-Ventilator Dyssynchrony: Clinical Significance and Implications for Practice. Crit Care Nurse 2009, 29:41-55.

4. Marjolein de, Sammy Pedram et al. Observational Study of Patient-Ventilator Asynchrony and Relationship to Sedation Level. J Crit Care 2009 March; 24(1): 74–80

5. Paolo Navalesi: On the imperfect synchrony between patient and ventilator. Critical Care 2011: 15:181

24. NEURALLY ADJUSTED VENTILATORY ASSIST (NAVA)

PS JAGANATHAN
Manager Clinical Application - Critical care
MAQUET Medical India (P) Ltd.

NAVA is a new exciting tool that has been recently introduced in clinical practice. The diaphragm is the principal respiratory muscle. The electrical activity generated by the diaphragm, as captured by the EAdi signal (as an expression of the neuronal activity of the respiratory center) is used to trigger the respiratory cycle and to deliver proportional assist in harmony with the patient's neural drive on a breath-to-breath basis. NAVA works as if, the ventilator is "connected" to the patient's own respiratory center.

There are two major differences between NAVA and conventional modes of ventilation. The first, rather than using pressure or flow triggering (where the ventilator detects a pressure or flow change in the circuit from patient effort), NAVA uses the neural signal of diaphragmatic electrical activity (EAdi) to initiate the mechanical offloading of respiratory muscles, referred to as neural triggering. The second difference is that, once initiated, a breath is assisted with pressure support in proportion to the amplitude of the EAdi signal. The EAdi signal is sampled every 16 milliseconds; such rapid sampling enables the ventilator to titrate support throughout the course of every breath as well as between breaths.

NAVA concept

Ideally, an assisted effort should be communicated to the ventilator as soon as neural signal from the central nervous system is initiated. However, technology has not developed to this level, yet! Currently, patient triggering goes through a series of pathways. Central nervous system initiates a signal and transmits it via phrenic nerve to the diaphragm promoting diaphragmatic excitation which in turn, contracts the diaphragm. The magnitude of diaphragmatic contraction is regulated by the breath demand determined by the metabolic requirements (Fig 24.1).

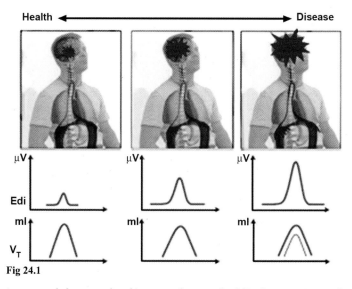

Fig 24.1

Fig 24.1: Showing normal, decreased and increased strength of diaphragmatic signal

In spontaneous breathing, contraction of the diaphragm decreases intrapleural pressure which causes intrapulmonary pressure to decrease and gas flows from atmosphere to the lungs. The same sequence provides a pressure drop in the circuit or flow removal from the circuit which triggers ventilator breath. This process of triggering takes up to 100 milliseconds before the ventilator delivers a breath. NAVA has shortened the pathway by capturing the diaphragmatic electrical signal via a special catheter and sent to the ventilator to cause inspiration (Fig 24.2).

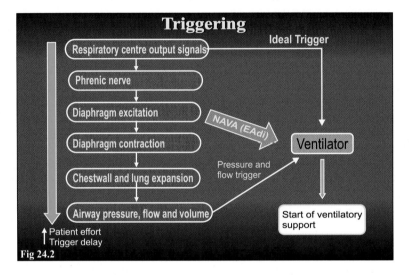

Fig 24.2

Fig 24.2: Neuro-ventilator coupling

The signal that excites the diaphragm is proportional to the integrated output of the respiratory center and thus controls the depth and cycling of the breath. The excitation of the diaphragm is independent of pneumatic influence and insensitive to the above problems associated with pneumatic triggering technologies.

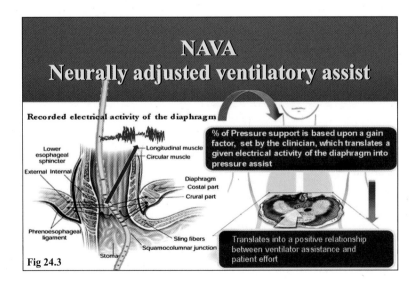

Fig 24.3

Neurally Adjusted Ventilatory Assist (NAVA)

By following diaphragm excitation and adjusting the support level in synchrony with the rise and fall of the electrical discharge, the ventilator and the diaphragm work with the same signal input. In effect, this allows the ventilator to function as an extra muscle, unloading extra respiratory work induced by the disease process. Electric trigger of NAVA is not affected by leaks and intrinsic PEEP.

Measurement of Diaphragmatic Electrical Signal

The EAdi signal is the sum of the electrical activity of the diaphragm, is expressed in microvolts (µV). The EAdi signal is measured trans esophageally by means of an EAdi catheter (doubles as a Naso-Gastric tube or Rice Tube), which has 8 bipolar microelectrodes mounted on the tip of a gastric tube.

It is positioned near the crural diaphragm, where the EAdi signal can be measured. For NAVA to work properly EAdi catheter should be properly placed to obtain an accurate EAdi signal.

EAdi signal capture can be affected in, major anatomical defect (diaphragmatic hernia); central apnea without respiratory drive (sedation, brain damage); or in the absence of electrical diaphragmatic activity (phrenic nerve damage, muscle relaxants).

NAVA catheter is not approved for MRI environments. If EAdi is not captured or absent, ventilator goes to backup pressure control or support mode.

The electrical discharge of the diaphragm is captured by an Edi Catheter fitted with an electrode array. The Edi catheter is positioned in the esophagus (Fig 24.4).

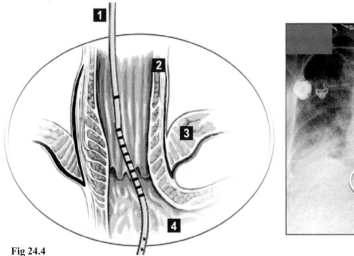
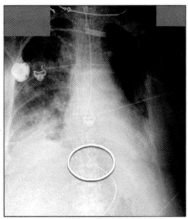

Fig 24.4

1. Edi catheter
2. Esophageal wall
3. Diaphragm
4. Stomach

Since NAVA uses the Edi to control the ventilator, it is important to understand what the signal represents.

Edi CATHETER

The Edi catheter is a single-use gastric feeding tube with an electrode array of ten electrodes. One electrode is a reference electrode and nine are measuring electrodes. The electrodes are made of stainless steel.

The table below provides guidelines for choosing the right Edi catheter for different patients.

Edi Catheter size	Inter electrode Distance, IED	Patient weight	Patient height
16 Fr 125 cm	16 mm		> 140 cm
12 Fr 125 cm	12 mm		75 – 160 cm
8 Fr 125 cm	16 mm		> 140 cm
8 Fr 100 cm	8 mm		45 – 85 cm
6 Fr 50 cm	6 mm	1.0 – 2.0 kg	<55 cm
6 Fr 49 cm	6 mm	0.5 – 1.5 kg	<55 cm

Before inserting the catheter we need to measure the NEX measurement and calculate the insertion distance by means of the tables for nasal or oral insertion respectively (Fig 24.5).

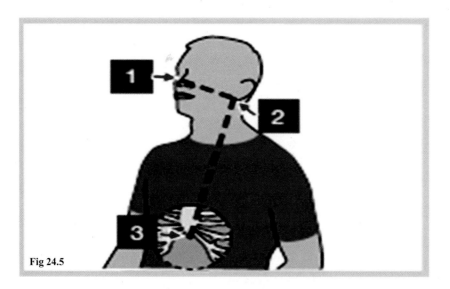

Fig 24.5

Insertion distance Y for oral insertion	
Fr/cm	Calculation of Y
16 Fr	NEX cm × 0.8 + 18 – Y cm
12 Fr	NEX cm × 0.8 + 15 – Y cm
8 Fr 125 cm	NEX cm × 0.8 + 18 – Y cm
8 Fr 100 cm	NEX cm × 0.8 + 8 – Y cm
6 Fr 50 cm	NEX cm × 0.8 + 3.5 – Y cm
6 Fr 49 cm	NEX cm × 0.8 + 2.5 – Y cm

Insertion distance Y for nasal insertion	
Fr/cm	Calculation of Y
16 Fr	NEX cm × 0.9 + 18 – Y cm
12 Fr	NEX cm × 0.9 + 15 – Y cm
8 Fr 125 cm	NEX cm × 0.9 + 18 – Y cm
8 Fr 100 cm	NEX cm × 0.9 + 8 – Y cm
6 Fr 50 cm	NEX cm × 0.9 + 3.5 – Y cm
6 Fr 49 cm	NEX cm × 0.9 + 2.5 – Y cm

Neurally Adjusted Ventilatory Assist (NAVA)

Verification of Proper Positioning of the Edi Catheter

After the insertion of Edi Catheter the position of the catheter can be seen on the screen. Verify the position by means of the ECG waveforms.

1. Verify that P and QRS waves are present in the top leads, and that the P waves disappear in the lower leads while QRS amplitude also decreases in the lower leads.
2. Verify that the Edi scale is fixed and set appropriately (greater than or equal to 0.5μV). Avoid clipping the Edi signal, i.e. avoid too low, an upper limit on the scale.
3. If Edi deflections are present, observe which leads are highlighted in blue.

If the leads highlighted in blue are in the center (i.e. second and third leads), secure the Edi catheter in this position (see below). Mark the Edi catheter (at its final position) and make a note of the final distance in cms (Fig 24.6).

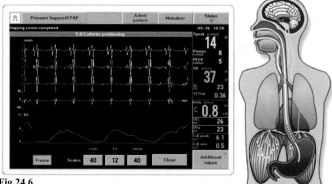

Fig 24.6

Inspect the regression of the P-wave amplitude on the four upper curves displayed in the positioning window. High amplitude of the P-wave in the uppermost curve, with a continuous regression to the lowest, which indicates a good position. Ideally, the P-wave in the lowest curve should be flat, as it is shown in this example. The leads highlighted in blue are in the center: the second and third leads. The Edi catheter is aligned correctly and ready for fixating.

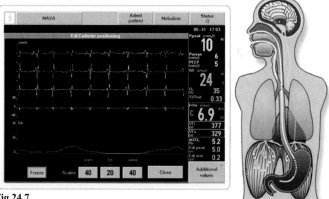

Fig 24.7

The Edi catheter is positioned too far down – the upper leads are highlighted in blue. Pull out the Edi catheter further in steps corresponding to the IED distance until the blue highlight appears in the center.

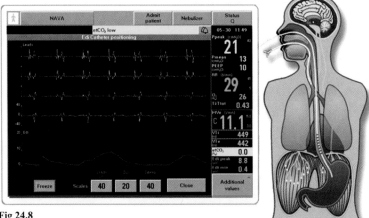

Fig 24.8

The Edi catheter is positioned too far up the bottom leads are highlighted in blue. Insert the Edi catheter in steps corresponding to the IED distance until the blue highlight appears in the center.

NAVA LEVEL

During NAVA, the amount of pressure delivered (in cmH$_2$O) is adjusted by multiplying the Edi signal (which is expressed in μV) by a proportionality factor, known as the NAVA level (expressed in cm H$_2$O/μV). The NAVA level expresses how many cm H$_2$O the patient will receive per μV Edi– the relationship is linear.

FORMULA FOR ESTIMATING PEAK PRESSURES DURING NAVA

Formula for Calculating the Pressure:

P_{peak} est. = NAVA level x (Edi_{peak} – Edi_{min}) + PEEP.

Eg: NAVA level = 2, Edi_{peak} = 8.0, Edi_{min} = 0.5, PEEP = 5 cm H$_2$O

Peak pressure = 2 × (8.0 – 0.5) + 5 = 20 cm H$_2$O

In the uppermost waveform, two curves are presented simultaneously (Fig 24.9). The gray curve shows the estimated pressure based on Edi and the set NAVA level, the yellow curve is the current patient airway pressure in the selected conventional mode (The colors are obvious on the monitoring screen).

If possible, perform an expiratory hold and verify that the positive Edi deflection coincides with a negative pressure deflection. Press "NAVA level" and use the main rotary dial to set the NAVA level. As a guide, the first NAVA level to be tried should be the same or a little below the pressure used in the current mode of ventilation.

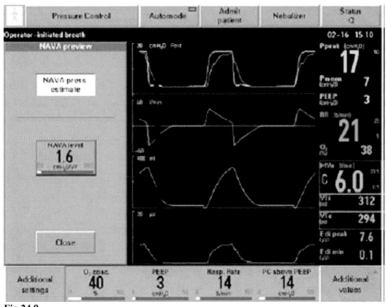

Fig 24.9

Press "Close" to save the NAVA level. The NAVA level will be transferred to the NAVA ventilation mode window. Note that the patient is still being ventilated in the conventional mode and that this is an estimate of the pressure to be delivered with NAVA. The "Set Ventilation mode" parameters window opens.

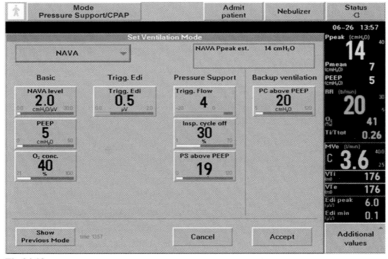

Fig 24.10

NAVA mode settings are NAVA level, PEEP O2%, Edi Trigg. 0.5 μV.
Pressure support, Insp. Cycle off, Trigg. Pressure/Flow,
Backup-PC above PEEP.

TRIGGER LEVEL

The NAVA "trigger" detects the increase in Edi and should be set to a level where random variability in the background noise does not exceed the trigger level. The variable background noise is typically less than 0.5 μV, which is the default value for Trigg. Edi.

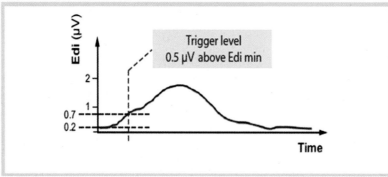

Fig 24.11

It is important to emphasize that NAVA is triggered by an increase in Edi from the Edi minimum rather than a specific level of Edi.

As a secondary source NAVA also employs the pneumatic trigger, based on flow or pressure, which operates in combination with the neural trigger on a first-come-first-served basis.

Triggered Breath Delivery

When the patient triggers a breath, gas flows into the lungs at a varying pressure proportional to the patient's Edi.

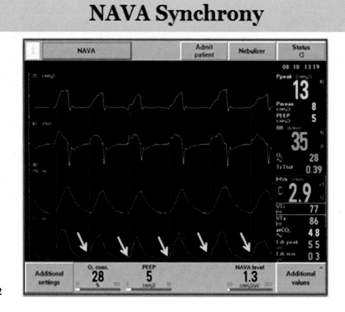

Fig 24.12

Neurally Adjusted Ventilatory Assist (NAVA)

Triggering of a breath is either Edi, flow or pressure trigger. Even if the breath is triggered on flow or pressure, the breath delivered to the patient remains proportional to the patient's Edi signal.

1. Edi triggered breath
2. Flow triggered breath

Breath Cycling–Expiration Begins

1. when the pressure increases 3 cm H_2O above the inspiratory target pressure;
2. when the Edi signal decreases below 70% of the peak value during the ongoing Inspiration. In case of low Edi signal the termination point is 40%.
3. when the maximum time limit for inspirations exceeded:
   a. For adults, 2.5 seconds;
   b. For infants, 1.5 seconds.

NAVA Respiratory Cycle in Assisted Spontaneous Ventilation

Mechanical inflation starts when the ventilator detects a deflection of the EAdi signal greater than the set threshold (mostly 0.5 µV). During the inspiratory phase of the respiratory cycle the mechanical assist is adapted to the instantaneous EAdi signal, which is measured every 16 ms and amplified by a set NAVA level. The NAVA level (set on the ventilator) dictates the amplification of the Edi signal when delivering assist to the patient. For example, if the NAVA level is set to 0.5 µV/cm H_2O and the EAdi for a specific breath is 20 µV, the maximum level of support for that breath is 10 cm H_2O (0.5 × 20=10 cm H_2O).

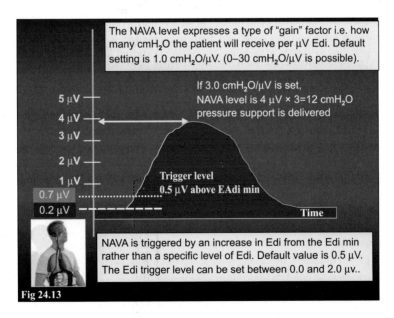

Fig 24.13

Reduce actual NAVA level by 0.2 µV/cmH_2O and evaluate after approximately 20 seconds whether or not the patient is still comfortable. If so, a further reduction in NAVA level can be made. If the patient becomes uncomfortable, return to the previous NAVA level. The usual NAVA level is between 0.5 and 3.0 µV/cmH_2O. In ARDS patients, the tidal volume should be taken into account (generally below 6 ml/kg predicted body weight).

Expiratory phase starts, if any one of the following three parameters is reached. EAdi signal reaches 40–70% of the peak EAdi signal, if the pressure increases 3 cmH$_2$O above the inspiratory target pressure or if the upper pressure limit is exceeded. The maximum time for inspiration in adults is 2.5 seconds and in infants 1.5 seconds.

Indications for NAVA

NAVA can be used in any patient who's Edi signals are intact. Any difficult weaning patient (failed weaning two or three times, COPD, ARDS), patient having asynchrony – fighting with the machine.

Contra-indications for NAVA

Esophageal, pharyngeal or maxilo-facial pathology or trauma preventing NG or OG tube insertion.

Brainstem or high spinal cord injury (above C$_3$).

Severe neuropathy (e.g. demyelination) affecting phrenic nerve signaling.

Raised intra-cranial pressure.

Analgesic/hypnotic dose causing total respiratory drive depression.

Patients receiving muscle relaxants.

Weaning from NAVA

Weaning with NAVA is done if the patient is settled, able to maintain Vt 6–8 ml/kg, respiratory rate in acceptable range, absence of hyperventilation, peak pressure and Edi$_{peak}$ should come down. We can come down on the NAVA level to 0.5 µv step by step. If the (peak pressure – PEEP) is 10 cm H$_2$O then patient can be extubated.

Monitoring of the Diaphragm Signal during Mechanical Ventilation and Weaning

Arguably the most important purpose of EAdi signal monitoring is the diagnosis of the diaphragmatic activity.

Monitoring this help in preventing development of diaphragmatic atrophy and avoid ventilator-induced diaphragm dysfunction.

EAdi monitoring helps determine the appropriate sedation depth, sedation titration and mechanical ventilation strategy. Weaning trials could explore whether a critical increase in the EAdi signal may serve as a predictive factor for weaning failure. On the other hand, a normalization of the EAdi signal might be predictive of successful weaning and extubation.

NAVA for NIPPV

The use of a pneumatic "cycle-on" in noninvasive ventilation is prone to air leakage, which is an important problem, commonly occurring around the face mask. Such leakage may induce patient-ventilator asynchrony and failure of the noninvasive ventilation.

The EAdi signal is not affected by air leakage and could therefore be used as an electrical "cycle-on" criterion, ensuring better patient-ventilator synchrony.

Conclusion

Clinical Benefits of NAVA

- Reduce work of Breathing
- Appropriate ventilation
- Variations in the amplitude of Edi prevent excessively high or low ventilation
- Adaptation to changes in metabolic demands
- Avoidance of diaphragmatic atrophy
- Reduced weaning time
- Shortened hospital stay

Fig 24.14

NAVA

- Measures the diaphragmatic EMG signal to control gas delivery
- A specifically designed nasogastric tube with series of EMC electrodes placed near the distal end, positioned across the diaphragm, is required
- By recognizing the neural signal at a higher level on the neural pathway controlling ventilation, the ventilator response and synchrony are improved
- The clinician sets only the pressure applied for each millivolt of EMG activity
- A portion of the ventilatory effort is provided by the ventilator
- Inspiration is terminated at a specific % of the peak EMG activity
- Contrary to PAV, NAVA greatly improves triggering
- In presence of severe air trapping or large leaks, triggering is not compromised

Fig 24.15

NAVA represents true assertion of brain over machine. NAVA's electrical trigger overcomes problems associated with auto-PEEP and leaks. NAVA delivers proportional support and improves patient-ventilator synchrony. NAVA results in noisy, natural breathing pattern.

★ ★ ★

EXTRACORPOREAL MEMBRANE OXYGENATION (ECMO)
A Non-Conventional Type of Ventilatory Support

Dr Kapil Zirpe. *MD. FICCM*
Director and HOD Neuro-trauma Unit
Dr. Sushma Patil, *DNB Anaesthesia, IDCCM*
Consultant, Neuro-trauma Unit
Ruby Hall Clinic, Pune, INDIA

Introduction

Extracorporeal Membrane Oxygenation can be applied as a bridge to treat patients with Life Threatening Respiratory and Cardiac Failure. ECMO is essentially a modification of cardiopulmonary bypass circuit which is routinely used in cardiac surgery. Blood is removed from the venous system either peripherally via cannulation of femoral vein or centrally via cannulation of the right atrium, oxygenated, carbon dioxide is extracted and then returned back to the body, either peripherally via a femoral artery or centrally via ascending aorta.

The use of ECMO was reported in 1950s when early attempts were made to use an artificial lung along with blood pump to support a patient of open heart surgery. In 1971 Hill Donald and Maury Bramson, of Santa Barbara reported use of ECMO. They attempted to support a 24-years male patient who had met with an accident and later developed ARDS. In 1975 Bartlett reported first neonatal survivor with respiratory failure caused due to Meconium Aspiration at University of California, Irvine.

The following scenario represents a clinical situation requiring maximal intervention to improve oxygenation.

Case: A 24-years male presented with breathlessness and intubated. The patient is placed on a mechanical ventilator in view of worsening respiratory symptoms. Other pertinent data revealed: PaO_2/FiO_2 or (P/F ratio) <100 with PEEP 10 cmH_2O on control ventilation. A chest radiogram showed extensive bilateral opacities.

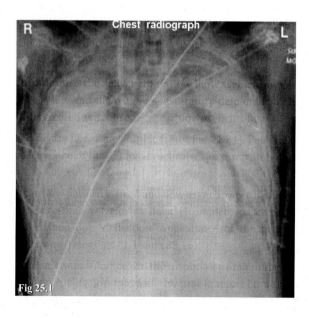

Fig 25.1

A $PaO_2/FiO_2 < 100$ mm Hg with PEEP ≥ 10 indicates severe ARDS. This condition will trigger "ARDS Protocol". The therapeutic Options are shown in (Fig 25.2).

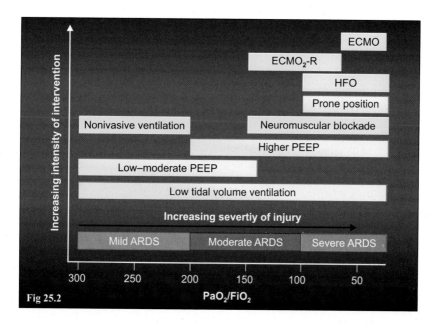

Fig 25.2

Figure 25.2 overviews the degree of severity of injury and corresponding intervention using ARDS net protocol.

According to current practice and documented literature survey, intervention techniques in progressively worsening lung condition, mild to severe ARDS, include invasive ventilation with low tidal volumes at low to moderate to high levels of PEEP. In the case above, a P/F ratio of < 100, with PEEP of >10 requires higher level of intervention. ECMO represents one of the highest level of intervention.

INDICATIONS for ECMO

Respiratory Distress Syndrome (RDS) patients from any precipitating cause, in severe condition, may require ECMO (Fig 25.3).

Respiratory Distress Syndrome

- Refractory cardiogenic shock
- Infections: Septicemia, Septic shock syndromes, Influenza, H_1N_1, Pneumonia (Swine flu)
- Cardiotoxicity
- Thoracic trauma involving lung contusion
- Resuscitation: Cardiac arrest, Cardiogenic shock, Cardiac trauma, Drug overdose, Hypothermia, Pulmonary edema, Pulmonary embolism
- Post cardiotomy, post heart transplant

Fig 25.3

In terms of cardiac failure the most common indications for ECMO are post cardiotomy (unable to get patient off cardiopulmonary by-pass following cardiac surgery), post-heart transplant and severe cardiac failure due to almost any other cause (acute coronary syndrome, decompensated cardiomyopathy, myocarditis, drug overdose causing cardiac failure).

Most importantly one must consider the likelihood of organ recovery.

CONTRA-INDCATIONS: (Fig 25.4)

- Prolonged mechanical ventilation
- Significant neurological injury
- Active bleeding/coagulation disorder
- Terminal disease with short life expectancy-disseminated malignancy
- Graft vs host disease
- Un-witnessed arrest or CPR for 30 minutes
- Uncontrollable metabolic acidosis
- Pulmonary fibrosis
- Immunosuppression
- Advanced age
- Technical problems-aortic dissection or aortic incompetence

Fig 25.4

CONFIGURATIONS FOR ECMO

ECMO can be inserted in veno-venous (VV) configuration which provides oxygenation to treat patients with refractory hypoxemia. It can also be applicable in a veno-arterial (VA) configuration providing both respiratory and cardiac support such as in **refractory cardiogenic shock**. Criteria for ECMO implantation are not clearly defined.

Figure 25.5 lists the difference between VV and VA configuration in ECMO.

Veno-arterial	Veno-venous
Higher PaO_2 achieved	Lower PaO_2 achieved
Lower perfusion rates required	Higher perfusion rates required
By-passes pulmonary circulation	Maintains pulmonary blood flow
Decreases PA pressures	Elevates mixed venous PaO_2
Provides cardiac support	No systemic criculatory assist
	ECMO configuration for acute respiratory failure should always be VV EXCEPT in the case of severe associated cardiogenic shock

Fig 25.5

Extracorporeal Membrane Oxygenation (ECMO)

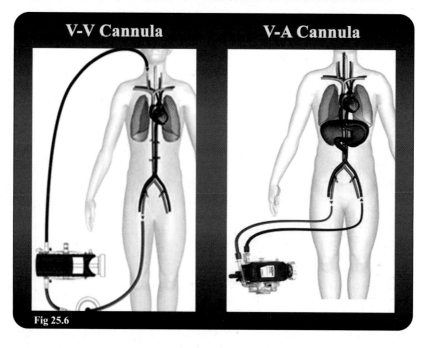

Figure 25.6: Veno-venous and Veno-arterial routes

CANNULAE SIZES and PREFERRED SITES:

According to Poiseuille's Law, Flow is proportional to the 4th power of radius and inversely proportional to tubing length and viscosity.

Preferred size of cannula:

"Venous": 25 and 29 Fr, 55 cm

"Arterial": 19 and 21 Fr, 15 cm

29/21 combination is preferred

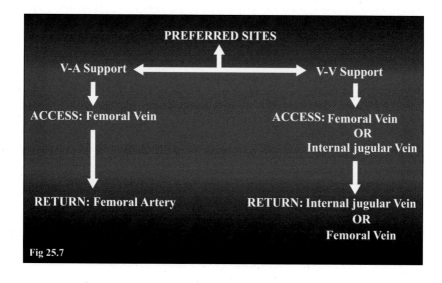

PLACEMENT OF CANNULAE:

- **In femoro-jugular configuration**

  Return cannula :- Close to the tricuspid valve

  Drainage cannula :- As central as possible and Not too close to the return cannula
- **The major limitation of VV ECMO is –RECIRCULATION**

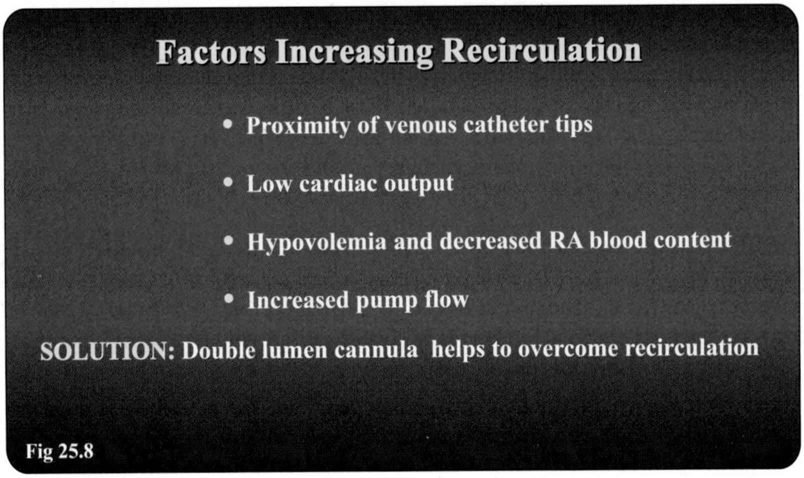

Factors Increasing Recirculation

- Proximity of venous catheter tips
- Low cardiac output
- Hypovolemia and decreased RA blood content
- Increased pump flow

SOLUTION: Double lumen cannula helps to overcome recirculation

Fig 25.8

COMPONENTS of ECMO

There are four basic components of ECMO

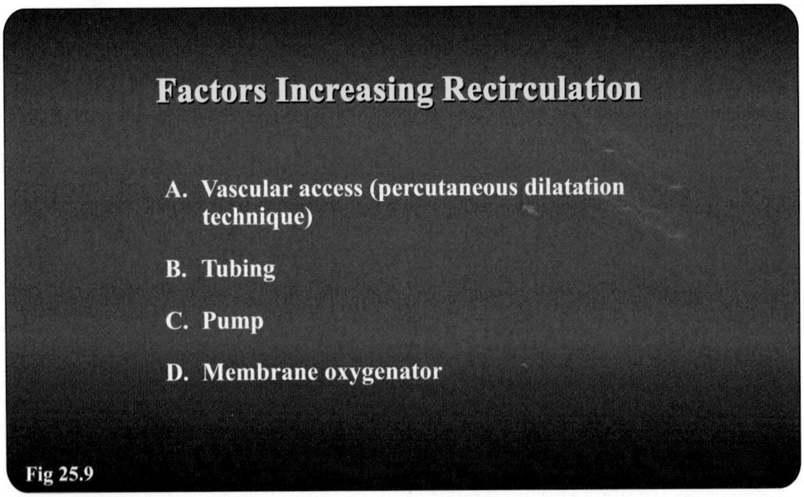

Factors Increasing Recirculation

A. Vascular access (percutaneous dilatation technique)

B. Tubing

C. Pump

D. Membrane oxygenator

Fig 25.9

A. VASCULAR ACCESS

1. Percutaneous (prefer ultrasono guidance)
2. Surgical

Extracorporeal Membrane Oxygenation (ECMO)

PERCUTANEOUS

1. Accessing a peripheral artery or vein via the minimal invasive "Seldinger Technique"/Ultrasono guided

2. The skin should form a tight seal around the cannulae

SURGICAL CUT

1. Accessing a peripheral artery or vein via a surgical incision, Direct visual cannulation of the vessel

2. Purse string for retention and sealing.

Fig 25.10

B. TUBING

PVC tubing circuit and polycarbonate connectors are required to form a circuit which has an arterial and venous limb. Lines and oxygenator are heparin-coated so the need for less anticoagulation and no heparin bolus is necessary at ECMO initiation.

C. PUMP

A driver or the pump is required to drive and control the blood circulation. Centrifugal Channel Pumps have cones or Flow which have very minimal contact or surface aiding lesser risk of Hemolysis, no heat generation due to friction and almost nil stagnant areas.

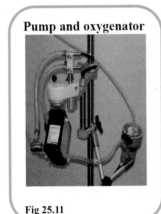
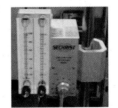

Pump and oxygenator | Oxygenator | Gas flow meter

Fig 25.11

Courtsey: Maquet-India

D. MEMBRANE OXYGENATOR OR THE ARTIFICIAL LUNG

Initial Silicon Rubber Membrane Oxygenators were replaced by Hollow Fiber polymethylpentene (PMP) membrane oxygenators. PMP aided in lesser Trans-membrane pressure drops, lesser priming volumes, quick and easy priming superior gas exchange performance, and integration of heat exchanger.

Circulation and Circuit

The Pump (centrifugal or roller) drives the deoxygenated blood from the access line–called the Venous line of the circuit into an Oxygenator. The gas exchanged blood is passed through a Heat Exchanger (sometimes integrated with Oxygenator–Cardiohelp) and returned back to patient called Arterial line

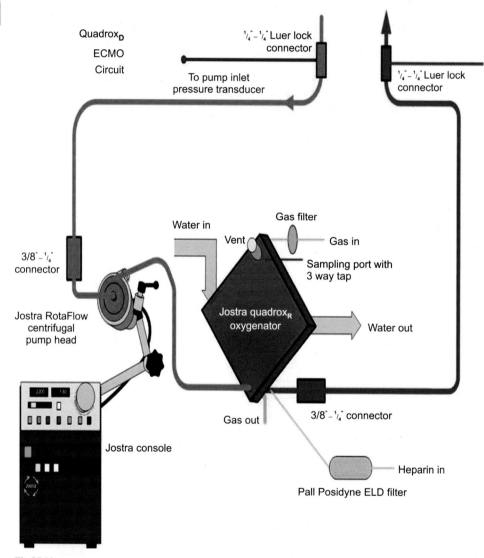

Fig 25.12

Courtesy: MAQUET

ECMO THERAPY: - APPLICATION PART

Before application of ECMO therapy all patients need to undergo pre-ECMO evaluation.

Pre-ECMO Evaluation

- Pre-ECMO Evaluation
- History (onset of symptoms, reversibility of diseases)
- Hemogram, Complete Coagulogram, Serum lactate, Serum Calcium, Magnesium
- Renal Function test, Liver function Test, ABG.
- 2DEcho, CT-Scan Brain
- APACHE IV score evaluation

Fig 25.13

The ECMO therapy is divided into 4 parts
1. Initiation
2. Maintenance
3. Weaning
4. Trouble shooting/complications

1. INITIATION:

After successful placement of cannulae, priming of ECMO circuit (tubing) is done with normal saline to remove the air from the tubing. The circuit is connected to the cannula. Systemic anticoagulation is given during cannulation, Heparin Bolus of 300 units/kg to achieve ACT >300 seconds. Initial ECMO settings and Patient Hemodynamic are as below:

CIRCUIT BLOOD FLOWS	2 TO 2.4 L/Min/Sq. meters
CIRCUIT GAS FLOW	Blood : Gas = 1:0.5 (initially) 1:2 (maximum)
PATIENT HEMODYNAMICS	Mean Arterial pressure >60 mmHg CVP = 10 to 14 mmHg

Fig 25.14

2. MAINTENANCE/MANAGEMENT:

Anticoagulation: Activated clotting times (ACT) are used to monitor heparin administration during ECMO. Heparin infusion rate is adjusted according to ACT.

Parameters of patient to monitor the adequacy of the support are:

> ABG and VBG every 4-6 hourly ($PaCO_2$ = 35-45%)
>
> Blood sugar level = Every 6 hourly (80-140 mg/dl)
>
> SvO_2 (maintained at 80-100% in VV ECMO and 65-75% in VA ECMO)
>
> SaO_2 (maintained at 95-100% in VA ECMO and 80-100% in VV ECMO)
>
> Urine output (0.5 to 1ml/kg), proper Input and Output Chart
>
> Arterial Blood Pressures (MAP > 60 mm Hg),
>
> Patient Temperature (35°–37° Celsius)
>
> Lung Protective ventilation/Lung rest setting
>
> ACT of 160-180 seconds maintained
>
> Nursing Management: Aseptic handling

Fig 25.15

During the patient is on ECMO, monitor following pressures :-

ECMO pressure to be monitored	
CIRCUIT PRESSURES	Pre-pump = <–80 mmHg Pre-membrane = <350 Hg Post-membrane = 300 mmHg Trans-membrane = <150 mmHg (pressure drop)
PATIENT HEMODYNAMICS	Arterial = >60 mm Hg (mean) CVP = 10 to 14 mm Hg
SPECIAL SITUATION	RRT in renal failure attach port pre-membrane and postpump

Fig 25.16

If Pre-pump Pressure> –80 mm Hg suspect Hypovolemia, Kink in the circuit tubing, Blockage of the tubing or sticking of the cannula to IVC wall.

If Premembrane>350 mm Hg anticipate hemolysis.

If Trans-membrane Pressure is > 150 mm Hg then suspect oxygenator block or hemolysis.

In case of Renal Failure RRT proximal port (towards dialyser) should be attached to Pre-Pump and distal port (postdialysis) should be drained in pre-membrane port.

Extracorporeal Membrane Oxygenation (ECMO)

3. **WEANING:**

Discontinuation of ECMO

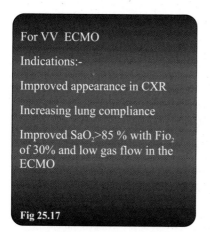

Fig 25.17

For weaning of VV ECMO support:-Prior to weaning, ventilation settings should be increased to desired settings-FiO$_2$ of 0.6 and moderate airway pressures. ECMO flow is reduced to 20-25 ml/kg, anticoagulation need to be increased depending on target blood flow gas flow and FiO$_2$ through Oxygenator is kept to minimum.

The ECMO circuit now acts as venous shunt. SvO$_2$ can be monitored to assess the adequacy of lung function.

4. **COMPLICATIONS/TROUBLE SHOOTING:**

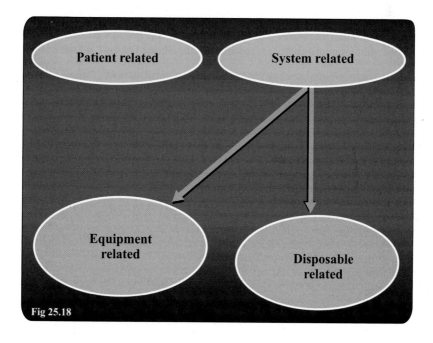

Fig 25.18

A. PATIENT RELATED COMPLICATIONS

- Bleeding
- Thrombo embolism: Visible thrombus in blood pump or cannulae
- Cannulation related complication-vessel damage
- HITT
- Pulmonary infarction, Limb ischemia
- Aortic thrombosis
- Coronary or cerebral hypoxia
- Infection and sepsis

Fig 25.19

B. EQUIPMENT RELATED COMPLICATIONS

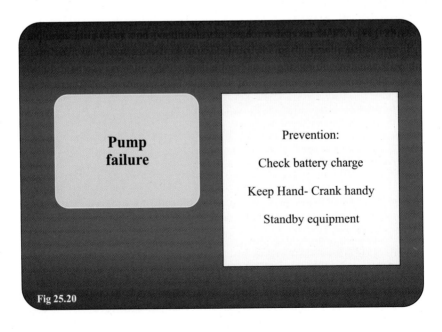

Pump failure

Prevention:
Check battery charge
Keep Hand- Crank handy
Standby equipment

Fig 25.20

C. DISPOSABLE RELATED COMPLICATIONS

Hemolysis	Use the largest possible cannula. Use centrifugal pump (with low hemolysis index) Use Oxygenator with least pressure drop Select appropriate sized tubing circuit Biocompatible coatings-uniform internal tubing surface
Air embolism	Life threatening and circuit emergency De-airing protocols
Circuit thrombosis/ Circuit rupture	Life threatening. Circuit/component change out

Fig 25.21

★ ★ ★

Suggested Reading

Chapter 1
1. Chatburn RL, Volsko TA. Mechanical Ventilators In Wilkins RL, Stoller JK, Kacmarek RM, (editors) Egon's Fundamentals of Respiratory Care Ed 9, St Louis 2009, Mosby.
2. Pierson DJ, Indication for mechanical ventilation in adults wuth acute respiratory failure, Respir Care 47:219;2002.
3. Slutsky AS. ACCP consensus conference: mechanical ventilation, Chest 104;1833;1933.

Chapter 2
1. Roussos C. Respiratory muscle fatigue and ventilator failure, Chest 97 (3 Suppl) 898; 1990.
2. Shapuro BA, Cane RD, Harrison RA, et al. changes in intrapulmonary shunting with administration of 1000% oxygen, chest 77:138;1980.

Chapter 5
1. Waugh JB Desphande VM, Brown MK, Harwood RJ. Rapid Interpretation of Ventilator Waveform Ed 2, Upper Saddle River NJ, 2007, Prentice Hall.

Chapter 6
1. Shelledy DC. Initiating and adjusting ventilator support in Wilkins RM JK, Kacmarck RM, (edition). Fgan's fundamentals of respiratory care ed 9, St Louis, 2009, Elsevier.

Chapter 7
1. Chatburn RL. Classification of ventilator models update and proposal for implementation, Respir Care 52;301;2007.
2. Rouby JJ, Ben Amewi M, Jawish D, et al. Continuous positive airway pressure (CPAP) vs intermittent mandatory pressure release ventilation (IMPRV) in patients with acute respiratory failure, Intensive Care med 18:69;1992.

Chapter 8
1. Amato MB, Barbas CSV, Medeiros DM, et al. Effect of a protective ventilation strategy on mortality in the acute respiratory distress syndrome, N Engl J Med 338;347: 1998.
2. Camppell PS, Davis BR. Pressure controlled versus volume-controlled ventilator, does it matter, Respir Care 47;416:2002.
3. Kacmarck RM, Hest D. Pressure – controlled inverse ratio ventilation. Panacea or auto-PEEP, Respire Care 35;945:1990 (editorial).
4. Marini JJ. Pressure—Targeted mechanical ventilation of acute lung injury, Sem Respir Med 14:262;1993.
5. Sasoon CSH. Mahutte CK. What you need to know about the ventilator in weaning, Respir Care 40:249;1995.

Chapter 12
1. Esteban A, protos F, Tobin MJ, et al. A comparison of four methods of weaning patients from mechanical ventilation(the Spanish lung failure collaborative group N Engl J Med 342–345;1995.
2. Hess d, Branson R. Ventilators and weaning modes part 11, Respir Care Clin N Am 6:407;2000.
3. Maclutyre NR. Weaning form mechanical ventilator support volume—assisting intermittent breathing versus pressure – assisting every breath, Respir Care 33;21–121;1988.
4. MacIntyre NR. Evidence-based ventilator weaning respire care 49:839;2004.
5. MacIntyre NR. Respiratory mechanics in the patient who is weaning form the ventilator, Respir Care 50;275;2005.
6. MacIntyre NR, Cook Dj, ELY EW Jr, et al. ACCP/AARC/SCCM task force evidence based guidelines for weaning and discontinuing mechanical ventilator support a collective task force felicitated by the American College of Chest Physicians ;the American Association for respiratory care and the American college of critical care Medicine, chest 120(Suppl 6);3758,2001; Respir care 47;69;2002.
7. Ross L, Pressnell Jl, Cade JF. Update in computer driven weaning from mechanical ventilation Anesth intensive Care 35(2):213-221;2007.

8. Ross L, Pressnell Jl, Cade JF. A randomized controlled trial of conventional versus automated weaning from mechanical ventilator using Smart care/PS, Intensive care Medicine, 34(10):1788–1795;2008.
9. Tobin MJ. Respiratory parameters for successful weaning, J Crit illness 6:819;1990.

Chapter 13

1. Sanra Blanch I. How to set positive end–expiratory pressure care 47: 279;2002.

Chapter 14

1. MacIntyre NR. Management of obstructive airway distress in MacItyre Nr, Branson RD editors mechanical ventilation 2nd edn, Philadelphia 2009, Saunders – Elsevier.
2. Mitnueter JC, reighley JE, Karetzkey MS. Response of the arterial PO_2 to oxygenation administration in chronic pulmonary diseases, Am inter Med 74:328;1971.
3. Wedzicha JA, Doualdson GC. Exacerbation of chronic obstructive pulmonary diseases, Respir Care 48;1204;2003.

Chapter 15

1. Brochard I. Mechanical ventilation invasive versus noninvasive, Eur Respir J Suppl 47:318;2003.
2. Hess D. Noninvasive pressure ventilation predictors of success and failure for adult acute care application. Respire Care 42; 424: 1997.
3. Hill NS, Brennam J, Gaspestad E, Navas. Non invasive ventilation in acute respiratory failure, Crit Care Med 35;2402–07; 2007.
4. Meduri GD, Fox RC, Ahou-Sbala N, et al. Non Invasive face mask mechanical ventilator in patients with acute hypescapnic respiratory failure, Cases 100–445;1991.

Chapter 16

1. ARPS net National heart, Lung and Blood Institute, National Institute of Health, Effects of Recruitment maneuvers in patients with acute lung injury and acute respiratory distress syndrome ventilated with high positive end–expiratory pressure, Crit Care Med 31:2592;2003.
2. Gattinoni L, Caizoni P, Cressoni M, et al. Lung recruitment with patients with acute respiratory distress syndrome, N Engl J Med 354;1755–1786;2006.
3. Gattinoni L, Pelosi P, et al. What has computed tomography tought us about the acute respiratory distress syndrome, Am J respire care Med 164:1701;2001.
4. Hapsma JJ Lachman PD, Lachman R. Lung protective ventilator in ARDS role of ventilators PEEP and surfactant, Monaldi Arch Chest Dis 59:108;2003.
5. Hes DR, Bigatello LM. Lung recruitment the role of recruitment maneuvers, Respir Care 47; 308, 2002.
6. Kallet Rh, Katz JA. Respiratory system mechanics in acute respiratory distress syndrome, Respir Care Clin N Am 9:297; 2003.
7. OptHoli TB. Ventilation for life determining lower and upper inflection points in setting PEEP and Vt in ARDS patients, AARC times 283;2004.
8. Respiratory distress syndrome network (ARDS network) ventilation with lower tidal volumes as compared with traditional tidal volumes for acute lung injury and acute respiratory distress syndrome N Engl J Med 342:1301; 2000.
9. Steinbers KP, Kacmarek RM. Should total Volume be 6 mL/Kg predicted body weight in virtually all patients with active respiratory failure, Respir Care 52 (5); 556–567;2007.
10. Villar J Perez Mendez L, Lopez J et al. An early Peep/PO_2 tidal sentines different degree of lung injury in patient with acute respiratory distress syndrome, Am J respire Crit care Med 176; 795–804;2002.

Chapter 17

1. American Association of Respiratory care AARC Evidence based clinical practice guideline care of the ventilator circuit and its relation to ventilator-associated pneumonia, Respir Care 48:865;2003.
2. Collared HR, Saint S, Matthay MA: Prevention of ventilator—associated pneumonia as evidence-based systematic review, Am internal Med 138;494:2003.
3. Dedek K, Keenaa S, Cook D, et al. Evidenced based clinical practice guideline for the prevention of ventilator associated pneumonia Am Inter Med 141.303,2004.

4. Littlewood K, Durbin CG. Evidenced-based airway management, Respir care 46; 1392: 2001.
5. Porzecanski T, Bowton DI. Diagnosis and treatment of ventilator associated pneumonia chest 130:597–604;2006.
6. Safdar N, Pezfulian C, Collard HR, et al. clinical and economical consequences of ventilator associated pneumonia a systematic review, Crit Care Med 33:2184–93; 2005.
7. Safdar N, Crnich CJ, Maki DG. The pathogenesis of ventilator associated pneumonia its relevance to developing effective strategies for prevention, Respir care (50) 6:725–741;2005.
8. Tolentino – Delos Reyes AF, Ruppert SD, Shiao SPK, evidence – based practice use of ventilator bundles to prevent ventilator associated pneumonia a Am J Crit Care 16:20–27;2007.

Chapter 18
1. Parthasarathy S, Jubran A, Tobin MJ. Assessment of neural inspiratory time in ventilator – supported patients, Am J respire Crit Care Med 162:546;200.

Chapter 19
1. Amato MS, Barbas CS, et al. Volume assured pressure support ventilation (VAPSV) a new approach for reducing muscle workload during acute respiratory failure, Chest 102: 1228;1992.
2. Davis KH, Johnson DJ, Branson RD, et al. Airway pressure release ventilation, Arch Surg 128:1348;1993.
3. Downs JB, Stock MC. Airway pressure release ventilation, a new approach in ventilator support during acute lung injury, Respir Care Clin N Am 32:517;1987.
4. Frawley PM, Habashi NM. Airway pressure release ventilation, theory and practice, AACN Clin Issue 12:234–246, 2001.
5. Havashi NM. Other approaches to open–lung ventilation: Airway pressure release ventilation. Crit Care Medicine 33 9 (Suppl): s228–s240;2005.
6. Kaliet RH. Patient-ventilator interaction during acute lung injury and the role of spontaneous breathing part 2, Airway Pressure release ventilation, Respir Care 56:190;2011.
7. Stock MC, Downs JB, Frolicher DA. Airway pressure release ventilation. Crit Care Med 13:462;1987.
8. Tobin MJ. Mechanical Ventilation. N Engl J Med 330:1056;1994.
9. Tobin MJ. Advances in mechanical ventilation N Engl J Med 344:1980;2001.
10. Younes M proportional assist ventilation, a new approach to ventilator support, Am Rev Respir 145:114;1992.
11. Younes M. Puddy A, Roberts D, et al. Proportional assist ventilation, results of an initial clinical trial, Am, rev respire 145:121; 1992.

Chapter 20
1. Barwing J Ambold M, Linden N, et al. Evaluation of the catheter positioning for neutrally adjusted ventilator assist, Inter care Med 35;1809:2009.
2. Sinderby C, Becz J. Nemally, adjusted ventilator assist NAVA, An update and summary of experiences, Netherlands J Crit care 11:243;2007.

Chapter 21
1. AARC Clinical practice guideline, Humidification during mechanical ventilation, American Association of Respiratory Care, Respir Care 37;887:1992.
2. Branson Rd, Campbell Rs. Humidification in the intensive care unit. Respir care Clin N Am 4:305;1998.
3. Branson RD, Campbell RS, Johannigman JA, et al. Comparison of conventional headed humidification and moisture exchanger in mechanically ventilated patient, Respir Care 44:912;1999.

Chapter 23
1. Nilsestnen JO, Hugette KD. Using ventilator graphics to indentify Patient-ventilator Asynchrony: Respir Care 50:202;2005.

Index

Academia 36
Acetylcholine (ACh) 282
Acidosis 317
Acute lung injury (ALI) 83, 102, 136, 186
Acute respiratory distress syndrome (ARDS) 5, 19, 83, 169, 216, 236, 292
Acute ventilatory failure 3, 26, 27, 28, 39
Adaptive support ventilation (ASV) 116, 153, 253, 260, 261
Adjunctive therapies 241
Afterload 323, 324, 325
Agitation 281, 332
Airway opening pressure (P_{awo}) 42, 43
Airway pressure 56, 98, 133
Airway resistance 11, 57, 63
Alarm settings 91, 93, 133
Albuterol 304
Alveolar hypoventilation 27, 224
Alveolar pressure 42, 56, 128
Alveolar ventilation 24
Anatomic disruption 290
Anemia 16
Anemic hypoxia 16
Anion gap 31, 32
Antagonists 249
Anti-cholinergic bronchodilators 303
Anti-inflammatory lipid profile 292
Apnea 7, 203
Apnea ventilation 206
Arterial pressure 329, 363
Artificial airways 244
Auto-triggering 202, 339, 340
Automode 116, 153
Auto-PEEP 54, 62, 102, 112, 136, 180

Barotraumas 240, 241
Benzodiazepines 277, 278
Bilevel positive airway pressure
BiPAP 100
Blood gas values 25, 40
Blood gases 40
Blood pressure 161
Bronchodilators 54, 57, 205, 295, 303

CaO_2 9, 17
Capnography monitoring 168, 169
Carbohydrate 28, 290
Carbon dioxide 356
Cardiac output 9, 162, 339, 368
Cardiogenic pulmonary edema 208
Cerebral perfusion 160
Chest curraise 42
Chest radiogram 356
Chest trauma 189, 196

Chest tube 58, 241, 275
Chest wall 41, 318, 346
CMV 301
Compliance 12, 57, 58, 60, 102, 128, 129
COPD 36, 162, 171, 172, 176
CPAP 64, 98, 216, 342
CPP 186, 188
Cuff pressure 132, 133

Deadspace ventilation 24, 142
Double triggering 335, 338
Dyssynchrony 202

EAdi 263–265, 346
ECMO (Extracorporeal membrane oxygenation) 230, 356, 357
Elastic recoil 57, 60
Electrolytes 286
End tidal carbon dioxide 268
Endotracheal tube 297, 301
Expiratory asynchrony 335
Expiratory flow 53, 175
Expiratory positive airway pressure (EPAP) 202
Expiratory time 47, 56, 124, 223, 333
Extubation 180

FiO_2 and PEEP 124, 167, 168
Flow asynchrony 335, 341
Flow-time 49, 52, 108
Flow-volume 50, 51
Fluid balance 162

Gas trapping 174
Guillain-Barré syndrome (GBS) 194

Hazards of mechanical ventilation 143, 233
Head and moisture exchanger (HME) 310
Head injury 186
Heated humidifiers 311
Heated wire 307
Hemodynamic monitoring 330
Hemoglobin 17
Humidification 205, 295, 300, 309, 312, 314, 315
Hyperkalemia 35
Hypertension 16
Hyperventilation 16, 18, 188
Hypokalemia 33, 35
Hypopnea 3
Hypothermia 357
Hypoventilation 27, 224, 333
Hypoxemia 10, 15, 17, 18, 20, 229, 243, 332

Ideal body weight (IBW) 120, 224, 286, 289
Impending respiratory failure 1
Inspiratory positive airway pressure (IPAP) 100

Inspiratory time 47, 56
Intermittent mandatory ventilation (IMV) 93, 152
Intracranial pressures (ICP) 187, 283
Intubation 41, 180, 308
Inverse ratio ventilation 222

Low tidal volume 220, 224, 328, 357
Lower inflection point (LIP) 59
Lung compliance 12, 13, 57, 58, 60, 128, 129, 131

Metabolic acidosis 32, 332, 358
Metabolic alkalosis 33–35, 333
Metered dose inhalers (MDI) 295, 298
Modes of mechanical ventilation 63, 64
Muscle fatigue 7
Myasthenia gravis 194

Nasal mask 181, 198, 200
Nasal passage 206
Negative pressure ventilators 42, 197
Neuromuscular 192, 194, 196, 281, 283
Noninvasive positive pressure ventilation (NPPV) 303
Nutritional support 285, 286

Oronasal mask 199
Oxygenation 10, 14, 144, 165, 227, 365

Pain 273, 280
Peak inspiratory pressure (PIP) 56, 127, 131, 132, 134
Peak inspiratory flow rates (PIFR) 62
Permissive hypercapnia 225
Phrenic nerve 257
Plateau pressure 57, 132, 180, 182, 224
Polymethylpentene (PMP) membrane 361
Positive end expiratory pressure (PEEP) 54, 59, 62, 112, 124, 130
Positive pressure ventilation 70, 100, 325
Pressure control ventilation (PCV) 113
Pressure cycled 46
Pressure limited 66, 80, 93
Pressure regulated volume control (PRVC) 112, 113, 115
Pressure support level 64, 98
Pressure-time 336, 341
Pressure-volume 105, 166
Prone position 228
Propofol or dexmedetomidine 278
Proportional assist ventilation (PAV) 204, 253, 260–262

Pulmonary artery wedge pressure 215
Pulmonary vascular resistance 159, 326
Pulse oximetry 210
Patient–ventilator asynchrony 204, 337, 343

Refractory hypoxemia 5, 7, 358
Renal failure 27, 364
Respiratory acidosis 5, 27
Respiratory frequency 46, 47
Respiratory muscles 85, 333
Respiratory rate 80, 86, 95, 112, 185, 225, 338
Restrictive airway disease 336

Sedation 203, 266, 276, 281
Sedative drugs 278
Shunting 19
SIMV 63, 65, 66
Sleep apnea 7
Spontaneous modes 63
Spontaneous respiratory rate 260
Spontaneous tidal volume 96, 268
Spontaneous ventilation 263, 353
Spontaneously breathing 182
Static lung compliance 129, 131
Stroke volume 325
Succinylcholine 282
Suctioning 58
Surfactants 222, 304
Synchronized intermittent mandatory ventilation 93, 152

Termination ventilator 70, 73
Trigger asynchrony 202, 335
Trigger level 352, 353
Triggered 88, 89, 113, 336

V/Q mismatch 174, 177, 191
VAPS 113
Venous return 161, 322
Ventilator assisted pneumonia (VAP) 244, 245, 247, 251
Vital capacity 147, 194
Vital signs 151, 210
Volume controlled ventilator (VCV) 74

Weaning 131, 143, 146, 152, 169, 212
Wedge pressure 215
Work of breathing 1, 60, 174, 255, 318, 341